Genetics Diagnosis, Inborn Errors of Metabolism and Newborn Screening: An Update

Editors

MICHAEL J. GAMBELLO
V. REID SUTTON

CLINICS IN PERINATOLOGY

www.perinatology.theclinics.com

Consulting Editor
LUCKY JAIN

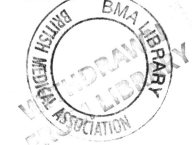

June 2015 • Volume 42 • Number 2

ELSEVIER

1600 John F. Kennedy Boulevard • Suite 1800 • Philadelphia, Pennsylvania, 19103-2899

http://www.theclinics.com

CLINICS IN PERINATOLOGY Volume 42, Number 2
June 2015 ISSN 0095-5108, ISBN-13: 978-0-323-35662-6

Editor: Kerry Holland
Developmental Editor: Casey Jackson

Clinics in Perinatology (ISSN 0095-5108) is published quarterly by Elsevier Inc., 360 Park Avenue South, New York, NY 10010-1710. Months of issue are March, June, September, and December. Business and Editorial Offices: 1600 John F. Kennedy Blvd., Ste. 1800, Philadelphia, PA 19103-2899. Customer Service Office: 3251 Riverport Lane, Maryland Heights, MO 63043. Periodicals postage paid at New York, NY and additional mailing offices. Subscription prices are $285.00 per year (US individuals), $445.00 per year (US institutions), $340.00 per year (Canadian individuals), $545.00 per year (Canadian institutions), $420.00 per year (international individuals), $545.00 per year (international institutions), $135.00 per year (US students), and $195.00 per year (Canadian and international students). International air speed delivery is included in all Clinics subscription prices. All prices are subject to change without notice. **POSTMASTER:** Send address changes to *Clinics in Perinatology*, Elsevier Health Sciences Division, Subscription Customer Service, 3251 Riverport Lane, Maryland Heights, MO 63043. **Customer Service: Telephone: 1-800-654-2452** (U.S. and Canada); **1-314-447-8871** (outside U.S. and Canada). **Fax: 1-314-447-8029. E-mail: journalscustomerservice-usa@elsevier.com** (for print support); **journalsonlinesupport-usa@elsevier.com** (for online support).

Reprints. For copies of 100 or more, of articles in this publication, please contact the Commercial Reprints Department, Elsevier Inc., 360 Park Avenue South, New York, NY 10010-1710. Tel. 212-633-3874; Fax: 212-633-3820; E-mail: reprints@elsevier.com.

Clinics in Perinatology is also pubilshed in Spanish by McGraw-Hill Interamericana Editores S.A., P.O. Box 5-237, 06500 Mexico D.F., Mexico.

Clinics in Perinatology is covered in *MEDLINE/PubMed (Index Medicus) Current Contents, Excepta Medica, BIOSIS and ISI/BIOMED.*

Contributors

CONSULTING EDITOR

LUCKY JAIN, MD, MBA
Richard W. Blumberg Professor and Executive Vice Chairman, Department of Pediatrics, Emory University School of Medicine; Executive Medical Director, Children's Healthcare of Atlanta Faculty Practices, Atlanta, Georgia

EDITORS

MICHAEL J. GAMBELLO, MD, PhD
Associate Professor, Department of Human Genetics and Pediatrics; Section Chief, Division of Medical Genetics, Department of Human Genetics, Emory University School of Medicine, Atlanta, Georgia

V. REID SUTTON, MD
Professor, Department of Molecular and Human Genetics, Baylor College of Medicine, Texas Children's Hospital, Houston, Texas

AUTHORS

MARGARET P. ADAM, MD
Professor of Pediatrics, Division of Genetic Medicine, Department of Pediatrics, University of Washington, Seattle, Washington

MARWAN ALI, MD
Clinical Fellow in Medical Genetics, Division of Genetics, Department of Pediatrics, University of California, San Francisco, San Francisco, California

ARUNKANTH ANKALA, PhD
Department of Human Genetics, Emory University School of Medicine, Atlanta, Georgia

SUSAN A. BERRY, MD
Department of Pediatrics, University of Minnesota, Minneapolis, Minnesota

COLLEEN P. COULTER, PT, DPT, PhD, PCS
Adjunct Assistant Professor of Rehabilitation Medicine, Emory University; Orthotics and Prosthetics Department, Children's Healthcare of Atlanta, Atlanta, Georgia

JASON R. COWAN, MS
Division of Developmental Biology, Cincinnati Children's Hospital Medical Center, Cincinnati, Ohio; Department of Pediatrics and Medical and Molecular Genetics, Herman B Wells Center for Pediatric Research, Indiana University School of Medicine, Indianapolis, Indiana

AYMAN W. EL-HATTAB, MD, FAAP, FACMG
Consultant and Chief, Division of Clinical Genetics and Metabolic Disorders, Pediatric Department, Tawam Hospital, Al-Ain, United Arab Emirates

STANLEY T. FRICKE, PhD
Professor, Department of Radiology; MR Physicist, Children's National Medical Center, Washington, DC

ANDREA L. GROPMAN, MD
Professor, Department of Neurology; Division Chief, Neurodevelopmental Disabilities and Neurogenetics, Children's National Medical Center, Washington, DC

J. AUSTIN HAMM, MD
Department of Genetics, The University of Alabama at Birmingham, Birmingham, Alabama

MADHURI R. HEGDE, PhD
Department of Human Genetics, Emory University School of Medicine, Atlanta, Georgia

KELLY L. JONES, MD
Acting Instructor, Division of Genetic Medicine, Department of Pediatrics, University of Washington, Seattle, Washington

BRIANNE E. KIRKPATRICK, MS
Geisinger Health System, Autism and Developmental Medicine Institute, Danville, Pennsylvania

DEBORAH KRAKOW, MD
Departments of Orthopaedic Surgery, Human Genetics and Obstetrics and Gynecology, David Geffen School of Medicine at UCLA, Los Angeles, California

DAVID H. LEDBETTER, PhD
Executive Vice President and Chief Scientific Officer, Geisinger Health System, Autism and Developmental Medicine Institute, Danville, Pennsylvania

CHRISTA LESE MARTIN, PhD
Director and Senior Investigator, Geisinger Health System, Autism and Developmental Medicine Institute, Danville, Pennsylvania

BONNIE McCANN-CROSBY, MD
Pediatric Endocrinology Fellow, Division of Pediatric Endocrinology, Baylor College of Medicine, Texas Children's Hospital, Houston, Texas

NATHANIEL H. ROBIN, MD
Departments of Genetics, Pediatrics, and Otolyngology, The University of Alabama at Birmingham, Birmingham, Alabama

MICHAEL L. SCHMITZ, MD
Chief, Orthopaedics and Rehabilitation Services, Children's Orthopaedics of Atlanta, Children's Healthcare of Atlanta, Atlanta, Georgia

ANNE SLAVOTINEK, MB.BS, PhD
Professor of Clinical Pediatrics, Division of Genetics, Department of Pediatrics, University of California, San Francisco, San Francisco, California

SUSAN E. SPARKS, MD, PhD
Clinical Geneticist, Department of Pediatrics, Carolinas Healthcare System, Charlotte, North Carolina; Adjunct Assistant Professor, Department of Pediatrics, University of North Carolina School of Medicine, Chapel Hill, North Carolina

V. REID SUTTON, MD
Professor, Department of Molecular and Human Genetics, Baylor College of Medicine, Texas Children's Hospital, Houston, Texas

STEPHANIE M. WARE, MD, PhD
Department of Pediatrics and Medical and Molecular Genetics, Herman B Wells Center for Pediatric Research, Indiana University School of Medicine, Indianapolis, Indiana

MATTHEW T. WHITEHEAD, MD
Assistant Professor, Department of Radiology; Director of Neuroradiology Education, Children's National Medical Center, Washington, DC

WILLIAM R. WILCOX, MD, PhD, FACMG
Professor, Department of Human Genetics, Emory University, Atlanta, Georgia

Contents

without cleft palate, esophageal atresia/tracheoesophageal fistula, congenital heart defects, ventral wall defects, and polydactyly.

Making the diagnosis of genetic syndromes in the neonatal period can be challenging, as limited information concerning growth and development is available. The pattern of dysmorphic features and malformations is therefore correspondingly more important in syndrome recognition. The authors provide specific examples of the differences in the presentation for selected syndromes between the newborn period and later childhood. The purpose is to describe the variation in presentation that can occur with chronologic age and to aid in the early diagnosis of these conditions.

Congenital limb deficiency disorders (LDDs) are birth defects characterized by the aplasia or hypoplasia of bones of the limbs. Limb deficiencies are classified as transverse, those due to intrauterine disruptions of previously normal limbs, or longitudinal, those that are isolated or associated with certain syndromes as well as chromosomal anomalies. Consultation with a medical geneticist is advisable. Long-term care should occur in a specialized limb deficiency center with expertise in orthopedics, prosthetics, and occupational and physical therapy and provide emotional support and contact with other families. With appropriate care, most children with LDDs can lead productive lives.

The skeletal dysplasias are a group of more than 450 heritable disorders of bone. They frequently present in the newborn period with disproportion, radiographic abnormalities, and occasionally other organ system abnormalities. For improved clinical care, it is important to determine a precise diagnosis to aid in management, familial recurrence, and identify those disorders highly associated with mortality. Long-term management of these disorders is predicated on an understanding of the associated skeletal system abnormalities, and these children are best served by a team approach to health care surveillance.

Craniofacial malformations are among the most common birth defects. Although most cases of orofacial clefting and craniosynostosis are isolated and sporadic, these abnormalities are associated with a wide range of genetic syndromes, and making the appropriate diagnosis can guide management and counseling. Patients with craniofacial malformation are best cared for in a multidisciplinary clinic that can coordinate the care delivered by a diverse team of providers.

Up to 14% of patients with congenital metabolic disease may show structural brain abnormalities from perturbation of cell proliferation, migration, and/or organization. Most inborn errors of metabolism have a postnatal onset. Abnormalities from genetic disease processes have a prenatal onset. Energy impairment, substrate insufficiency, cell membrane receptor and cell signaling abnormalities, and toxic byproduct accumulation are associations between genetic disorders and structural brain anomalies. Collective imaging patterns of brain abnormalities can provide clues to the underlying etiology. We review selected metabolic diseases associated with brain malformations and highlight characteristic clinical and imaging manifestations that help narrow the differential diagnosis.

Neonatal hypotonia is a common problem in the neonatal intensive care unit. The genetic differential diagnosis is broad, encompassing primary muscular dystrophies, chromosome abnormalities, neuropathies, and inborn errors of metabolism. Recognition of hypotonia is relatively straightforward, but determining the cause can be challenging. It is important for the neonatologist to have an organized approach to the assessment of neonatal hypotonia. Physical examination and history alongside basic laboratory testing and imaging aid in the differential diagnosis. Identification of the cause is essential for determining prognosis, associated morbidities, and recurrence risk. The prevailing therapeutic modality is physical, occupational, speech/feeding, and respiratory therapy.

Congenital heart defects (CHDs) are structural abnormalities of the heart and great vessels that are present from birth. The presence or absence of extracardiac anomalies has historically been used to identify patients with possible monogenic, chromosomal, or teratogenic CHD causes. These distinctions remain clinically relevant, but it is increasingly clear that nonsyndromic CHDs can also be genetic. This article discusses key morphologic, molecular, and signaling mechanisms relevant to heart development, summarizes overall progress in molecular genetic analyses of CHDs, and provides current recommendations for clinical application of genetic testing.

Disorders of sexual development (DSDs) are a group of disorders in which there is discordance between anatomic or hormonal sex and sex chromosome complement. These disorders present with ambiguity in the newborn period and require prompt evaluation to determine the underlying cause for treatment and appropriate sex assignment of the infant. Neonatologists should confer with a multidisciplinary team for the diagnostic evaluation and management of patients with DSDs. This article provides a review of normal sexual development, algorithms used for evaluating infants with ambiguous genitalia, and conditions that can present with ambiguous genitalia in the newborn period.

Inborn errors of metabolism (IEM) are individually rare but collectively common. Approximately 25% of IEMs can have manifestations in the neonatal period. Neonates with IEM are usually healthy at birth; however, in hours to days after birth they can develop nonspecific signs that are common to several other neonatal conditions. Therefore, maintaining a high index of suspicion is extremely important for early diagnosis and the institution of appropriate therapy, which are mandatory to prevent death and ameliorate complications from many IEMs.

Newborn screening is a major aspect of public health success. Babies in every state are tested for a recommended uniform screening panel of conditions not otherwise immediately evident in the first days of life. With the goal of reducing morbidity and mortality, conditions should be added to newborn screening panels using a scientific, evidence-based process. Newborn screening is a system involving partners at many levels; neonatologists have a special role in ensuring that their vulnerable patients also receive this life-saving test. Careful attention to the social, legal, and ethical aspects will help increase the scope of newborn screening.

PROGRAM OBJECTIVE
The goal of *Clinics in Perinatology* is to keep practicing perinatologists, neonatologists, obstetricians, practicing physicians and residents up to date with current clinical practice in perinatology by providing timely articles reviewing the state of the art in patient care.

TARGET AUDIENCE
Perinatologists, neonatologists, obstetricians, practicing physicians, residents and healthcare professionals who provide patient care utilizing findings from *Clinics in Perinatology*.

LEARNING OBJECTIVES
Upon completion of this activity, participants will be able to:
1. Review the many types of genetic testing for neonatal care.
2. Discuss genetics and genetic testing in the newborn, and the roll of genetics in perinatology in the 21st century.
3. Recognize syndromes in the newborn period.

ACCREDITATION
The Elsevier Office of Continuing Medical Education (EOCME) is accredited by the Accreditation Council for Continuing Medical Education (ACCME) to provide continuing medical education for physicians.

The EOCME designates this enduring material for a maximum of 15 *AMA PRA Category 1 Credit*(s)™. Physicians should claim only the credit commensurate with the extent of their participation in the activity.

All other health care professionals requesting continuing education credit for this enduring material will be issued a certificate of participation.

DISCLOSURE OF CONFLICTS OF INTEREST
The EOCME assesses conflict of interest with its instructors, faculty, planners, and other individuals who are in a position to control the content of CME activities. All relevant conflicts of interest that are identified are thoroughly vetted by EOCME for fair balance, scientific objectivity, and patient care recommendations. EOCME is committed to providing its learners with CME activities that promote improvements or quality in healthcare and not a specific proprietary business or a commercial interest.

The planning committee, staff, authors and editors listed below have identified no financial relationships or relationships to products or devices they or their spouse/life partner have with commercial interest related to the content of this CME activity:
Margaret P. Adam, MD; Marwan Ali, MD; Arunkanth Ankala, PhD; Susan A. Berry, MD; Colleen P. Coulter, PT, DPT, PhD, PCS; Jason R. Cowan, MS; Ayman W. El-Hattab, MD, FAAP, FACMG; Anjali Fortna; Stanley T. Fricke, PhD; Michael J. Gambello, MD, PhD; Andrea L. Gropman, MD; J. Austin Hamm, MD; Madhuri R. Hegde, PhD; Kerry Holland; Lucky Jain, MD, MBA; Kelly L. Jones, MD; Brianne E. Kirkpatrick, MS; Deborah Krakow, MD; Bonnie McCann-Crosby, MD; Palani Murugesan; Nathaniel H. Robin, MD; Michael L. Schmitz, MD; Megan Suermann; V. Reid Sutton, MD; Stephanie M. Ware, MD, PhD; Matthew T. Whitehead, MD; William R. Wilcox, MD, PhD, FACMG.

The planning committee, staff, authors and editors listed below have identified financial relationships or relationships to products or devices they or their spouse/life partner have with commercial interest related to the content of this CME activity:
David H. Ledbetter, PhD is a consultant/advisor for, with stock ownership in, Natera, Inc.
Christa Lese Martin, PhD is a consultant/advisor for Mead Johnson & Company, LLC; Nestlé; and Alcresta, and has research support from Abbott Nutritional and Alcresta.
Anne Slavotinek, MB.BS, PhD receives royalties/patents from UpToDate, under a division of Wolters Kluwer; and Oxford University Press, is a consultant/advisor for Amgen Inc; and has research support from the National Institutes of Health.
Susan E. Sparks, MD, PhD is a consultant/advisor for Sarepta Therapeutics; has research support from Eli Lilly and Company; BioMarin Pharmaceutical Inc; and Genzyme Corporation, a Sanofi Company; and has an employment affiliation with Genzyme, a Sanofi Company.

UNAPPROVED/OFF-LABEL USE DISCLOSURE
The EOCME requires CME faculty to disclose to the participants:
1. When products or procedures being discussed are off-label, unlabelled, experimental, and/or investigational (not US Food and Drug Administration [FDA] approved); and

2. Any limitations on the information presented, such as data that are preliminary or that represent ongoing research, interim analyses, and/or unsupported opinions. Faculty may discuss information about pharmaceutical agents that is outside of FDA-approved labelling. This information is intended solely for CME and is not intended to promote off-label use of these medications. If you have any questions, contact the medical affairs department of the manufacturer for the most recent prescribing information.

TO ENROLL
To enroll in the *Clinics in Perinatology* Continuing Medical Education program, call customer service at 1-800-654-2452 or sign up online at http://www.theclinics.com/home/cme. The CME program is available to subscribers for an additional annual fee of $235 USD.

METHOD OF PARTICIPATION
In order to claim credit, participants must complete the following:
1. Complete enrolment as indicated above.
2. Read the activity.
3. Complete the CME Test and Evaluation. Participants must achieve a score of 70% on the test. All CME Tests and Evaluations must be completed online.

CME INQUIRIES/SPECIAL NEEDS
For all CME inquiries or special needs, please contact elsevierCME@elsevier.com.

CLINICS IN PERINATOLOGY

THE CLINICS ARE AVAILABLE ONLINE!
Access your subscription at:
www.theclinics.com

Erratum

An error was made in the March 2012 issue of *Clinics in Perinatology* (Volume 39, Issue 1, p. 1–268) on page 76.

Under the subheading "Adverse effects," beginning in the fifth line down, a sentence states:

"Cidofovir is contraindicated in patients with a serum creatinine of *less than* 1.5 mg/dL, …"

This sentence should correctly read: "Cidofovir is contraindicated when a patient's serum creatinine is *greater than* 1.5 mg/dL."

Clin Perinatol 42 (2015) xv
http://dx.doi.org/10.1016/j.clp.2015.04.003
perinatology.theclinics.com
0095-5108/15/$ – see front matter © 2015 Elsevier Inc. All rights reserved.

Foreword

The Future of Personalized and Precision Perinatal Medicine

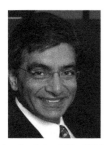

Lucky Jain, MD, MBA
Consulting Editor

Advances in the discovery of variations in the human genome that code for common diseases have been nothing short of spectacular. Introduction of new and cheaper sequencing methods has put the entire genome and exome (**Fig. 1**) well within the reach of patients and clinicians.[1] For busy clinicians who have been observing these developments from the sideline, it may be time to do two things: (1) get to know the common terms used in genetic testing along with the information they provide, and (2) be prepared to engage in a meaningful discussion about the clinical application of these tests.[2–4]

First, a word about terminology.[2,3] The 23 chromosomes that constitute our diploid genome carry close to 23,500 protein-coding genes. The coding information within these genes is carried in small segments called exons. These 180,000 or so exons collectively occupy just 1% of the genome and are referred to as the "exome." The "genome" is much larger and contains approximately 3.2 billion nucleotides. Scientists and commercial ventures have been exploring ways to make this information accessible to the lay public. It started with gene chips to study single-nucleotide polymorphisms, which eventually led to the introduction of genome-wide association studies. Many of these methods are limited in their value and in the extent of genetic variability they can uncover. This is in contrast to whole-genome sequencing, which can shed light on the complete spectrum of genetic determinants comprising an individual's heritable makeup.

These nomenclature and methodology issues notwithstanding, it is the second aspect of genetic testing that generates the most confusion and alarm among clinicians who are not geneticists: how do we manage the mountain of information which will eventually become available?[4] Which method will give us the most reliable information about DNA variation? Should parents have access to genetic information about diseases that may not manifest until the third or fourth decade? Should society have a say in how we use information that has a high public health impact (and potential

Clin Perinatol 42 (2015) xvii–xix
http://dx.doi.org/10.1016/j.clp.2015.04.002   **perinatology.theclinics.com**
0095-5108/15/$ – see front matter © 2015 Published by Elsevier Inc.

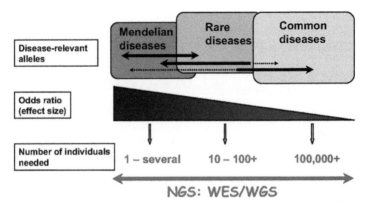

Fig. 1. Roadmap for the application of next generation sequencing technologies for the identification of disease-relevant genomic variations. NGS, next generation sequencing; WES, whole exome sequencing; WGS, whole exome sequencing. (*Adapted from* Majewski J, Schwartzentruber J, Lalonde E, et al. What can exome sequencing do for you? J Med Gen 2011;48:581; with permission.)

resource use)? Can we create panels of information (and/or testing) that become accessible to teams (clinicians, patient, parent) only when it is deemed most useful? These and other burning questions need to be answered before the train leaves the platform.

In many ways, this issue of the *Clinics in Perinatology* dedicated to perinatal genetics could not have come at a better time. Not only do the superb articles selected by Drs Gambello and Sutton familiarize us with the "gamut" of genetic testing for perinatal-neonatal care but also they provide us with a strong framework for future conversations about the most efficient application of new technologies. For clinicians who are responsible for ordering and managing genetic testing, this charge comes with a bigger responsibility that goes beyond the initial test (**Fig. 2**).[5] We have to be good stewards of resources that may be needed once the information becomes available and be mindful about how and where the information is housed. I can't thank

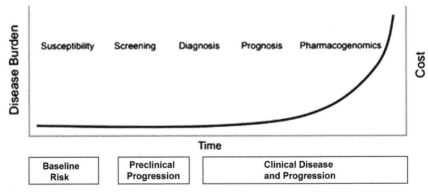

Fig. 2. The course of a chronic disease over time, illustrating opportunities over time to use various molecular and clinical tools to refine risk of developing disease and interventions. (*Adapted from* Ginsbug GS, Willard HF. Genomic and personalized medicine: foundations and applications. Transl Res 2009;154:281; with permission.)

Drs Gambello and Sutton enough for their effort and the publication team at Elsevier (Kerry Holland and Casey Jackson) for their attention to every detail.

Lucky Jain, MD, MBA
Department of Pediatrics
Emory University School of Medicine and
Children's Healthcare of Atlanta
2015 Uppergate Drive
Atlanta, GA 30322, USA

E-mail address:
ljain@emory.edu

REFERENCES

1. Majewski J, Schwartzentruber J, Lalonde E, et al. What can exome sequencing do for you? J Med Genet 2011;48:580–9.
2. Khoury MJ, McBride CM, Schully SD, et al. The Scientific Foundation for personal genomics: recommendations from a National Institutes of Health-Centers for Diseases Control and Prevention multidisciplinary workshop. Genet Med 2009; 11:559–67.
3. Marian AJ. Sequencing your genome: what does it mean? Methodist Debakey Cardiovasc J 2014;10:3–6.
4. Feero WG. Clinical application of whole-genome sequencing: proceed with care. JAMA 2014;311:1017–8.
5. Ginsburg GS, Willard HF. Genomic and personalized medicine: foundations and applications. Transl Res 2009;154:277–87.

Preface

Genetics in the Twenty-First Century

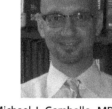
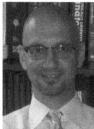

Michael J. Gambello, MD, PhD   V. Reid Sutton, MD
Editors

Genetic disorders constitute a significant portion of admissions to neonatal intensive care units. Studies of admissions to pediatric hospitals have documented that up to 71% of admissions have an underlying disorder with a significant genetic component. Moreover, those patients with a significant genetic contribution had longer hospital stays and greater hospital charges.[1] Given this high health care burden, genetics is a very important component of neonatal care. Moreover, as genetic technologies have advanced rapidly over the past decade, a much higher percentage of individuals who are evaluated for a genetic condition receive a definitive diagnosis compared with a decade ago. Studies have shown that array comparative genomic hybridization identified chromosomal abnormalities in about 12% of cases where routine chromosome studies are normal. In addition, whole-exome sequencing, which has become clinically available in the past few years, achieves a diagnosis in approximately 25% of individuals. This rate will continue to increase as gene discovery continues. This issue reviews common genetic disorders encountered in the newborn period, including well-established chromosomal disorders, single-gene syndromes, and inborn errors of metabolism, and incorporates information about new and emerging technologies and diagnoses.

Michael J. Gambello, MD, PhD
Department of Human Genetics and Pediatrics
Emory University School of Medicine
615 Michael Street, Suite 301
Atlanta, GA 30322, USA

Clin Perinatol 42 (2015) xxi–xxii
http://dx.doi.org/10.1016/j.clp.2015.04.001
0095-5108/15/$ – see front matter © 2015 Published by Elsevier Inc.

V. Reid Sutton, MD
Department of Molecular & Human Genetics
Baylor College of Medicine
& Texas Children's Hospital
6701 Fannin Street, Suite 1560
Houston, TX 77030, USA

E-mail addresses:
mgambel@emory.edu (M.J. Gambello)
vrsutton@texaschildrens.org (V.R. Sutton)

REFERENCE

1. McCandless SE, Brunger JW, Cassidy SB. The burden of genetic disease on inpatient care in a children's hospital. Am J Hum Genet 2004;74(1):121–7.

Gamut of Genetic Testing for Neonatal Care

Arunkanth Ankala, PhD, Madhuri R. Hegde, PhD*

KEYWORDS

- Genetic testing • Perinatal diagnostics • Clinical genetics • Neonatal diagnostics
- Exome sequencing

KEY POINTS

- The choice of genetic testing will depend upon history, physical examination, and differential diagnosis.
- A molecular diagnosis is important for management, natural history, and future studies.
- Consultation with a medical geneticist can facilitate the selection of the appropriate genetic tests.
- This article discusses the clinical utility and indications for each of a host of genetic testing options available for a referring neonatologist.

INTRODUCTION

There are over 3500 known monogenic genetic diseases, most of which present during the first 28 days of life.[1] Despite the fact that these are monogenic Mendelian disorders, clinical diagnosis of most of these conditions is complicated in several ways, including pleiotropy (1 gene presenting multiple phenotypes), clinical heterogeneity (symptoms overlapping with other disorders), and genetic heterogeneity (multiple genes associated with the same phenotype or disease). Moreover, with the rapid advances in sequencing technologies, the identification of new genetic diseases and novel genes associated with known diseases makes it difficult for clinicians to maintain an up-to-date knowledge of clinical genetics. Although a treatment or management protocol may not be available for many genetic diseases, timely diagnosis is nonetheless important for natural history, management decisions, and recurrence risks. The appropriate choice of genetic testing can provide an accurate and usually rapid diagnosis.

Rapid and cost-effective genetic testing is currently available in multiple forms. Genetic technologies have evolved dramatically to offer a wide variety of tests,

Disclosure statement: The authors declare that they do not have any conflicts of interest.
Department of Human Genetics, Emory University School of Medicine, 615 Michael Street, Atlanta, GA 30322, USA
* Corresponding author.
E-mail address: mhegde@emory.edu

Clin Perinatol 42 (2015) 217–226
http://dx.doi.org/10.1016/j.clp.2015.02.001   perinatology.theclinics.com

each with increasing clinical utility and yields (**Fig. 1**).[2–4] Although conventional G-banded karyotyping and fluorescence in situ hybridization (FISH) are still used extensively, chromosomal microarray (CMA) testing is the most widely used cytogenetic diagnostic tool. CMA is also considered the first-tier clinical diagnostic test for individuals with developmental disabilities or congenital anomalies.[4] Biochemical genetic testing includes enzymatic assays, chromatography methods, and mass spectrometry assays. Biochemical testing is the mainstay of newborn screening programs leading to the definitive diagnosis of inborn errors of metabolism. Current molecular genetic testing encompasses targeted mutation testing, single-gene sequencing, next-generation sequencing (NGS)-based multigene panel testing, whole-exome sequencing, and whole-genome sequencing. With the availability of so many different testing options, clinicians need guidance when trying to select the best diagnostic test for their patients with potential genetic conditions. Therefore, general recommendations and consensus statements are needed to help clinicians make the best choice for their patients.[3,4] This article discusses the full gamut of genetic testing, along with the clinical utilities and indications for each test type, in the context of neonatal care. Although a brief introduction to the different cytogenetic tests available is provided, the major focus of the article is a discussion of the strengths and limitations of the available clinical molecular genetic tests.

CYTOGENETIC TESTING

The peripheral blood karyotype (also called a G-banded karyotype for the Giemsa stain used to visualize the chromosome bands) and fluorescent in situ hybridization

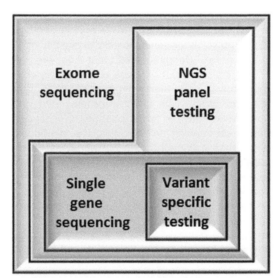

Fig. 1. Pictorial representation of the clinical utilities of the various molecular genetic tests currently available. While variant specific testing interrogates known and highly frequent variant associated with a disease for rapid diagnosis, single-gene sequencing by Sanger method interrogates the entire gene implicated with a disease, more specifically when the disease has high allelic heterogeneity. NGS panel testing involves sequencing of multiple genes, all of which are known to be associated with a specific disorder or phenotype. ES interrogates all genes (more specifically exons) in the human genome regardless of the phenotype and is often the preferred diagnostic test when the clinical presentation is atypical, complex or nonspecific, or when a disease specific panel is not clinically available.

(FISH) were the foundation of cytogenetic analysis until the development of the more sensitive array-based chromosome microarray. A karyotype is only recommended for suspected whole-chromosome aneuploidy (trisomies 13, 18, 21) or a balanced trans-location (suspected because of an unbalanced translocation in a child). Although a karyotype can identify deletions or duplications of 5 Mb or greater, array-based chromosome microarrays have a much higher resolution. FISH has been the standard technology for detecting recurrent known chromosomal anomalies such as Williams syndrome or 22q11.2 deletion syndrome.

MICROARRAY-BASED CHROMOSOMAL MICROARRAY

Array-based comparative genomic hybridization (aCGH) or chromosome microarray has revolutionized the fields of cytogenetics and molecular genetics.[5,6] Chromosome microarrays are used to detect chromosome deletions or duplications as small as 50 kb or less,[7,8] a much higher resolution than that of the conventional karyotype. Today, array-based genomic copy number analyses are performed in multiple ways and under various names, depending on the resolution and design of the assay. Chromosomal microarray (CMA), also referred to as molecular karyotyping, is most often available as aCGH that is designed using oligonucleotide probes or as a single nucleotide polymorphism array (SNP array) that interrogates known SNPs.[9,10] While CMAs are genome-wide arrays used frequently in cytogenetics, there are gene-specific molecular arrays that target a specific gene, such as *DMD* or multiple genes of interest.[11] CMA is currently the first-tier clinical diagnostic test for individuals with developmental disabilities or multiple congenital anomalies.[4] Although CMA testing has significantly improved the diagnostic ability, from 3% for G-banded karyotyping to 15% to 20%, most cases remain undiagnosed.[4] Molecular genetic testing is usually sought for the diagnosis of a majority of these cases.

COMPENDIUM OF MOLECULAR GENETIC TESTING ASSAYS

Molecular genetic testing began in the mid-1980s in research laboratories exploring linkage analysis to aid disease gene discovery. With the identification of novel disease-causing genes, molecular genetic tests became available and were launched in both academic and commercial settings. Today, many molecular tests are available for neonatal diagnostics. These assays include conventional polymerase chain reaction (PCR)-based assays, Southern blotting, multiplex ligation-dependent probe amplification (MLPA) assays, Sanger sequencing assays, aCGH, and NGS-based assays, specifically multigene panels and exome sequencing (ES) and genome sequencing (GS). A variety of these assays is discussed in detail here, with reference to their clinical utilities and the indications for ordering each.

Variant-Specific Assays

As indicated, these tests interrogate a single variant or a group of specific known pathogenic variants in a gene or genes associated with a certain disease or phenotype. Here, note that the term pathogenic variants is being used throughout this text to refer to any disease-causing mutation, in keeping with the current practice in molecular genetics. A classic example of a variant-specific assay is the US Food and Drug Administration (FDA)-approved clinical assay for cystic fibrosis (CF), which targets a set of 23 or more variants known to contribute to most CF cases regardless of ethnicity. Although over 1300 pathogenic variants have been found in *CFTR*, the gene associated with CF, any newborn with a positive CF screen is recommended for follow-up testing for the 23 most common variants.[12] This is a very efficient genetic test, because it is cost-effective while having a very high clinical yield of 57% to 97% in certain ethnicities.[13,14] There are similar assays for other disorders, such as MCADD (medium-chain acyl-coenzyme A dehydrogenase) deficiency, in which approximately 40% to 50% of affected individuals are either homozygous or heterozygous for a single common pathogenic variant, c.985A>G (p.K304E).[15]

Single-Gene Sanger Sequencing Assays

Single-gene testing is preferred when a patient's clinical features are typical for a particular disorder; the disorder is strongly associated with 1 or 2 specific genes, and there are no well-defined common mutations. The clinical sensitivity of a single-gene test is high only if the clinical findings strongly suggest associated disease, and there is no genetic heterogeneity (other genes causing same phenotype). Much like the variant-specific assays, single-gene Sanger sequencing assays are more appropriate for monogenic disorders with a clearly distinguishable phenotype. However, unlike the variant-specific assays discussed previously, genes indicated for this test type often have high allelic heterogeneity, meaning the pathogenic variants can be all along the length of the gene, without a specific hotspot or high recurrence of a single variant. There are a number of such monogenic disorders such as neonatal Marfan and CHARGE (coloboma heart defect, atresia choanae, retarded growth and development, genital abnormality, and ear anomalies) syndromes.[16] Neonatal Marfan syndrome is a severe and rapidly progressing phenotype characterized by congenital contractures, dilated cardiomyopathy, congestive heart failure, pulmonary emphysema, and mitral or tricuspid valve regurgitation in the newborn period.[17] FBN1 is the major gene associated with Marfan syndrome; however, there have been several hundred pathogenic variants reported within this gene. Similarly, CHD7 is the major gene associated with CHARGE syndrome, accounting for over 90% of typical affected cases.[18] Sanger sequencing of the single gene in question will establish a molecular diagnosis in most of these cases.

Molecular Deletion/Duplication Array Tests

Targeted molecular arrays are routinely used in clinical laboratories to detect deletions and duplications within a gene in an individual. As indicated previously, although the clinical application may be different (interrogating intragenic deletions and duplications for molecular testing vs larger intergenic, multigenic, or chromosomal deletions and duplications for cytogenetic testing), the basic technology for array testing is the same for molecular arrays and CMA. Although the test is applicable to any and all known genes, the clinical yield is limited. This is because of the variant spectra of disease-associated genes. Although certain genes like DMD and PMP22 have a high frequency of deletions and duplications contributing to the disease, most other genes occasionally have intragenic deletions and duplications. Therefore for most genes, molecular arrays are usually preferred only when the clinical suspicion for mutations in that gene is strong despite negative sequencing results or when a single sequence variant is detected in an autosomal-recessive condition. Because every negative test adds to the pressure of urgency, understanding the clinical yields of each test is helpful.

Targeted Disease-Specific or Phenotype-Specific Multigene Panel Assays

Unlike certain diseases with a distinctive phenotype, most disorders have significantly high clinical variability and genetic locus heterogeneity, such that a multigene panel approach is deemed appropriate for an efficient and timely molecular diagnosis. NGS-based multigene panel tests usually involve targeted enrichment of a group of genes known to be associated with a disease or phenotype and simultaneous sequencing and analysis of all these genes in 1 single assay.[19] The obvious difference in the number of genes included in the panels depends on the stringency of inclusion criteria practiced by each testing laboratory. Although some laboratories tend to include genes that have even the slightest association with a disease or phenotype, to increase diagnostic yield, other laboratories may aim for high test specificity by including only those genes with strong established evidence for disease causality.[3] This is because the specificity of the assay may be compromised when variants are found in multiple genes in a test. This rationale holds true for preferring targeted panels over ES or GS. Besides the diagnostic specificity of a targeted multigene panel approach discussed previously, a panel approach, because it targets and sequences only a specific set or subset of genes (more precisely exons), has an added advantage over ES: high coverage. Coverage refers to the number of times a particular nucleotide is interrogated or sequenced in the assay, and higher coverage means greater confidence that a detected variant is a true positive. The multigene panel testing approach has not only increased the analytical sensitivity of DNA diagnostic testing, but also simplified the decision-making process for ordering physicians.[20] This is clearly evident from the dramatic increase in the number and variety of disorders for which multigene panel tests are being offered and ordered.

The different indications for multigene panel testing include high genetic heterogeneity, where multiple genes cause the same phenotype or disease, clinical heterogeneity, where the clinical presentation of a disease has high overlap with several other completely different diseases, or the presence of 1 or 2 nonspecific symptoms that are characteristic of multiple otherwise different disorders. Neonatal diabetes is another good example of a disease for which a targeted multigene panel test is appropriate and clinically available. Unlike Apert syndrome or Marfan syndrome, neonatal diabetes can be caused by many genes, among them ABCC8, KCNJ11, INS, ZFP57, GCK, IPF1, EIF2AK3, and others.[21] In diseases like this, where multiple genes can be causative of a phenotype, oftentimes only the most frequent, well-known, or well-established genes are tested, and after 1 or 2 negative results, the pursuit of a molecular diagnosis is given up. Establishing a molecular diagnosis is important in several ways, including patient management and disease treatment. For instance, the recommended treatment for neonatal diabetes caused by pathogenic variants in ABCC8 or KCNJ11 is sulfonylurea, while neonatal diabetes caused by INS variants is treated with insulin replacement.[22,23] Therefore, for clinically heterogeneous diseases or in scenarios in which multiple genes are suspected, a targeted multigene panel should be the first-tier test.

Mitochondrial Genome Testing

When discussing human inherited disorders, it is important to remember mitochondrial disorders and the molecular genetic testing available for their clinical diagnosis. Mitochondrial diseases are a special group of rare inherited disorders that have extreme phenotypic heterogeneity and can be transmitted by any mode of inheritance. Prematurity, intrauterine growth retardation and hypotonia necessitating ventilatory support, neonatal seizures, elevated lactate levels, and hyperammonemia are characteristic of mitochondrial disorders. The phenotypic overlap with other neurologic and metabolic disorders makes it difficult to clinically diagnose a mitochondrial disease. Furthermore, mitochondrial diseases are caused not only by variants in the mitochondrial genome, but also by pathogenic variants in more than 100 of 1200 nuclear genes that encode mitochondrial targeted proteins.[24–26] Therefore, when a mitochondrial disorder is suspected in a neonate, either targeted mitochondrial mutation testing, whole mitochondrial genome sequencing, or a panel test that interrogates both the mitochondrial genome and nuclear genes known to be associated with mitochondrial disorders is appropriate. Honzik and colleagues[27] have proposed a detailed algorithm for molecular genetic testing of mitochondrial disorders in neonates. This is a gene-by-gene approach. However, in the interest of time, whole mitochondrial sequencing or comprehensive mitochondrial panel testing (which includes nuclear genes) may be preferred.[28,29] In fact, NGS-based sequencing for mitochondrial disease diagnosis in a patient cohort of infants suspected of mitochondrial disease has been shown to have a high diagnostic yield of 25% to 50%[30] versus 16% by sequential single-gene sequencing and deletion analysis.[31] Taken together, NGS-based mitochondrial sequencing or panel testing that includes nuclear genes associated with mitochondrial diseases may be preferable for rapid diagnosis of infantile or neonatal mitochondrial diseases.

Testing for Epigenetic Variations

Along with DNA-based molecular genetic testing goes epigenetic testing, which mostly involves DNA methylation analysis. Alterations in DNA methylation (epigenetic signature) of certain genes and genomic regions can lead to silencing or inappropriate expression of genes, thereby causing disease. Beckwith-Wiedemann syndrome (BWS) and Russell-Silver syndrome are among some of the disorders that present neonatally. Diagnosis of BWS and treatment of neonatal hypoglycemia are highly critical for survival of the neonate. Additionally, Prader-Willi and Angelman syndromes, which frequently present with congenital or neonatal hypotonia, are also diagnosable by methylation analysis.[32] In fact, methylation testing is the first test recommended for these disorders. Therefore methylation test should be preferred whenever these disorders are suspected in a neonate.

Exome Sequencing

ES is a fascinating diagnostic tool made possible with the advent of NGS technology. ES interrogates the exome, which refers to the comprehensive coding region of the human genome, represents less than 1.5% of the entire genetic material, and yet accounts for over 80% to 85% of disease-causative variants. Even though ES has been a game changer, it is hotly debated whether ES/GS approaches, as they interrogate the complete genome and not just the genes possibly associated with the disease phenotype, should be the last resort for diagnosis after all known targeted single-gene and panel tests have been exhausted.[33] Nevertheless, 1 way to look at it is that, basically, interrogation of the whole genome of an individual with nondescript developmental delay or congenital anomalies has been in practice since the early days of cytogenetics in the form of G-banded karyotyping, and most recently chromosomal microarrays, but that ES/GS provides significantly enhanced resolution, resolution to the level of nucleotides or single nucleotide variants. Neonatal diagnostics is complicated by the fact that most of the neonates and infants do not have a fully developed phenotype, and the underlying disease may not be completely recognizable until later. Thus, ES may be chosen immediately after an initial impression of a genetic component to a confounding or unusual presentation. In fact, in certain cases, having ES results may prompt re-evaluation to better correlate and understand the clinical presentation (**Case 1**). Experts opine that, even if a diagnosis may not be made immediately, early integration of genomic information would further the clinical investigation of such phenotypes that demand ongoing evaluation of disease presentation.[34] Recently a multidisciplinary unit performing comprehensive exome sequence analysis has claimed that about 80% of cases referred from neonatal intensive care units and pediatric subspecialty clinics could be molecularly diagnosed.[34] A second rationale against opting ES as the first-tier test is that it may miss variants (that would otherwise be detected by targeted multigene panel testing) in disease-specific genes because of a lack of coverage. As pointed out by some recent reports,[3] for certain well-characterized diseases ES may be part of a 2-tier approach, with a disease-specific targeted multigene panel test being the first test, followed by ES, if negative. Such an approach would allow one to characterize new diseases or better understand the neonatal presentation of already known diseases.[35] Regardless, a timely diagnosis facilitated by ES allows

1. Mitigating uncertainty and enabling prospective management
2. Preventive management before onset of all disease symptoms
3. Diagnosis of multiple disorders that confound clinical investigation and diagnosis
4. Avoidance of futile intensive care expenses
5. Enabling stem cell transplantation (for example in neonates with severe combined immunodeficiency [SCID]).
6. Offering reproductive choices for the future

Genome Sequencing

GS is 1 single comprehensive test that has the proven potential to replace most other current-day genetic tests, including CMA, multigene panel testing, and ES. GS is designed to interrogate every single nucleotide in the entire human genome and detect single nucleotide variants, as well as large-scale genomic rearrangements. Because GS involves analysis of both exonic and intronic regions of every single gene in the human genome, it can resolve large deletions, duplications, and transloca-tions to the nucleotide level and help one understand the complete consequence of such events.[36] However, there is still a long way to go before the true potential of the technology can be brought to bear for clinical diagnostics. The most successful application of GS for neonatal diagnostics has been demonstrated by Saunders and colleagues[1] who established a molecular diagnosis in multiple neonates within 5 days. However, the authors of the study do accept that a reasonable and time-sensitive assay for diagnosis could only be performed through an abridged version of GS, where the analysis was restricted to phenotype-associated genes. A complete and thorough analysis of the entire genome is highly demanding in terms of interpre-tive input, time, and cost. The most compromising aspect of GS is the sequence coverage, which is very low when compared with that of ES. Efforts are being made to develop better sequencing chemistries and higher throughput instruments, and studies are ongoing to explore the clinical utility of GS both for neonatal diagnostics and clinical genetics in general. Therefore, while some overly optimistic individuals may argue in favor of offering GS for neonatal diagnostics, the referring clinician who is making the decision still needs to exercise caution.

SUMMARY

With genomic technologies improving rapidly, new diseases are being identified, and many more of the 20,000 or more genes of the human genome are being implicated in genetic diseases. As current clinical practice is shifting from clinical diagnosis first to mo-lecular evaluation first, physicians are beginning to experience the true potential of personalized genomics. In this era of genomic medicine, clinicians and allied subspecial-ists all play an important role in bridging the gap between traditional evidence-based medicine and the emerging personalized medicine. Furthermore, with such complemen-tary efforts, genotype–phenotype correlations that have remained a black box for many genetic conditions will finally be apparent and improve the treatment of genetic disease.

Case 1

Confounding phenotype clarified by exome sequencing

This is a neonatal case reported by Golder N. Wilson.[37] The individual was diagnosed with arthrogryposis and joint contractures of all extremities, pulmonary hypoplasia, cryptorchidism, and inguinal hernia. After negative chromosomal microarray testing, ES was performed. As per the report, the clinical impression prior to ES was non-syndromic arthrogryposis with respiratory complications exacerbated by prematurity (delivered after 32-week gestation period). ES detected 4 heterozygous variants in different genes related to the clinical phenotype. Post-ES clinical reinterpretation by Wilson indicated that the confounding clinical presentation in the neonate was in fact contributed by more than one disease. A diagnosis of hyperekplexia 3 was established by the de novo variant in *SLC6A5* and that of Stickler syndrome by a maternally inherited variant in the *COL2A1* gene. Moreover, based on the maternal inheritance of the *COL2A1* variant, the mother of the infant, who herself had a history of arthritis and joint laxity, was clinically examined and diagnosed to have Stickler syndrome. These diagnoses in the infant and subsequently in the mother also potentially explained the cause of oligohydramnios and premature delivery of the neonate.[37] This example clearly demonstrates the roles of molecular geneticists (and the technology) and clinicians in complementing each other to successfully establish rapid and timely diagnosis in current-day clinics.

REFERENCES

1. Saunders CJ, Miller NA, Soden SE, et al. Rapid whole-genome sequencing for genetic disease diagnosis in neonatal intensive care units. Sci Transl Med 2012;4(154):154ra135.
2. Ankala A, Hegde M. Genomic technologies and the new era of genomic medicine. J Mol Diagn 2014;16(1):7–10.
3. Xue Y, Ankala A, Wilcox WR, et al. Solving the molecular diagnostic testing conundrum for Mendelian disorders in the era of next-generation sequencing: single-gene, gene panel, or exome/genome sequencing. Genet Med 2014. [Epub ahead of print].
4. Miller DT, Adam MP, Aradhya S, et al. Consensus statement: chromosomal microarray is a first-tier clinical diagnostic test for individuals with developmental disabilities or congenital anomalies. Am J Hum Genet 2010;86(5):749–64.
5. Slavotinek AM. Novel microdeletion syndromes detected by chromosome microarrays. Hum Genet 2008;124(1):1–17.
6. Vissers LE, Stankiewicz P. Microdeletion and microduplication syndromes. Genomic structural variants. New York: Springer; 2012. p. 29–75.
7. Askree SH, Chin EL, Bean LH, et al. Detection limit of intragenic deletions with targeted array comparative genomic hybridization. BMC Genet 2013; 14:116.
8. Selzer RR, Richmond TA, Pofahl NJ, et al. Analysis of chromosome breakpoints in neuroblastoma at sub-kilobase resolution using fine-tiling oligonucleotide array CGH. Genes Chromosomes Cancer 2005;44(3):305–19.
9. Rauch A, Ruschendorf F, Huang J, et al. Molecular karyotyping using an SNP array for genomewide genotyping. J Med Genet 2004;41(12):916–22.
10. Vermeesch JR, Rauch A. Reply to Hochstenbach et al. 'Molecular karyotyping'. Eur J Hum Genet 2006;14(10):1063–4.
11. Hegde MR, Chin EL, Mulle JG, et al. Microarray-based mutation detection in the dystrophin gene. Hum Mutat 2008;29(9):1091–9.
12. Watson MS, Cutting GR, Desnick RJ, et al. Cystic fibrosis population carrier screening: 2004 revision of American College of Medical Genetics mutation panel. Genet Med 2004;6(5):387–91.

13. Grody WW, Cutting GR, Klinger KW, et al. Laboratory standards and guidelines for population-based cystic fibrosis carrier screening. Genet Med 2001;3(2): 149–54.

14. Palomaki GE, Haddow JE, Bradley LA, et al. Updated assessment of cystic fibrosis mutation frequencies in non-Hispanic Caucasians. Genet Med 2002;4(2):90–4.

15. Gregersen N, Winter V, Curtis D, et al. Medium-chain acyl-CoA dehydrogenase (MCAD) deficiency: the prevalent mutation G985 (K304E) is subject to a strong founder effect from northwestern Europe. Hum Hered 1993;43(6):342–50.

16. Ghandi Y, Zanjani KS, Mazhari-Mousavi SE, et al. Neonatal Marfan syndrome: report of two cases. Iran J Pediatr 2013;23(1):113–7.

17. Jacobs AM, Toudjarska I, Racine A, et al. A recurring FBN1 gene mutation in neonatal Marfan syndrome. Arch Pediatr Adolesc Med 2002;156(11):1081–5.

18. Bergman JE, Janssen N, Hoefsloot LH, et al. CHD7 mutations and CHARGE syndrome: the clinical implications of an expanding phenotype. J Med Genet 2011; 48(5):334–42.

19. Valencia CA, Ankala A, Rhodenizer D, et al. Comprehensive mutation analysis for congenital muscular dystrophy: a clinical PCR-based enrichment and next-generation sequencing panel. PLoS One 2013;8(1):e53083.

20. Ankala A, da Silva C, Gualandi F, et al. A comprehensive genomic approach for neuromuscular diseases gives a high diagnostic yield. Ann Neurol 2015;77: 206–14.

21. Molven A, Njolstad PR. Role of molecular genetics in transforming diagnosis of diabetes mellitus. Expert Rev Mol Diagn 2011;11(3):313–20.

22. Sagen JV, Raeder H, Hathout E, et al. Permanent neonatal diabetes due to mutations in KCNJ11 encoding Kir6.2: patient characteristics and initial response to sulfonylurea therapy. Diabetes 2004;53(10):2713–8.

23. Zung A, Glaser B, Nimri R, et al. Glibenclamide treatment in permanent neonatal diabetes mellitus due to an activating mutation in Kir6.2. J Clin Endocrinol Metab 2004;89(11):5504–7.

24. Schon EA, DiMauro S, Hirano M. Human mitochondrial DNA: roles of inherited and somatic mutations. Nat Rev Genet 2012;13(12):878–90.

25. Ylikallio E, Suomalainen A. Mechanisms of mitochondrial diseases. Ann Med 2012;44(1):41–59.

26. Tucker EJ, Compton AG, Thorburn DR. Recent advances in the genetics of mitochondrial encephalopathies. Curr Neurol Neurosci Rep 2010;10(4):277–85.

27. Honzik T, Tesarova M, Magner M, et al. Neonatal onset of mitochondrial disorders in 129 patients: clinical and laboratory characteristics and a new approach to diagnosis. J Inherit Metab Dis 2012;35(5):749–59.

28. Dames S, Chou LS, Xiao Y, et al. The development of next-generation sequencing assays for the mitochondrial genome and 108 nuclear genes associated with mitochondrial disorders. J Mol Diagn 2013;15(4):526–34.

29. Dinwiddie DL, Smith LD, Miller NA, et al. Diagnosis of mitochondrial disorders by concomitant next-generation sequencing of the exome and mitochondrial genome. Genomics 2013;102(3):148–56.

30. Calvo SE, Compton AG, Hershman SG, et al. Molecular diagnosis of infantile mitochondrial disease with targeted next-generation sequencing. Sci Transl Med 2012;4(118):118ra110.

31. McCormick E, Place E, Falk MJ. Molecular genetic testing for mitochondrial disease: from one generation to the next. Neurotherapeutics 2013;10(2):251–61.

32. Nicholls RD, Saitoh S, Horsthemke B. Imprinting in Prader–Willi and angelman syndromes. Trends Genet 1998;14(5):194–200.

33. Lerner-Ellis JP. The clinical implementation of whole genome sequencing: a conversation with seven scientific experts. J Inherit Metab Dis 2012;35(4):689–93.
34. Katsanis N, Cotten M, Angrist M. Exome and genome sequencing of neonates with neurodevelopmental disorders. Future Neurol 2012;7(6):655–8.
35. Murali C, Lu JT, Jain M, et al. Diagnosis of ALG12-CDG by exome sequencing in a case of severe skeletal dysplasia. Mol Genet Metab Rep 2014;1:213–9.
36. Talkowski ME, Ordulu Z, Pillalamarri V, et al. Clinical diagnosis by whole-genome sequencing of a prenatal sample. N Engl J Med 2012;367(23):2226–32.
37. Wilson GN. Exome analysis of connective tissue dysplasia: death and rebirth of clinical genetics? Am J Med Genet A 2014;164A(5):1209–12.

Copy Number Variants, Aneuploidies, and Human Disease

Christa Lese Martin, PhD*, Brianne E. Kirkpatrick, MS,
David H. Ledbetter, PhD

KEYWORDS

- Copy number variant • CNV • Chromosomal microarray
- Noninvasive prenatal testing • Genomic databases • Aneuploidy • Prenatal
- Neonatal

KEY POINTS

- Copy number variants (CNVs) are a common cause of a wide range of human disorders, accounting for ~15% of neurodevelopmental disorders, cardiac abnormalities, and other congenital anomalies.
- Various methods are available to detect CNVs, including those that can identify CNVs across the entire genome and those that only target specific regions of the genome (eg, the common aneuploidies involving chromosomes 13, 18, 21, X, and Y).
- Accurate clinical interpretation of CNVs requires incorporation of genotype plus phenotype information.
- Identifying a genetic cause for a patient's phenotype can help to define targeted interventions and clinical management.

INTRODUCTION

In the perinatal setting, chromosome abnormalities span a wide range of genomic imbalance, from polyploidy (the presence of 3 [triploidy] or 4 [tetraploidy] copies of every chromosome), to whole-chromosome aneuploidy (typically involving only a single chromosome), to submicroscopic deletions and duplications that can only be detected by DNA-based copy number methods, such as fluorescence *in situ* hybridization (FISH) or chromosomal microarray (CMA). As technologies have improved to

Disclosure: D.H. Ledbetter is a consultant to Natera, Inc.
This work was supported in part by NIH grants RO1 MH074090 and U41 HG006834 (both to C.L. Martin and D.H. Ledbetter).
Geisinger Health System, Autism & Developmental Medicine Institute, 120 Hamm Drive, Lewisburg, PA 17837, USA
* Corresponding author.
E-mail address: clmartin1@geisinger.edu

detect smaller and smaller copy number variants (CNVs) across the genome, clinicians are learning the high frequency and important role that this type of genomic variation plays in human health and development.

CNVs have been identified as a common cause of several human diseases, many of which present in the neonatal period and/or early childhood. These diseases include neurodevelopmental disorders (such as autism, intellectual disability, and epilepsy), congenital heart defects, and other congenital anomalies.[1-3] However, not all CNVs are disease causing: some CNVs have been identified in apparently normal individuals.[4,5] Whether a CNV is disease causing or not depends on many factors, such as gene content (eg, a CNV that is gene rich is more likely to cause a phenotype than one containing few or no genes).[6] Therefore, understanding the corresponding phenotypic effects of particular CNVs is becoming increasingly important in clinical medicine so clinicians can define which CNVs cause a clinical phenotype versus those that are part of normal variation.

This article highlights key aspects of copy number detection during the prenatal and neonatal periods. Many infants presenting to neonatology services for a possible genetic diagnosis may have had prenatal testing; it is important to understand which test was performed to interpret the results and know whether additional genetic testing is warranted. In contrast, if prenatal testing was not done, then decisions need to be made about which genetic tests are most appropriate to order. To make informed test ordering decisions, it is important for neonatologists and other providers to understand the limitations and benefits of the various laboratory technologies. Therefore, this article compares methods for CNV detection. It also explores some of the most common CNVs associated with disease and how interpretation of CNVs is accomplished through the use of various resources, including online genomic databases. Given that CNVs are now appreciated as one of the most frequent causes of a broad spectrum of human disorders, early diagnosis and accurate interpretation is important to implement timely interventions and targeted clinical management.

METHODS FOR THE DETECTION OF COPY NUMBER VARIANTS

Various methods have been developed over the years for the detection of chromosomal deletions, duplications, and rearrangements. As shown in **Fig. 1**, some of these methods allow genomewide analyses, in which the entire chromosome complement is being interrogated, whereas others are targeted analyses and only examine specific regions of the genome. In addition, methods differ in their level of resolution (ie, how small an imbalance can be detected) and the type of sample that can be analyzed. **Table 1** summarizes the most commonly used cytogenetic methods for the detection of chromosome abnormalities and compares the benefits and limitations of each.

Of the techniques listed in **Table 1**, Giemsa-banded (G-banded) chromosome analysis and CMA are the only ones that are considered genomewide analyses, in which the entirety of each chromosome is being analyzed. However, the resolution of CMA far exceeds that of G-banding; genomic imbalances that could only be approximated by G-banding analysis can now be measured with precision by CMA based on the ability to link the probes contained on a microarray with the underlying DNA sequence coordinates. For these reasons, and others detailed later, CMA has become the first-tier test for clinical cytogenetic testing in the pediatric setting.

Most genomewide microarrays used for clinical CMA now also include single-nucleotide polymorphism (SNP) probes in addition to probes used for copy number detection. The addition of SNP probes offers several advantages. For example, SNP probes allow the detection of triploidy and some cases of tetraploidy.[7] These

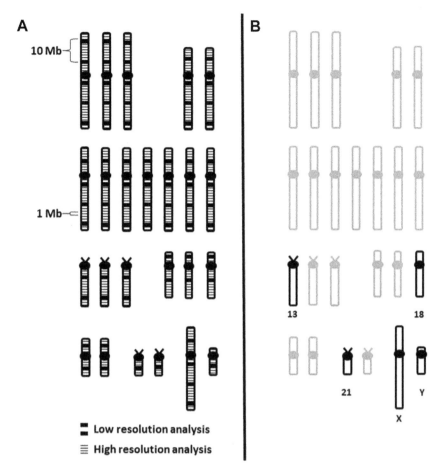

Fig. 1. Comparison of genomewide versus targeted analyses for CNV detection using a schematic diagrams of a human karyotype. (*A*) Genomewide analysis by G-banding or CMA. The thick black lines correspond with the lower resolution obtained from traditional G-banding analysis, whereas the thin black lines correspond with the higher resolution from newer techniques, like CMA. This example shows that CMA can detect an imbalance of 1 Mb that would be missed by G-banding. G-banding could only detect larger imbalances, such as the 10 Mb abnormality shown. (*B*) Targeted analysis. The only chromosomes being analyzed by targeted analysis are shown in black. The gray chromosomes would not be analyzed by targeted tests.

abnormalities are usually not detectable by copy number analyses alone, but are important to identify in the prenatal setting because both are common causes of fetal loss. In addition, genomic regions with an absence of heterozygosity (AOH) may be detected. AOH can suggest the presence of uniparental disomy (UPD), in which homologous chromosomes are both inherited from the same parent, instead of 1 from each parent. UPD for certain chromosomes has been associated with genetic disorders, such as Prader-Willi syndrome, when both chromosomes 15 are inherited from the mother in about 20% to 25% of cases. AOH can also distinguish genomic regions that are identical by descent, which could increase risk for an autosomal recessive disorder if a deleterious mutation is present. The use of SNP arrays for these indications is not a diagnostic test; however, both of these findings could prompt

Table 1
Benefits and limitations of tests used to detect copy number variation

Test Type	Test Evaluates	Test Benefits	Test Limitations
G-banded chromosome analysis	Genomewide large-scale deletions, duplications, and structural rearrangements[a], aneuploidy	Can detect balanced rearrangements	Cannot detect small imbalances (<3–5 Mb) May miss low-level mosaic cases
Chromosomal microarray analysis	Genomewide deletions and duplications; aneuploidy	Can detect small deletions and duplications not detected by G-banded karyotype; can be done using DNA isolated from uncultured cells	Cannot detect balanced rearrangements (eg, translocations or inversions); does not give information about the mechanism of an imbalance; may miss low-level mosaic cases
Chromosomal microarray analysis, with SNPs	Genomewide deletions and duplications; aneuploidy	Able to detect some uniparental disomies; can detect regions of AOH and consanguinity	Cannot detect balanced rearrangements (eg, translocations or inversions); does not give information about the mechanism of an imbalance; may miss low-level mosaic cases
Interphase FISH for aneuploidy	Aneuploidy of specific chromosomes (13, 18, 21, X, Y)	Performed on uncultured cells	Limited to certain regions of the genome
NIPS	Aneuploidy of specific chromosomes (13, 18, 21, X, Y)	Performed using a blood sample from the mother	Limited to certain regions of the genome

Abbreviations: AOH, absence of heterozygosity; NIPS, noninvasive prenatal screening; SNP, single-nucleotide polymorphism.
[a] Structural rearrangements are translocations, inversions, supernumerary chromosomes, and so forth.

targeted diagnostic testing for UPD or sequencing of a specific autosomal recessive gene based on the patient's clinical phenotype.[8]

In contrast with genomewide methods, targeted methods for the detection of cytogenetic aberrations are used to examine specific regions of the genome, such as aneuploidy for a single chromosome or deletion/duplication of a region associated with a known genetic syndrome. With the adoption of CMA, most targeted tests for microdeletion or microduplication syndromes are not used anymore, because many of these syndromes lack distinctive phenotypic findings and CMA can test for multiple regions in 1 assay instead of testing for 1 disorder at a time.[1]

Targeted tests are still predominantly used for aneuploidy testing of the chromosomes most frequently involved in human disorders, including 13, 18, 21, X, and Y, particularly in the prenatal setting or when a trisomy is suspected in a neonate based on clinical features. **Table 1** compares 2 targeted methods for aneuploidy detection: FISH and noninvasive prenatal screening (NIPS; discussed later in more detail).

PRENATAL DIAGNOSIS OF COPY NUMBER VARIANTS

As mentioned earlier, infants presenting to neonatology services for a possible genetic diagnosis may or may not have had prenatal testing. It is important for providers to understand these laboratory tests and their results to accurately determine whether any additional genetic testing is necessary. For example, if the mother had an amniocentesis with chromosome analysis during pregnancy and that test was normal, has a chromosome abnormality been ruled out or should other genetic testing be pursued?

Amniocentesis was first shown to be a safe and accurate method for prenatal diagnosis of genetic anomalies in the early 1970s.[9] Since that time, approaches to prenatal screening and diagnosis for chromosomal aberrations have quickly evolved based on new technologies and emerging practices. When considering results from prenatal testing, it is important to understand the difference between diagnostic and screening tests, and between genomewide versus targeted testing, because different levels of information are obtained.

Diagnostic tests provide an accurate representation of the fetal chromosome complement; currently, all prenatal diagnostic tests require an invasive procedure, such as amniocentesis or chorionic villi sampling, to obtain a sample directly from the fetus or placenta. In contrast, screening tests have risks for false-positive and false-negative results, because the sample is not being directly obtained from the fetus. Some commonly used noninvasive screening tests for aneuploidy, which are performed on a blood sample from the mother of the fetus, include maternal serum screening and NIPS.

G-banded chromosome analysis has historically been the gold-standard for detecting genomewide prenatal chromosome abnormalities. However, several large studies have now compared the diagnostic yield of G-banding with genomewide CMA for prenatal diagnosis and have shown that a significant proportion of clinically relevant chromosome aberrations are missed by G-banding alone.[10,11] Callaway and colleagues[11] (2013) recently performed a systematic review of the literature, including more than 12,000 prenatal cases that had CMA after a normal karyotype. This analysis revealed clinically significant CNVs in 2.4% of cases, with the highest yield in cases ascertained for abnormal ultrasonography (6.5%). However, even cases referred because of increased maternal age or for other reasons, such as abnormal serum screening or parental anxiety, had significant yields of 1.0% and 1.1%, respectively. Despite these data, in the prenatal setting, array is still not considered standard of care for all pregnancies. The most recent recommendations from the American Congress of

Obstetricians and Gynecologists (ACOG), published in 2013, allow CMA to replace a G-banded karyotype when ultrasonography anomalies are detected and invasive testing is being pursued. Either a karyotype or CMA can be used in patients undergoing invasive testing with a structurally normal fetus.[12] Therefore, if only a G-banded karyotype is performed prenatally and is normal, CMA should be ordered in a neonate presenting with features suggestive of a chromosomal disorder. **Box 1** lists some of the most common clinical features that should prompt consideration of a chromosomal disorder; the presence of more than 1 of these findings in a patient raises the suspicion for a genetic cause proportionately.

A rapidly evolving field in prenatal diagnosis is NIPS, also referred to as noninvasive prenatal testing. Even though a recent study showed no increased risk for fetal loss caused by invasive procedures,[13] the misperception that any invasive test carries some increased risk for fetal loss still exists. In addition, some women do not want invasive testing, independent of the risk for fetal loss. These two issues have been the main driving factors for technological developments for noninvasive screening methods and the uptake of noninvasive testing by patients. With the advent of NIPS in 2011, the number of amniocentesis and chorionic villi sampling procedures has significantly decreased, as shown by data from several maternal-fetal medicine centers.[14–17] NIPS is based on the detection of cell-free fetal DNA in maternal plasma using next-generation sequencing or other methods for fetal DNA assessment.[14,18] At this time, NIPS is mainly used for the targeted detection of common aneuploidies (13, 18, 21, X, and Y; shown in **Fig. 1**B). However, the technology is already being refined to detect common microdeletion/duplication syndromes as well as genome-wide CNVs.[19] Because NIPS is currently only a targeted screening test, a complete evaluation of the fetal genome is not obtained and clinically significant chromosome abnormalities could be missed. In addition, several cases of discordant results between NIPS and diagnostic cytogenetic testing have been reported.[20,21] Therefore, in the context of a neonate presenting with features suggestive of a chromosomal disorder, if the only result from prenatal genetic testing is a normal NIPS test, additional genetic testing is warranted.

COPY NUMBER DETECTION IN THE NEONATAL PERIOD

Although some chromosome abnormalities may be suspected and tested for in the prenatal period because of ultrasonography abnormalities or other clinical indications, most are not suspected until birth when dysmorphic features, congenital

---

Box 1
Selected clinical features that suggest the presence of a chromosomal disorder

Congenital anomalies
   Examples: structural abnormalities of the heart, renal system, skeletal system, and/or brain

Dysmorphic features

Hypotonia

Intrauterine growth retardation

Failure to thrive

Microcephaly

Seizures

Ambiguous genitalia

malformations, or other anomalies are observed. Early studies of the frequency of chromosome abnormalities in newborns estimated the rate to be ~4% from chromosome analysis.[22,23] Aneuploidies of chromosomes 21, X, and Y were the most common abnormalities detected, with trisomy of chromosomes 13 or 18, unbalanced rearrangements, and supernumerary chromosomes occurring less frequently.

With the advent of CMA it was hypothesized that the contribution of chromosomal imbalances in neonates was being underestimated. This hypothesis was proved to be correct by a large study of 638 neonates with various birth defects who were referred for clinical CMA.[24] Clinically significant imbalances were detected in 17.1% of patients, most of which would not have been identified by G-banding analysis. Although there were various reasons for referral for CMA testing among the samples with abnormal findings, the highest diagnostic yield was observed in the author-defined category "possible chromosome abnormality ± other birth defect" (66.7%). Other high-yield clinical indications were "ambiguous genitalia ± other birth defect" (33.3%), "dysmorphic features with multiple congenital anomalies ± other birth defect" (24.6%), and "congenital heart disease ± other birth defect" (21.8%). Overall, 2.5% of abnormal cases had whole-chromosome aneuploidies, whereas 12.7% had deletions or duplications.

Importantly, at the time of this study, high-resolution genomewide CMA analysis had not yet been developed for clinical testing. The arrays used in this study were targeted arrays (containing coverage over known clinically relevant regions of the genome, such as microdeletion/duplication syndromes, telomeres, and centromeres) with only low-resolution coverage across the rest of the genome, corresponding with approximately 1 targeted region per chromosome band at the 650-band level of resolution (~5–10 Mb). Even with coverage at a lower resolution than used in currently available clinical arrays, this study still identified abnormalities in a significant number (17.1%) of neonates. With the higher resolution arrays currently being used, this diagnostic yield is predicted to be even greater, showing the importance of CMA in the clinical care of neonates.

Because congenital heart defects (CHDs) are among the most common birth defects, and also a common indication for cytogenetic testing in the neonatal period, many studies have focused on the contribution of CNVs to isolated CHDs and CHDs with other associated defects. A recent review including data from 20 studies examined the diagnostic yield of CMA in CHDs.[3] Clinically relevant CNVs were reported in 3% to 25% of patients with CHDs plus other associated defects, with many of these studies in the 17% to 20% range. Even in cases with isolated CHDs, the diagnostic yield was still significant, with 3% to 10% of cases having a clinically relevant CNV. Thus most CHDs, whether observed in the context of additional phenotypic findings or as isolated defects, warrant consideration of CMA to detect pathogenic CNVs.

The most common submicroscopic CNV associated with CHDs is a deletion of 22q11.2. This CNV is estimated to occur in 1 in 2000 to 1 in 4000 live births. In addition to CHDs, the most common being conotruncal defects, individuals with a 22q11.2 deletion can show various clinical features, including palatal abnormalities, hypocalcemia, immune deficiency, and a range of neurodevelopmental disorders.[25] In ~10% of cases, this deletion is inherited from an affected parent who usually has a more mild presentation than the proband; therefore, parental testing to determine inheritance is important for recurrence risk estimates and familial genetic counseling.

More broadly, the implementation of high-resolution genomewide CMA for other common postnatal indications, such as developmental delay, intellectual disability, autism spectrum disorder, or multiple congenital anomalies, has also shown a diagnostic yield that far surpasses that of G-banding. A systematic literature review of 33 CMA studies of these patient populations estimated that ~15% to 20% have a clinically relevant CNV, compared with a yield of only ~3% from G-banding (the 3% estimate excluded Down syndrome and other recognizable chromosomal syndromes).[1] These data ultimately resulted in CMA being recommended as the first-tier clinical test for individuals with developmental disorders or congenital anomalies by several groups, including the American College of Medical Genetics and Genomics (ACMG).[1,26]

CLINICAL INTERPRETATION OF COPY NUMBER VARIANTS

The use of CMA has obvious advantages compared with previous cytogenetic methods for diagnostic yield. Another invaluable benefit of CMA as a diagnostic test is the ability to immediately link the genomic coordinates from the DNA probes contained on the array to the human genome sequence to evaluate size, gene content, and other elements that make up the architecture of the human genome. With the wide range of copy number variation present in the human genome, clinicians are still learning which variation in individuals is causative of disease and which has a benign or negligible impact. Cataloging both benign and pathogenic regions of the genome is imperative to aid in the clinical interpretation of CNVs.

Recurrent and Nonrecurrent Copy Number Variants

The collection of CNVs from across the genome allows the comparison of overlapping CNVs to determine underlying mechanisms and the resulting phenotypic effects. Although it has been estimated that most (~75%) CNVs occur at nonrecurrent sites across the genome, ~25% of CNVs are mediated by nonallelic homologous recombination between flanking sequences of shared DNA sequence homology (commonly referred to as segmental duplications or genomic hotspots) and make up a class of CNVs termed recurrent CNVs.[27,28] Because these CNVs, which contain identical unique genomic regions of imbalance across patients, recur because of their underlying mechanism, they are frequently encountered during CMA analysis.

Table 2 lists some of the most frequently observed recurrent CNVs that are encountered during clinical CMA testing. Some of these CNVs (eg, Prader-Willi/Angelman syndromes and 22q11.2 deletion syndrome) have been described for some time now because they were associated with a specific syndrome and detected either through high-resolution G-banding or FISH analyses. Other CNVs, with more variable phenotypes (eg, deletions and duplications of 1q21.1 and 16p11.2), have only emerged recently because of the ability to detect smaller imbalances across the genome via CMA. Targeted research studies comparing the phenotype of individuals with many of these recurrent CNVs are now underway to better define the deleterious impact of each CNV.[29,30]

Interpretation Guidelines

The technical definition of a CNV is "a segment of DNA that is ≥ 1 kilobase (kb) in size that differs in copy number compared with a representative reference genome."[31] However, most CNVs that are less than ~400 kb are observed frequently in cohorts of apparently normal control individuals, and are therefore not thought to have appreciable effects on human health and/or development.[32] Because of this, for the purposes of detecting CNVs as part of clinical testing, several organizations have recommended a resolution of greater than or equal to 400 kb across the genome to avoid detection of these common, benign CNVs.[1,33] Some array designs used by clinical laboratories contain higher resolution coverage ($\sim$20–50 kb) over known disease-causing genes in order to detect single gene deletions or duplications.

Note that the term CNV must be qualified with additional information in order to understand the clinical relevance of the finding: (1) a CNV must be designated as a deletion or duplication, and (2) a CNV should have a defined category of clinical significance.

As outlined in **Table 3**, the ACMG has defined 5 categories for interpreting the clinical significance of CNVs and examples of each are listed. CNVs included on clinical reports should be classified into one of these categories so that clinicians can review the laboratory findings and correlate with their patient's clinical phenotype. It is common ($\sim$10% of cases) for a CNV to be reported as of uncertain clinical significance based on the limited information that the laboratory had at the time of testing, but when a clinician reviews the CNV detected and pairs it with more detailed phenotypic data from the patient, a more definitive interpretation of "pathogenic" can often be made. This example highlights the critical need for coordinated communication between clinical laboratories and clinicians for accurate interpretation of genomic testing.

When a CNV is identified, several characteristics of the genomic region that is either deleted or duplicated need to be considered in interpreting its significance. The following bulleted list documents some of the basic questions to investigate:

1. Is the CNV included in databases of normal variation? If so, the CNV is considered a benign variant. If not, then the potential pathogenicity needs to be evaluated.
2. Does the CNV contain a region of the genome known to cause a genomic syndrome when deleted or duplicated (eg, a recurrent CNV region associated with a particular phenotype)? If so, then the CNV would be consistent with causing the syndrome that corresponds with either a deletion or duplication of that region, depending on the CNV finding.
3. Does the CNV contain a gene that is known to cause a syndrome as a result of haploinsufficiency (deletion) or triplosensitivity (duplication)? If so, then the CNV that encompasses the entire gene would be consistent with causing the syndrome that corresponds with either a deletion or duplication of that gene, depending on the CNV finding.
4. If the CNV does not overlap a known region or gene, what is the gene content and size of the CNV? In general, a larger imbalance with high gene content is more likely to be considered pathogenic.
5. Is the CNV *de novo*? In general, a *de novo* CNV is more likely to be pathogenic than one inherited from a parent with an apparently normal phenotype.
6. Is the CNV inherited? If a CNV is inherited, then it is important to evaluate the phenotype of the parent carrying the same CNV. The parent could be affected with the same clinical phenotype as the proband. Alternatively, the parent could have more subtle phenotypic effects than the proband caused by variable expressivity of the CNV. The CNV could also be a benign variant if it is observed frequently in the general population.

Genomic Resources for Copy Number Variant Curation

Even though new genomic discoveries are made and published every day, the interplay between genomic variants and their impact on various systems involved in human development and function are still not known. Because many genomic variants are

Table 2
Frequently observed recurrent CNVs identified among clinical populations referred for CMA testing

CNV[a]	Copy Number	Syndrome	Size (Mb)	Genomic Coordinates (hg19)
Highly Penetrant Phenotype				
7q11.23 (*ELN*)	Deletion	Williams	1.4	chr7:72744455-74142513
8p23.1 (*SOX7, CLDN23*)	Deletion	—	3.6	chr8:8119296-11765719
8p23.1 (*SOX7, CLDN23*)	Duplication	—	3.6	chr8:8119296-11765719
15q11.2q13 BP2-3 (*UBE3A*)	Deletion	Prader-Willi or Angelman	4.8	chr15:23758391-28557186
17p11.2 (*RAI1*)	Deletion	Smith-Magenis	3.5	chr17:16757112-20219651
17p11.2 (*RAI1*)	Duplication	Potocki-Lupski	3.5	chr17:16757112-20219651
17q21.31 (*MAPT, KANSL1*)	Deletion	Koolen-de Vries	—	—
22q11.2 (*TBX1, HIRA*)	Deletion	DiGeorge/velocardiofacial	2.9	chr22:18661726-21561514
Variable Clinical Phenotype				
1q21.1 (*GJA5*)	Deletion	—	0.8	chr1:146577487-147394506
1q21.1 (*GJA5*)	Duplication	—	0.8	chr1:146577487-147394506
7q11.23 (*ELN*)	Duplication	—	1.4	chr7:72744455-74142513
15q11.2q13 BP2-3 (*UBE3A*)	Duplication	—	4.8	chr15:23758391-28557186
15q13.3 BP4-5 (*KLF13, CHRNA7*)	Deletion	—	1.3	chr15:31137105-32245408
15q13.3 BP4-5 (*KLF13, CHRNA7*)	Duplication	—	1.3	chr15:31137105-32245408

16p11.2 (TBX6)	Deletion	—	0.6	chr16:29649997-30199855
16p11.2 (TBX6)	Duplication	—	0.6	chr16:29649997-30199855
16p11.2 distal (SH2B1)	Deletion	—	—	—
16p11.2 distal (SH2B1)	Duplication	—	—	—
16p12.1 (CDR2, EEF2K)	Deletion	—	—	—
16p13.11 (MYH11)	Deletion	—	—	—
17q12 (HNF1B)	Deletion	Renal cysts and diabetes	—	—
17q12 (HNF1B)	Duplication	—	—	—
22q11.2 (TBX1, HIRA)	Duplication	—	2.9	chr22:18661726-21561514

The list is divided into CNVs that have a highly penetrant phenotype and those with more variable phenotypic presentations. Within each category, the CNVs are listed in chromosomal order. The CNV list was compiled from multiple sources, but should not be considered exhaustive: DECIPHER syndrome list (https://decipher.sangeer.ac.uk/syndromes#overview), Clinical Genome Resource (ClinGen) pathogenic list (http://www.ncbi.nlm.nih.gov/dbvarstudy ID nstd45), and also Refs.[27,38-41]

Abbreviation: BP, breakpoint.

[a] Genes in the CNV region are included as landmarks for genomic location and are not necessarily known to be causative of phenotype.

Table 3
ACMG recommended categories for defining the clinical significance of a CNV

Category	Definition	Example
Pathogenic	CNV is documented as clinically significant consistently and in multiple publications and/or case databases	22q11.2 deletion syndrome (DiGeorge/velocardiofacial syndrome)
Uncertain (no subclassification)	Clinical significance not know at time of reporting but CNV meets the laboratory reporting criteria; expected that CNVs in this category will shift toward pathogenic or benign over time	500-kb deletion of chromosome 3 that contains 5 genes but the inheritance of the deletion is not known and there is nothing known about the 5 genes in the deleted interval
Subclassifications		
Uncertain: likely pathogenic	Some evidence to increase the likelihood that the CNV is pathogenic	500-kb de novo deletion of chromosome 3 that contains 5 genes and there is a single case report in the literature that has similar breakpoints and shares a distinct phenotype
Uncertain: likely benign	Some evidence to increase the likelihood that the CNV is benign	500-kb deletion of chromosome 3 that does not contain any genes but is not found in any control databases
Benign	CNV is documented as benign consistently and in multiple publications and/or control databases or represents a common polymorphism (present in >1% of the population)	2q37.3 telomere polymorphism (~200 kb in size and well documented as benign in multiple studies)

Adapted from Kearney HM, Thorland EC, Brown KK, et al. Working Group of the American College of Medical Genetics Laboratory Quality Assurance Committee. American College of Medical Genetics standards and guidelines for interpretation and reporting of postnatal constitutional copy number variants. Genet Med 2011;13(7):680–85.

rare, community efforts are needed to assist in deciphering the clinical significance of genomic variants in an evidence-based manner. Toward the goal of curating genome-wide CNVs, multiple online genome resources, as detailed by de Leeuw and colleagues[34] (2012), have been garnered from large-scale data sharing and are now publically available.

Table 4 lists some of the online resources for CNVs and their corresponding phenotypes that are most commonly used for interpreting clinical significance. The table includes 3 different types of tools that can be used to aid in CNV interpretation: (1) genome browsers, in which the genomic coordinates of a particular CNV can be entered and the browser used to view its genomic content; (2) databases of CNVs submitted from case and control cohorts, which can be used to compare individual cases with other previously observed CNVs; (3) catalogs of phenotypic information collected from the literature or written by experts that provide overviews of well-described syndromes or gene/disease associations. All of these resources are dynamic and evolving at a rate that largely depends on the discovery, data submission, and curation efforts of researchers, clinical laboratories, clinicians, and others.

Table 4
Online, publically available genome resources with CNV and phenotype data

Database	Web Address	Case CNV Data	Control CNV Data	Phenotype Data
Genome Browsers				
dbVar	http://www.ncbi.nlm.nih.gov/dbvar/	X[a]	X[a]	X[a]
Ensembl	http://www.ensembl.org	X[a]	X[a]	X[a]
UCSC Genome Browser	https://genome.ucsc.edu/	X[a]	X[a]	X[a]
Databases of CNVs Submitted from Case and Control Cohorts				
ClinVar[b]	http://www.ncbi.nlm.nih.gov/clinvar/	X	—	X
DECIPHER	https://decipher.sanger.ac.uk/	X	—	X
DGV	http://dgv.tcag.ca/dgv/app/home	—	X	—
ECARUCA	http://ecaruca.net	X	—	X
Catalogs of Phenotypic Information				
GeneReviews	http://www.genetests.org/resources/genereviews.php	—	—	X
MedGen	http://www.ncbi.nlm.nih.gov/medgen	—	—	X
OMIM	http://www.omim.org/	—	—	X
Orphanet	http://www.orpha.net/	—	—	X

Abbreviation: dbVar, Database of Genomic Structural Variation; DECIPHER, Database of Chromosomal Imbalance and Phenotype in Humans Using Ensembl Resources; DGV, Database of Genomic Variation; ECARUCA, European Cytogeneticists Association Register of Unbalanced Chromosome Aberrations; OMIM, Online Mendelian Inheritance in Man.
[a] Displays data in browser format that is derived from several of the CNV and phenotype resources listed later.
[b] Main submission portal for data from the groups previously known as the International Standards for Cytogenomic Arrays and the International Consortium for Clinical Genomics, which are now integrated into ClinGen.

SUMMARY

CNVs provide a genetic cause for a wide range of disorders diagnosed in the prenatal and neonatal periods. There are a growing number of examples in which knowing a genetic cause leads to genome-directed clinical care and improved medical management. For example, in neonates with 22q11.2 deletions, not only is it important to assess for all of the congenital anomalies associated with this CNV, it is also important to monitor neonatal calcium levels. A recent study showed that neonatal seizures and neonatal hypocalcemia were predictors of a more severe level of intellectual disability. The investigators thus concluded that early monitoring of calcium levels before seizure onset might improve outcomes in these patients by preventing damage to neurons caused by seizures.[35]

The continuing evolution of genomic technologies for the detection of CNVs and aneuploidy in the perinatal setting will allow earlier diagnosis of these conditions in fetuses and neonates. Next-generation whole-exome sequencing (WES) and whole-genome sequencing (WGS) methods are already being used to detect CNVs in postnatal samples and the feasibility of using WGS for noninvasive sequencing of a human fetus by analyzing parental blood samples was recently reported.[36,37] As the decreasing costs of WES and WGS make broader adoption possible, an era of genomic medicine can be envisioned in which it is feasible to routinely perform these genomewide methods for variant detection on neonatal, or ultimately prenatal, samples collected noninvasively. Through increasing understanding of the interplay between genomic variants and health, there is the potential to realize the full benefits of personalized genomic medicine, resulting in earlier interventions and improved outcomes.

ACKNOWLEDGMENTS

The authors thank Erin Rooney Riggs, MS, for critically reviewing this article and Thomas Challman, MD, and Eli Williams, PhD, for useful discussions about selected information presented.

REFERENCES

1. Miller DT, Adam MP, Aradhya S, et al. Consensus statement: chromosomal microarray is a first-tier clinical diagnostic test for individuals with developmental disabilities or congenital anomalies. Am J Hum Genet 2010;86(5):749–64.
2. Mefford HC, Yendle SC, Hsu C, et al. Rare copy number variants are an important cause of epileptic encephalopathies. Ann Neurol 2011;70(6):974–85.
3. Lander J, Ware SM. Copy number variation in congenital heart defects. Curr Genet Med Rep 2014;2:168–78.
4. Iafrate AJ, Feuk L, Rivera MN, et al. Detection of large-scale variation in the human genome. Nat Genet 2004;36(9):949–51.
5. Sebat J, Lakshmi B, Troge J, et al. Large-scale copy number polymorphism in the human genome. Science 2004;305(5683):525–8.
6. Coe BP, Girirajan S, Eichler EE. A genetic model for neurodevelopmental disease. Curr Opin Neurobiol 2012;22(5):829–36.
7. Lathi RB, Massie JA, Loring M, et al. Informatics enhanced SNP microarray analysis of 30 miscarriage samples compared to routine cytogenetics. PLoS One 2012;7:e31282.
8. South ST, Lee C, Lamb AN, et al. Working group for the American College of medical genetics and genomics laboratory quality assurance committee. ACMG

standards and guidelines for constitutional cytogenomic microarray analysis, including postnatal and prenatal applications: revision 2013. Genet Med 2013; 15(11):901–9.

9. Nadler HL, Gerbie AB. Role of amniocentesis in the intrauterine detection of genetic disorders. N Engl J Med 1970;282(11):596–9.

10. Wapner RJ, Martin CL, Levy B, et al. Chromosomal microarray versus karyotyping for prenatal diagnosis. N Engl J Med 2012;367(23):2175–84.

11. Callaway JL, Shaffer LG, Chitty LS, et al. The clinical utility of microarray technologies applied to prenatal cytogenetics in the presence of a normal conventional karyotype: a review of the literature. Prenat Diagn 2013;33(12):1119–23.

12. American College of Obstetricians and Gynecologists Committee on Genetics. Committee opinion no. 581: the use of chromosomal microarray analysis in prenatal diagnosis. Obstet Gynecol 2013;122:1374–7.

13. Akolekar R, Beta J, Picciarelli G, et al. Procedure-related risk of miscarriage following amniocentesis and chorionic villus sampling: a systematic review and meta-analysis. Ultrasound Obstet Gynecol 2014;45:16–26.

14. Lo JO, Cori DF, Norton ME, et al. Noninvasive prenatal testing. Obstet Gynecol Surv 2014;69(2):89–99.

15. Beamon CJ, Hardisty EE, Harris SC, et al. A single center's experience with noninvasive prenatal testing. Genet Med 2014;16:681–7.

16. Louis-Jacques A, Burans C, Robinson S, et al. Effect of commercial cell-free fetal DNA tests for aneuploidy screening on rates of invasive testing. Obstet Gynecol 2014;123(Suppl 1):67S.

17. Pettit KE, Hull AD, Korty L, et al. The utilization of circulating cell-free fetal DNA testing and decrease in invasive diagnostic procedures: an institutional experience. J Perinatol 2014;34:750–3.

18. Bianchi DW, Platt LD, Goldberg JD, et al. Genome-wide fetal aneuploidy detection by maternal plasma DNA sequencing. Obstet Gynecol 2012;119(5):890–901.

19. Yu SC, Jiang P, Choy KW, et al. Noninvasive prenatal molecular karyotyping from maternal plasma. PLoS One 2013;8:e60968.

20. Pan M, Li FT, Li Y, et al. Discordant results between fetal karyotyping and noninvasive prenatal testing by maternal plasma sequencing in a case of uniparental disomy 21 due to trisomic rescue. Prenat Diagn 2013;33(6):598–601.

21. Gao Y, Stejskal D, Jiang F, et al. False-negative trisomy 18 non-invasive prenatal test result due to 48, XXX, +18 placental mosaicism. Ultrasound Obstet Gynecol 2014;43(4):477–8.

22. Hook EB. Chromosome abnormalities: prevalence, risks and recurrence. In: Brock DJ, Rodeck CH, Ferguson-Smith MA, editors. Prenatal diagnosis and screening. Edinburgh (United Kingdom): Churchill Livingstone; 1992. p. 351.

23. Jacobs PA, Browne C, Gregson N, et al. Estimates of the frequency of chromosome abnormalities detectable in unselected newborns using moderate levels of banding. J Med Genet 1992;29(2):103–8.

24. Lu XY, Phung MT, Shaw CA, et al. Genomic imbalances in neonates with birth defects: high detection rates by using chromosomal microarray analysis. Pediatrics 2008;122(6):1310–8.

25. McDonald-McGinn DM, Emanuel BS, Zackai EH. 22q11.2 deletion syndrome. In: Pagon RA, Adam MP, Ardinger HH, et al, editors. GeneReviews [Internet]. University of Washington; 2013.

26. Manning M, Hudgins L. Professional practice and guidelines C. Array-based technology and recommendations for utilization in medical genetics practice for detection of chromosomal abnormalities. Genet Med 2010;12(11):742–5.

27. Kaminsky EB, Kaul V, Paschall J, et al. An evidence-based approach to establish the functional and clinical significance of copy number variants in intellectual and developmental disabilities. Genet Med 2011;13(9):777–84.

28. Sharp AJ, Locke DP, McGrath SD, et al. Segmental duplications and copy-number variation in the human genome. Am J Hum Genet 2005;77(1):78–88.

29. Hanson E, Bernier R, Porche K, et al. The cognitive and behavioral phenotype of the 16p11.2 deletion in a clinically ascertained population. Biol Psychiatry 2014 [pii: S0006-3223(14)00427-2].

30. Bassett AS, McDonald-McGinn DM, Devriendt K, et al. Practical guidelines for managing patients with 22q11.2 deletion syndrome. J Pediatr 2011;159(2):332–9.

31. Kearney HM, Thorland EC, Brown KK, et al, Working Group of the American College of Medical Genetics Laboratory Quality Assurance Committee. American College of Medical Genetics standards and guidelines for interpretation and reporting of postnatal constitutional copy number variants. Genet Med 2011; 13(7):680–5.

32. Redon R, Ishikawa S, Fitch KR, et al. Global variation in copy number in the human genome. Nature 2006;444(7118):444–54.

33. Kearney HM, South ST, Wolff DJ, et al. American college of medical genetics recommendations for the design and performance expectations for clinical genomic copy number microarrays intended for use in the postnatal setting for detection of constitutional abnormalities. Genet Med 2011;13(7):676–9.

34. de Leeuw N, Dijkhuizen T, Hehir-Kwa JY, et al. Diagnostic interpretation of array data using public databases and internet sources. Hum Mutat 2012. [Epub ahead of print].

35. Cheung EN, George SR, Andrade DM, et al. Neonatal hypocalcemia, neonatal seizures, and intellectual disability in 22q11.2 deletion syndrome. Genet Med 2014;16(1):40–4.

36. Zhao M, Wang Q, Wang Q, et al. Computational tools for copy number variation (CNV) detection using next-generation sequencing data: features and perspectives. BMC Bioinformatics 2013;14(Suppl 11):S1.

37. Kitzman JO, Snyder MW, Ventura M, et al. Noninvasive whole-genome sequencing of a human fetus. Sci Transl Med 2012;4(137):137ra76.

38. Cooper GM, Coe BP, Girirajan S, et al. A copy number variation morbidity map of developmental delay. Nat Genet 2011;43(9):838–46.

39. Moreno-De-Luca D, Sanders SJ, Willsey AJ, et al. Using large clinical data sets to infer pathogenicity for rare copy number variants in autism cohorts. Mol Psychiatry 2013;18(10):1090–5.

40. Rosenfeld JA, Coe BP, Eichler EE, et al. Estimates of penetrance for recurrent pathogenic copy-number variations. Genet Med 2013;15(6):478–81.

41. Ledbetter DH, Riggs ER, Martin CL. Clinical applications of whole-genome chromosomal microarray analysis. In: Ginsburg GS, Willard HF, editors. Genomic and personalized medicine, vol. 1. 2nd edition. New York: Academic Press; 2013. p. 133.

Evaluation and Diagnosis of the Dysmorphic Infant

Kelly L. Jones, MD, Margaret P. Adam, MD*

KEYWORDS

- Aplasia cutis congenita • Holoprosencephaly • Asymmetric crying facies
- Preauricular tags • Cleft lip with or without cleft palate • Congenital heart defects
- Ventral wall defects • Polydactyly

KEY POINTS

- Congenital anomalies are a significant cause of neonatal intensive care unit (NICU) admissions.
- Congenital anomalies may be genetic in etiology or may be the result of teratogenic exposure or multifactorial inheritance (the interaction of both genetic and environmental factors).
- The presence of a particular congenital anomaly may necessitate evaluation for the presence of other specific associated anomalies or genetic syndromes.
- Most genetic syndromes are defined by a specific pattern of congenital anomalies.
- Some congenital anomalies may be inherited within families as an isolated trait, highlighting the importance of taking a family history and of examining parents for similar anomalies, when appropriate.

INTRODUCTION

Congenital anomalies are present in at least 10% of all NICU admissions, many of whom have an underlying genetic condition.[1] Neonatologists are often the first physicians to evaluate these infants and consequently need to be familiar with various physical differences to pursue further screening for occult malformations, perform diagnostic testing, and appropriately counsel families. The purpose of this article is review the dysmorphology examination with particular attention to anomalies that are readily apparent in the neonatal period.

Disclosure: None.
Division of Genetic Medicine, Department of Pediatrics, University of Washington, 4800 Sand Point Way Northeast, OC.9.850, Seattle, WA 98105, USA
* Corresponding author. Division of Genetic Medicine, 4800 Sand Point Way Northeast, PO Box 5371/OC.9.850, Seattle, WA 98105.
E-mail address: margaret.adam@seattlechildrens.org

Clin Perinatol 42 (2015) 243–261
http://dx.doi.org/10.1016/j.clp.2015.02.002   **perinatology.theclinics.com**

An anomaly is a structural defect that deviates from the normal standard and can be categorized as major or minor. A major anomaly has surgical, medical, or cosmetic importance and may be a marker for other occult malformations. A minor anomaly has no significant surgical or cosmetic importance; however, many genetic syndromes are recognized based on the pattern of minor anomalies present. Anomalies arise from 1 of 3 mechanisms, each of which has different diagnostic and inheritance implications. The first mechanism is termed a malformation, which is a structural defect arising from an intrinsically abnormal developmental process. Malformations include anomalies like congenital heart defects and cleft lip and palate. These types of anomalies are more likely associated with a genetic condition or predisposition. A deformation is an abnormality arising from prenatal mechanical forces on otherwise normally formed fetal structures. Deformations can include clubfeet, overlapping toes, and unusual head shape (although these disorders may also be malformations). Deformations are rarely genetic and recurrence risks are typically low. Lastly, disruptions are structural defects resulting from the destruction or interruption of intrinsically normal tissue. Examples of disruptive anomalies include limb reduction defects from amniotic band sequence and certain types of intestinal atresias due to vascular insufficiency.[2] Anomalies due to this mechanism are much less likely due to a genetic condition or to recur in a future pregnancy.

BIRTH PARAMETERS

Both increased and decreased birth parameters are associated with multiple genetic and nongenetic etiologies. Fetal macrosomia may be defined as a birth weight greater than 4000 g or more than 2 SDs above the mean of a reference population, whereas fetal-growth restriction is defined as a birth weight less than 2 SDs below the mean for gestational age in a reference population. The differential diagnoses for both fetal macrosomia and fetal growth restriction are broad and include chromosomal abnormalities and teratogenic exposures. Chromosomal abnormalities have varying phenotypes depending on the size of the chromosomal segment involved and the individual genes in that segment. Consequently, it is beneficial to evaluate for congenital anomalies in those who have macrosomia or growth restriction. In both instances, a chromosomal microarray should be considered. If the physical examination indicates features of a well-characterized genetic syndrome, such as a trisomy or Beckwith-Wiedemann syndrome, then testing can be tailored to that particular syndrome (**Tables 1** and **2**).[3–8]

Although abnormal birth parameters in the presence of congenital anomalies frequently indicate a genetic syndrome, this is not always the case. For example, infants of diabetic mothers are commonly macrosomic (although growth restriction can also occur) and may display congenital malformations at a frequency of 2 to 4 times the general population rate. Consequently, it may be difficult to distinguish between diabetic embryopathy and a genetic syndrome.[4] In the absence of confirmed maternal diabetes and one of the more specific anomalies seen in diabetic embryopathy, such as caudal regression syndrome or tibial hemimelia with preaxial polydactyly (**Fig. 1**), this diagnosis should be considered a diagnosis of exclusion and the clinician should consider further genetic testing, such as a chromosomal microarray, to evaluate for a chromosome abnormality.[2,3]

Similarly, fetal growth restriction can be due to nongenetic causes, such as placental insufficiency, maternal hypertension, multiple gestation (ie, twinning), and maternal preeclampsia. Most of these conditions result in asymmetric growth restriction as a result of inadequate nutrient transfer to the fetus.[9] Placental insufficiency has also been associated with an increased risk of hypospadias in male infants[10]; therefore, not all birth

Table 1
Overgrowth in the neonatal period and associated conditions

Differential Diagnosis	Associated Features	Potential Evaluations	Potential Genetic Studies
Beckwith-Wiedemann syndrome	Macroglossia Abdominal wall defects Hemihyperplasia Neonatal hypoglycemia Visceromegaly Posterior helical ear pits Anterior linear ear lobe creases	Blood glucose level monitoring Abdominal ultrasound α-Fetoprotein level	Methylation analysis of 11p15
Chromosomal abnormalities	Congenital heart defects Ophthalmologic abnormalities Genitourinary abnormalities	Echocardiogram Ophthalmologic evaluation Renal ultrasound	Chromosomal microarray
Infant of a diabetic mother	HPE Spina bifida Congenital heart defects Neonatal small left colon Vertebral defects Tibial hemimelia with preaxial polydactyly Caudal regression syndrome	Cranial ultrasound or head MRI Echocardiogram Renal ultrasound Sacral ultrasound AP and lateral radiographs of the entire spine	None

Abbreviation: AP, anterior-posterior.

defects associated with growth restriction are genetic. As with diabetic embryopathy, however, this type of teratogenic mechanism should remain a diagnosis of exclusion and chromosomal microarray in such infants should be considered.

APLASIA CUTIS CONGENITA

Aplasia cutis congenita (ACC) is congenital absence of the skin. Although ACC can occur on any part of the body, it most commonly affects the scalp (70%–80% of

Table 2
Fetal growth restriction and associated genetic conditions

Differential Diagnosis	Associated Features	Potential Evaluations	Potential Genetic Studies
Chromosomal abnormalities	(See **Table 1**)	(See **Table 1**)	(See **Table 1**)
Trisomy 13	HPE Microphthalmia/colobomas Congenital heart defects Cutis aplasia	Head ultrasound Ophthalmologic evaluation Echocardiogram Renal ultrasound	Routine chromosome analysis
Trisomy 18	Prominent occiput Micrognathia Congenital heart defects Horseshoe kidney Overlapping fingers	Echocardiogram Renal ultrasound	Routine chromosome analysis

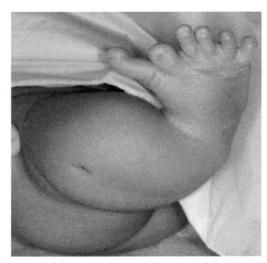

Fig. 1. Tibial hemimelia with proximally placed preaxial polydactyly of the right foot in an infant born to a women with poorly controlled insulin-dependent diabetes. Note the short and bowed lower extremity with a dimple around the knee. (*From* Adam MP, Hudgins L, Carey JC, et al. Preaxial hallucal polydactyly as a marker for diabetic embryopathy. Birth Defects Res A Clin Mol Teratol 2009;85:14; with permission.)

cases). A majority of cases are sporadic solitary scalp lesions but 15% to 30% of scalp ACC cases are associated with defects in the underlying bone and dura.[11] ACC may be associated with etiologic factors, including birth trauma, intrauterine infections with varicella zoster or herpes viruses, fetus papyraceous, and teratogens, like cocaine and methimazole.[11,12] ACC has also been associated with multiple genetic conditions, including trisomy 13 and Adams-Oliver syndrome (AOS), a condition characterized by ACC and terminal limb defects. AOS can be inherited in either an autosomal dominant or an autosomal recessive fashion (**Table 3**).[7,11,13] Complications of ACC include

Table 3			
Aplasia cutis congenita and associated genetic conditions			
Differential Diagnosis	**Associated Features**	**Potential Evaluations**	**Potential Genetic Studies**
AOS	Limb defects Cutis marmorata telangiectasia congenita CNS abnormalities Cardiovascular abnormalities	Brain imaging Limb radiographs Echocardiogram	Sequencing of *ARHGAP31,* *DOCK6, RBPJ,* *EOGT*
Scalp or midline back ACC (without multiple anomalies)	May have underlying bony or neural tube defects	Infectious work-up Skull radiograph Head MRI Spinal ultrasound or MRI	None
Trisomy 13	(See **Table 2**)	(See **Table 2**)	(See **Table 2**)

Abbreviation: CNS, central nervous system.

infection, meningitis, bleeding, and superior sagittal sinus thrombosis. Mortality for those with ACC is 20% to 50% and depends on the size of the lesion and any associated defects. Solitary scalp ACC that is small in size and lateral to the midline usually does not require further diagnostic evaluation per se; however, if a scalp or back defect is midline or membranous in quality, a brain MRI or a spine ultrasound or MRI to evaluate for an underlying neural tube defect should be considered. Treatment of ACC is usually conservative.[11] After healing, areas of scalp affected by ACC do not grow any hair (**Fig. 2**).

HOLOPROSENCEPHALY

Holoprosencephaly (HPE) is a structural brain abnormality resulting from the incomplete cleavage of the forebrain into the right and left hemispheres during the third to fourth week of gestation. HPE consists of a continuum of brain malformations with alobar HPE (a single ventricle and no separation of the cerebral hemispheres [**Fig. 3A**]) at one end of the spectrum to very mild midbrain fusion (see **Fig. 3B**) at the other end of the spectrum.

HPE may be associated with a range of craniofacial abnormalities, including cyclopia, microcephaly, hypotelorism, depressed nasal bridge, single maxillary incisor, and midline cleft lip with or without cleft palate (CLP) (**Fig. 4**). Some affected individuals also have pituitary dysfunction and feeding difficulties. The HPE phenotype is variable among simplex cases and among members of the same family with an inherited form of HPE; consequently, subtle facial features may be overlooked in mildly affected family members. In any infant for whom HPE is considered, first-degree relatives should be questioned and examined to identify those with microcephaly, hypotelorism, or a single central incisor. Due to variable expressivity of the phenotype, affected first-degree family members may be mildly affected. Because some cases of HPE are inherited in an autosomal dominant fashion, identifying other affected family members has implications for genetic testing and recurrence risks.[14,15]

The etiologies for both syndromic and nonsyndromic HPE are heterogeneous and include maternal diabetes mellitus, single gene disorders (often inherited in an autosomal dominant manner), and chromosomal abnormalities (**Table 4**).[3,7,16] Chromosomal abnormalities are present in up to 50% of patients with HPE and include trisomy 13, trisomy 18, and a variety of other copy number variants. Determining which laboratory testing to perform depends on family history and the presence of other

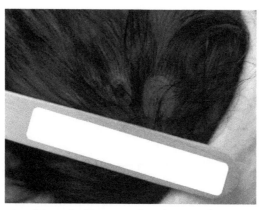

Fig. 2. ACC on the vertex of the scalp. (*Courtesy of* Heather Brandling-Bennett, MD, Seatle, WA.)

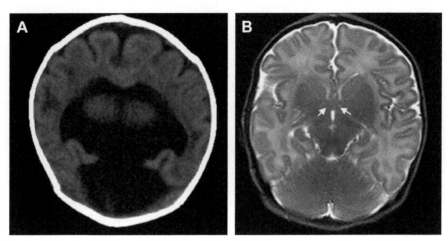

Fig. 3. (A) Brain MRI of an infant with alobar HPE, the most severe form of HPE, demonstrating a single large ventricle. (B) Brain MRI of an infant with a milder form of HPE in which there is subtle fusion of the thalami (arrows).

abnormalities. Testing may include routine chromosome analysis (if trisomy 13 or 18 is suspected) or chromosomal microarray analysis. Further single gene testing may be considered in those with a family history suggestive of an inherited form of HPE, with mutations in SHH accounting for up to 30% to 40% of familial cases.[16] Treatment is multidisciplinary and may include pituitary hormone replacement, antiepileptic medications, and surgical repair of midline CLP in those who are more mildly affected.[15]

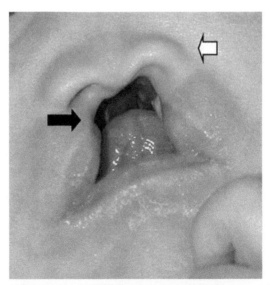

Fig. 4. This infant with HPE has microcephaly, hypotelorism, a hypoplastic nose, and a midline cleft of the lip and palate. The white arrow points to hypoplastic nares and the black arrow points to the large midline cleft lip and palate.

Table 4
Holoprosencephaly and associated conditions

Differential Diagnosis	Associated Features	Potential Evaluations	Potential Genetic Studies
Chromosomal abnormalities	(See **Table 1**)	(See **Table 1**)	(See **Table 1**)
Infant of diabetic mother	(See **Table 1**)	(See **Table 1**)	(See **Table 1**)
Single gene disorder	Microcephaly Hypotelorism Nasal hypoplasia Midline CLP Single central incisor	Head MRI imaging Dental evaluation in those where teeth have erupted	Sequencing of *SHH, ZIC2, SIX3, TGIF1, GLI2, PTCH*
Trisomy 13	(See **Table 2**)	(See **Table 2**)	(See **Table 2**)
Trisomy 18	(See **Table 2**)	(See **Table 2**)	(See **Table 2**)

ASYMMETRIC CRYING FACIES

Aysmmetric crying facies (ACF) is a minor anomaly, which presents with drooping of the corner of the mouth on the unaffected side when crying or grimacing. Asymmetric crying facies is typically due to congenital absence of the depressor anguli oris muscle (DAOM). Individuals with ACF have preservation of the nasolabial fold depth bilaterally and retain the ability to wrinkle the forehead and to close both eyes equally well, all of which distinguishes this anomaly from the less common facial nerve palsy.[2] ACF has been associated with other congenital anomalies in 20% to 70% of cases. Most anomalies are found in the head/neck and cardiovascular systems but they can also involve the skeletal, genitourinary, and gastrointestinal systems. In particular, ACF has been associated with the 22q11 deletion syndrome (also known as velocardiofacial or DiGeorge syndrome); consequently, individuals with ACF should be evaluated for signs of velocardiofacial syndrome, including dysmorphic facial features, congenital heart defects, and long fingers/toes. Long-term follow-up should focus on evaluation of growth and development and standard treatment of associated anomalies, if present (**Table 5**).[17,18]

Table 5
Asymmetric crying facies and associated conditions

Syndromes/ Conditions to Consider	Associated Features	Potential Evaluations	Potential Genetic Studies
Isolated congenital absence or hypoplasia of DAOM	Congenital heart defects	Echocardiogram	None
22q11 Deletion	Laterally built-up nose Aplasia/hypoplasia of thymus Hypocalcemia Congenital heart defects Long fingers and toes Renal anomalies	Ionized calcium and intact parathyroid hormone levels Thyroid function tests Immunology evaluation Echocardiogram Hearing screen Renal ultrasound Ophthalmologic evaluation	Chromosomal microarray or FISH for 22q11 deletion

PREAURICULAR EAR TAGS AND PITS

Preauricular ear tags and pits are frequent findings on routine neonatal physical examinations. Preauricular tags are small, skin-colored nodules that can be found anywhere along a line drawn from the tragus to the angle of the mouth (**Fig. 5**). Preauricular pits are small openings at the anterior margin of the crus of the helix. Both of these anomalies can be found in isolation or as part of a genetic syndrome. All patients with a preauricular tag or pit should have a hearing assessment because abnormalities of the external ear may be associated with middle or inner ear abnormalities and hearing loss. Furthermore, these patients should be examined for any other malformations, which may indicate an underlying genetic syndrome like craniofacial microsomia or branchio-oto-renal syndrome (**Tables 6** and **7**).[2,19,20] The association of preauricular ear tags and pits with urinary tract anomalies has also been studied previously.[20,21] Wang and colleagues[21] suggested renal ultrasound only when ear tags or pits are associated with other malformations or dysmorphic features or if there is a family history of hearing loss, ear anomalies, or maternal gestational diabetes or teratogen exposure. In the absence of these findings, the preauricular tags and pits are presumed isolated and no further evaluation is needed.

OROFACIAL CLEFTING

Orofacial clefts, including CLP and cleft palate only (CP), are the most common craniofacial birth defects in humans, with an incidence of 1 in 700 to 1 in 1000 live births. Subclinical phenotypes may occur and include microform clefts, bifid uvula, submucous CP, and velopharyngeal insufficiency. Most orofacial clefts occur in

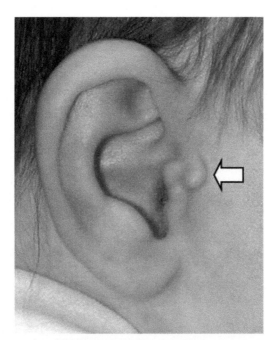

Fig. 5. Arrow pointing to small isolated right preauricular skin tag. (*From* Adam M, Hudgins L. The importance of minor anomalies in the evaluation of the newborn. NeoReviews 2003;4:e99–104.)

Table 6
Conditions associated with preauricular ear tags

Differential Diagnosis	Associated Features	Potential Evaluations	Potential Genetic Studies
Craniofacial microsomia	External ear anomalies Hearing loss Cleft palate Maxillary and/or mandibular hypoplasia Renal anomalies	Audiology evaluation Renal ultrasound	Chromosomal microarray
Isolated	May have a positive family history	Audiology evaluation	None

isolation, presumably due to the combined effect of genetic and environmental factors. Approximately 30% of CLP and 50% of CP are associated, however, with other malformations, most commonly cerebral, dental, and cardiovascular anomalies.[22] The risk of associated anomalies is even higher in the presence of bilateral clefts. Hearing loss also commonly occurs. The constellation of anomalies may indicate an underlying genetic syndrome, which may require further evaluation (**Tables 8** and **9**).[7,15,18,23–27]

The management of a neonate with an orofacial cleft is multidisciplinary with priority given to respiratory and nutritional support. The cleft itself is treated with orthodontic and surgical interventions. Other services, such as speech therapy, and interventions may be required depending on the clinical presentation (see article by Robin and Hamm elsewhere in this issue for a more detailed discussion).[27]

CARDIAC DEFECTS

Congenital heart disease (CHD) is the most common major congenital anomaly seen by neonatologists and a major cause of neonatal morbidity and mortality. There are multiple etiologies for CHD. Isolated CHD is thought to be the result of multifactorial inheritance with both genetic and environmental factors contributing to the malformation. Other CHDs are due to teratogenic effects of infections (eg, rubella and influenza), maternal factors (eg, diabetes mellitus and phenylketonuria), and prenatal exposures (eg, anticonvulsants and alcohol).[3,28,29]

Genetic etiologies are significant causes of CHD and include trisomies; 45,X (Turner syndrome); chromosomal deletions and/or duplications; and single gene disorders. Although no single cardiac defect is pathognomonic for a particular genetic syndrome, there are certain cardiac defects that are more prevalent in specific syndromes. For example, the 22q11 deletion is present in approximately 50% to 90% of neonates

Table 7
Conditions associated with preauricular ear pits

Differential Diagnosis	Associated Features	Potential Evaluations	Potential Genetic Studies
Branchio-oto-renal syndrome	External ear anomalies Brachial cleft fistulae Renal anomalies	Audiology evaluation Renal ultrasound	Sequencing of *EYA1, SIX5, SIX1*
Craniofacial microsomia	(See **Table 6**)	(See **Table 6**)	(See **Table 6**)

Table 8
Cleft palate with or without cleft lip associated genetic conditions

Differential Diagnosis	Associated Features	Potential Evaluations	Potential Genetic Studies
HPE (if cleft is midline)	(See **Table 4**)	(See **Table 4**)	(See **Table 4**)
Isolated cleft lip/palate	None	Audiology evaluation Feeding assessment	None
Trisomy 13	(See **Table 2**)	(See **Table 2**)	(See **Table 2**)
Van der Woude	Lower lip pits	Feeding assessment	Sequencing of IRF6

with an interrupted aortic arch but it is also present in neonates with tetralogy of Fallot, truncus arterious, and ventricular septal defects. Furthermore, many of the patients with CHD and an underlying genetic syndrome have other associated features that help guide further evaluation and testing (**Table 10**).[18,29–33]

Table 9
Cleft palate without cleft lip and associated conditions

Differential Diagnosis	Associated Features	Potential Evaluations	Potential Genetic Studies
22q11 Deletion	(See **Table 5**)	(See **Table 5**)	(See **Table 5**)
CHARGE	Coloboma Ear anomalies Cardiac defects Choanal atresia Genitourinary abnormalities Omphalocele	Audiology evaluation ENT evaluation Echocardiogram Ophthalmologic evaluation Renal ultrasound	Sequencing of CHD7
Isolated cleft palate	None	None	None
Smith-Lemli-Optiz	Microcephaly Characteristic facial features Cataracts Hypospadias Postaxial polydactyly 2–3 Toe syndactyly	7-Dehydrocholesterol and total cholesterol levels Echocardiogram Ophthalmologic evaluation	Sequencing DHCR7
Stickler	Myopia Cataract Retinal detachment Hearing loss Spondyloephiphyseal dysplasia	Audiology evaluation Ophthalmologic evaluation	Sequencing of COL2A1, COL9A1, COL9A2, COL11A1, and COL11A2
Treacher-Collins	Lower eyelid abnormalities Microtia and other external ear abnormalities Zygomatic bone hypoplasia	Airway and feeding evaluations Audiology evaluation	Sequencing of TCOF1, POLR1C, and POLR1D

Abbreviation: ENT, ear, nose, and throat.

ESOPHAGEAL ATRESIA/TRACHEOESOPHAGEAL FISTULA

Esophageal atresia (EA) is a developmental defect of the foregut characterized by the discontinuity of the esophagus. It is frequently associated with a tracheoesophageal fistula (TEF) and in approximately half of affected individuals, the EA/TEF anomalies are associated with other congenital anomalies.[34,35] There is a broad spectrum of anomalies associated with EA/TEF, including microcephaly, single umbilical artery, and duodenal atresia. Vertebral, anorectal, cardiac, and genitourinary anomalies are some of the most frequent and are a part of the VACTERL association. VACTERL (Vertebral defects, Anal atresia, Cardiac defects, Tracheo-Esophageal fistula, Renal anomalies and Limb abnormalities) association is considered when at least 3 features of the association are present. The genetic etiology of VACTERL has not been elucidated and it is thought to be multifactorial, although some cases may be due to teratogenic exposure, such as maternal diabetes. Therefore, VACTERL association is not considered a genetic syndrome and should be considered a diagnosis of exclusion. In individuals for whom a diagnosis of VACTERL association is entertained, chromosomal microarray and chromosomal breakage studies for Fanconi anemia should be considered. Other genetic syndromes associated with EA/TEF include CHARGE syndrome, Down syndrome, trisomy 18, and other chromosomal abnormalities (**Table 11**).[3,7–9,25,34–37]

VENTRAL WALL DEFECTS

Omphalocele and gastroschisis are the most common congenital ventral wall defects. Omphalocele is a midline defect characterized by eviscerated abdominal contents, which are covered by a protective sac. Omphalocele is associated with other anomalies in up to 90% of cases. Chromosomal abnormalities, including aneuploidies, occur in approximately 20% of cases.[38,39] Beckwith-Wiedemann syndrome, CHARGE syndrome, and VACTERL association are the most common genetic conditions associated with omphalocele (**Table 12**).[5–7,25,36] In infants with omphalocele, careful examination for other anomalies, including cardiac, renal, and ophthalmologic, should be considered. In the absence of findings that point to a specific syndrome (ie, Beckwith-Wiedemann syndrome), chromosomal microarray testing should be considered.

In contrast, the viscera in gastroschisis are not covered by a sac and protrude through a defect typically located just to the right of the umbilicus. Occasionally the sac covering an omphalocele can rupture, giving the appearance of gastroschisis, but the location of the ventral wall defect can be used to determine whether the most likely diagnosis is a ruptured omphalocele or gastroschisis. Gastroschisis is associated with young maternal age and maternal exposure to tobacco, alcohol, and ibuprofen. Gastroschisis may be associated with intrauterine growth restriction and prematurity.[40] Gastroschisis often occurs as an isolated defect but can have associated anomalies in up to one-third of cases. The most common associated anomalies are intestinal atresias, although musculoskeletal, cardiac, urogenital, and other gastrointestinal defects may be present.[39] For infants who have apparently isolated gastroschisis or gastroschisis associated only with intestinal atresia, genetic testing is typically normal and recurrence risks are low.

POLYDACTYLY

Polydactyly is a common congenital anomaly and can occur on the ulnar (postaxial) or the radial (preaxial) aspects of the extremities. Of the 2 types, postaxial polydactyly is

Table 10
Cardiac defects and associated genetic syndromes

Cardiac Defect	Genetic Syndrome	Associated Features	Potential Evaluations	Potential Genetic Studies
Atrial septal defect	Holt-Oram	Upper limb malformation Cardiac conduction disease	Upper limb radiographs Echocardiogram	Sequencing of *TBX5*
Atrioventricular canal	Down (trisomy 21)	Up-slanting palpebral fissures 5th-Finger clinodactyly Single transverse palmar creases Increased gap between 1st and 2nd toes	Audiology evaluation Complete blood cell count Ophthalmologic evaluation Thyroid function tests	Routine chromosome analysis
Coarctation of the aorta	Kabuki	Long palpebral fissures Large ears Spinal column abnormalities Postnatal growth deficiency	Ophthalmologic evaluation Renal ultrasound Spine radiographs	Sequencing of *KMT2D* and *KDM6A*
	Turner	Webbed posterior neck Broad chest with wide-spaced nipples Lymphedema of hands and feet	Audiology evaluation Renal ultrasound Thyroid function tests	Routine chromosome analysis
Hypoplastic left heart syndrome	Turner	Webbed posterior neck Broad chest with wide-spaced nipples Lymphedema of hands and feet	Audiology evaluation Renal ultrasound Thyroid function tests	Routine chromosome analysis
Interrupted aortic arch	22q11 Deletion	(See **Table 5**)	(See **Table 5**)	(See **Table 5**)
Peripheral pulmonary artery stenosis	Alagille	Bile duct paucity Butterfly vertebrae Posterior embryotoxon	Abdominal ultrasound Chest radiographs Liver function tests Ophthalmologic evaluation	Sequencing of *JAG1*

Pulmonary valve stenosis	Noonan	Tall forehead Hypertelorism Down-slanting palpebral fissures Low-set, posteriorly rotated ears Excess nuchal skin Low posterior hairline	Ophthalmologic evaluation Renal ultrasound	Molecular testing: at least 12 genes, including *PTPN11* (multigene panel testing available)
Supravavular aortic stenosis	Williams	Hypercalcemia Hypotonia Peripheral pulmonic stenosis Failure to thrive Renal artery stenosis	Bladder and kidney ultrasound Calcium level Ophthalmologic evaluation	Microarray or deletion testing for 7q11.23
Tetralogy of Fallot	22q11 Deletion	(See **Table 5**)	(See **Table 5**)	(See **Table 5**)
Ventricular septal defect	Down (trisomy 21)	(See previously)	(See previously)	(See previously)
	22q11 Deletion	(See **Table 5**)	(See **Table 5**)	(See **Table 5**)

Table 11
Tracheoesophageal fistula and associated conditions

Differential Diagnosis	Associated Features	Potential Evaluations	Potential Genetic Studies
Infant of a diabetic mother	(See Table 1)	(See Table 1)	(See Table 1)
Down (trisomy 21)	(See Table 10)	(See Table 10)	(See Table 10)
CHARGE	(See Table 9)	(See Table 9)	(See Table 9)
Chromosomal abnormalities	(See Table 1)	(See Table 1)	(See Table 1)

Fanconi anemia	Microcephaly
	Short stature
	Pigmentary abnormalities
	Thumb abnormalities (absent/
	  hypoplastic, bifid, duplicated, etc.)
	Other upper extremity abnormalities
	Lower extremity abnormalities
	Genitourinary abnormalities
	Pancytopenia
		Hematologic studies including complete
		  blood count and bone marrow aspirate
		Renal ultrasound
			Chromosomal breakage studies
			Molecular testing; at least 16 genes,
			  including *FANCA* and *BRCA2*

Trisomy 18	(See Table 2)	(See Table 2)	(See Table 2)
VACTERL association	Vertebral defects Anal atresia/imperforate anus Cardiac defects TEF Limb anomalies Renal anomalies	Abdominal radiographss AP and lateral radiographs of the entire spine Echocardiogram Radiographs of affected limbs Renal ultrasound	None

Abbreviation: AP, anterior-posterior.

Table 12
Ventral wall defects and associated conditions

Type of Defect	Genetic Syndrome	Associated Features	Potential Evaluations	Potential Genetic Studies
Omphalocele	Beckwith-Wiedemann	(See **Table 1**)	(See **Table 1**)	(See **Table 1**)
	CHARGE	(See **Table 9**)	(See **Table 9**)	(See **Table 9**)
	Trisomy 13	(See **Table 2**)	(See **Table 2**)	(See **Table 2**)
	Trisomy 18	(See **Table 2**)	(See **Table 2**)	(See **Table 2**)
	VACTERL	(See **Table 11**)	(See **Table 11**)	(See **Table 11**)
Gastroschisis	None	Cardiac anomalies Intestinal atresia Genitourinary anomalies Musculoskeletal anomalies	Abdominal radiographs Echocardiogram Renal ultrasound Skeletal radiographs	None

the most common. Postaxial polydactyly can manifest as a fully developed digit (type A) or as a rudimentary cutaneous appendage (type B). Type B polydactyly generally occurs as an isolated autosomal dominant condition with reduced penetrance. It is more common in African American individuals, with a prevalence of 1 in 143 live births versus 1 in 1339 in white infants. Type B polydactyly frequently occurs bilaterally. It is commonly treated in the nursery with suture ligation.[41–43]

In contrast, preaxial polydactyly is less common, with a prevalence of up to 1 in 3000 live births but occurs more frequently in white infants. It also is associated with an increased incidence of systemic conditions, such as Fanconi anemia, chromosomal abnormalities, and VACTERL association (**Table 13**).[36,37] Therefore, the finding of preaxial polydactyly should prompt a thorough evaluation for other congenital anomalies and consideration of genetic testing for Fanconi anemia (chromosomal breakage studies) at a minimum.[41,42]

Table 13
Preaxial polydactyly and associated conditions

Differential Diagnosis	Associated Features	Potential Evaluations	Potential Genetic Studies
Fanconi anemia	Microcephaly Short stature Pigmentary abnormalities Thumb abnormalities (absent/hypoplastic, bifid, duplicated, etc.) Other upper extremity abnormalities Lower extremity abnormalities Genitourinary abnormalities Pancytopenia	Hematologic studies including complete blood count and bone marrow aspirate Renal ultrasound	Chromosomal breakage studies Molecular testing; at least 16 genes, including *FANCA* and *BRCA2*
VACTERL association	(See **Table 11**)	(See **Table 11**)	(See **Table 11**)

SUMMARY

Neonatologists often have the unique opportunity to be the first to identify abnormalities in the neonate. Once a particular anomaly has been identified in a patient, a thorough examination with particular attention to other associated anomalies should be pursued, taking into consideration a patient's age, gender, race, and family history. **Tables 1–13** summarize the anomalies discussed in this review, possible associated syndromes and findings, and suggested investigations. The ability to recognize anomalies and their associated conditions can be the key to the diagnosis and management of a patient and to appropriate recurrence risk counseling for the family.

Best Practices

What is the current practice?

Chromosomal microarray is the recommended first-line test for infants with dysmorphic features that are not specific to a well-recognized genetic syndrome.[44] A genetics consultation should also be considered.

What changes in current practice are likely to improve outcomes?

Making a diagnosis in a child with dysmorphic features enables providers to recognize occult malformations and provide surveillance for complications that may develop over time. It also provides families information regarding the prognosis for their child and recurrence risks for future pregnancies.[2]

Major Recommendations

Whenever a dysmorphic feature is recognized, a comprehensive examination for the presence of other anomalies must be undertaken. If there are other features of a well-delineated syndrome present, further evaluation, including a detailed family history, diagnostic studies, and genetic testing, should be pursued (refer to **Tables 1–13** for examples and further information).

If features of a well-delineated syndrome are not recognized but there are at least 3 minor anomalies present, further evaluation, including a detailed family history and a chromosomal microarray, should be obtained. Also, the patient should be evaluated for the presence of an occult major malformation, because the presence of 3 or more minor anomalies is associated with a significantly increased risk of the occurrence of an occult major malformation.[2]

Rating for the Strength of the Evidence

Chromosomal microarray is the first-line test for infants with dysmorphic features that are not specific to a well-recognized genetic syndrome per the ACMG guidelines.[44] This test has a diagnostic yield of 15% to 20%.[8]

Bibliographic Sources

Adam M, Hudgins L. The importance of minor anomalies in the evaluation of the newborn. Neoreviews 2003;4:e99–104.

Manning M, Hudgins L. Array-based technology and recommendations for utilization in the medical genetics practice for detection of chromosomal abnormalities. Genet Med 2010;12:742–5.

Miller DT, Adam MP, Aradhya S, et al. Consensus statement: chromosomal microarray is a first-tier clinical diagnostic test for individuals with developmental disabilities or congenital anomalies. Am J Hum Genet 2010;86:749–64.

Summary statement

Whenever a dysmorphic feature is recognized, a comprehensive evaluation for the presence of other dysmorphic features and a possible underlying genetic syndrome must be undertaken to help guide management and provide appropriate counseling to the family.

REFERENCES

1. Synnes AR, Berry M, Jones H, et al. Infants with congenital anomalies admitted to neonatal intensive care units. Am J Perinatol 2004;21:199–207.
2. Adam M, Hudgins L. The importance of minor anomalies in the evaluation of the newborn. Neoreviews 2003;4:e99–104.
3. Hay WW. Care of the infant of the diabetic mother. Curr Diab Rep 2012;12:4–15.
4. Adam M, Hudgins L, Carey J, et al. Preaxial hallucal polydactyly as a marker for diabetic embryopathy. Birth Defects Res A Clin Mol Teratol 2009;85:13–9.
5. Pettenati M, Haines J, Higgins R, et al. Wiedemann-Beckwith syndrome: presentation of clinical and cytogenetic data on 22 new cases and review of the literature. Hum Genet 1986;74:143–54.
6. Weksberg R, Shuman C, Smith AC. Beckwith-Wiedemann syndrome. Am J Med Genet C Semin Med Genet 2005;137C:12–23.
7. Carey J. Trisomy 18 and 13 syndromes. In: Cassidy S, Allanson J, editors. Management of genetic syndromes. 3rd edition. New York: John Wiley & Sons; 2010. p. 807–23.
8. Miller DT, Adam MP, Aradhya S, et al. Consensus statement: chromosomal microarray is a first-tier clinical diagnostic test for individuals with developmental disabilities or congenital anomalies. Am J Hum Genet 2010;86:749–64.
9. American College of Obstetricians and Gynecologists. ACOG practice bulletin no. 134: fetal growth restriction. Obstet Gynecol 2013;121:1122–33.
10. Shih EM, Graham JM. Review of genetic and environmental factors leading to hypospadias. Eur J Med Genet 2014;57(8):453–63.
11. Tollefson MM. Aplasia cutis congenita. Neoreviews 2012;13:e285–92.
12. Yoshihara A, Noh J, Yamaguchi T, et al. Treatment of graves' disease with antithyroid drugs in the first trimester of pregnancy and the prevalence of congenital malformation. J Clin Endocrinol Metab 2012;97:2396–403.
13. Cohen I, Silberstein E, Perez Y, et al. Autosomal recessive Adams-Oliver syndrome caused by homozygous mutation in EOGT, encoding an EGF domain-specific O-GlcNAc transferase. Eur J Hum Genet 2014;22:374–8.
14. Olsen CL, Hughes JP, Youngblood LG, et al. Epidemiology of holoprosencephaly and phenotypic characteristics of affected children: New York State, 1984–1989. Am J Med Genet 1997;73:217–26.
15. Gropman AL, Muenke M. Holoprosencephaly. In: Cassidy S, Allanson J, editors. Management of genetic syndromes. 3rd edition. New York: John Wiley & Sons; 2010. p. 441–60.
16. Nanni L, Ming JE, Bocian M, et al. The mutational spectrum of the sonic hedgehog gene in holoprosencephaly: SHH mutations cause a significant proportion of autosomal dominant holoprosencephaly. Hum Mol Genet 1999;8:2479–88.
17. Shapira M, Borochowitz ZU. Asymmetric crying facies. Neoreviews 2009;10:e502–9.
18. Cancrini C, Puliafito P, Digilio MC, et al. Clinical features and follow-up in patients with 22q11.2 deletion syndrome. J Pediatr 2014;164:1475–80.
19. Heike CL, Hing AV, Aspinall CA, et al. Clinical care in craniofacial microsomia: a review of current management recommendations and opportunities to advance research. Am J Med Genet C Semin Med Genet 2013;163C:271–82.
20. Kugelman A, Tubi A, Bader D, et al. Pre-auricular tags and pits in the newborn. J Pediatr 2002;141:388–91.
21. Wang RY, Earl DL, Ruder RO, et al. Syndromic ear anomalies and renal ultrasounds. Pediatrics 2001;108:E32.

22. Setó-Salvia N, Stanier P. Genetics of cleft lip and/or cleft palate: association with other common anomalies. Eur J Med Genet 2014;57(8):381–93.

23. Battaile KP, Steiner RD. Smith-Lemli-Opitz syndrome: the first malformation syndrome associated with defective cholesterol synthesis. Mol Genet Metab 2000; 71:154–62.

24. Dixon MJ, Marazita ML, Beaty TH, et al. Cleft lip and palate: understanding genetic and environmental influences. Nat Rev Genet 2011;12:167–78.

25. Bergman JE, Janssen N, Hoefsloot LH, et al. CHD7 mutations and CHARGE syndrome: the clinical implications of an expanding phenotype. J Med Genet 2011; 48:334–42.

26. Robin N, Moran R, Warman M, et al. Stickler syndrome. In: Pagon R, Adam M, Ardinger H, et al, editors. GeneReviews. 2011. Available at: http://www.ncbi. nlm.nih.gov/books/NBK1116/. Accessed July 30, 2014.

27. Tighe D, Petrick L, Cobourne MT, et al. Cleft lip and palate: effects on neonatal care. Neoreviews 2011;12:e315–24.

28. Jenkins KJ, Correa A, Feinstein JA, et al. Noninherited risk factors and congenital cardiovascular defects: current knowledge: a scientific statement from the American Heart Association Council on Cardiovascular Disease in the Young: endorsed by the American Academy of Pediatrics. Circulation 2007;115:2995–3014.

29. Beck A, Hudgins L. Congenital cardiac malformations in the neonate: isolated or syndromic. Neoreviews 2003;4:e105–10.

30. Sybert VP, McCauley E. Turner's syndrome. N Engl J Med 2004;351:1227–38.

31. Bull MJ, Committee on Genetics. Health supervision for children with Down syndrome. Pediatrics 2011;128:393–406.

32. Pierpont ME, Basson CT, Benson DW, et al. Genetic basis for congenital heart defects: current knowledge: a scientific statement from the American Heart Association Congenital Cardiac Defects Committee, Council on Cardiovascular Disease in the Young: endorsed by the American Academy of Pediatrics. Circulation 2007; 115:3015–38.

33. Roberts AE, Allanson JE, Tartaglia M, et al. Noonan syndrome. Lancet 2013;381: 333–42.

34. De Jong EM, Felix JF, Deurloo JA, et al. Non-VACTERL-type anomalies are frequent in patients with esophageal atresia/tracheo-esophageal fistula and full or partial VACTERL association. Birth Defects Res A Clin Mol Teratol 2008;82:92–7.

35. Brosens E, Ploeg M, van Bever Y, et al. Clinical and etiological heterogeneity in patients with tracheo-esophageal malformations and associated anomalies. Eur J Med Genet 2014;57(8):440–52.

36. Solomon BD, Baker LA, Bear KA, et al. An approach to the identification of anomalies and etiologies in neonates with identified or suspected VACTERL (vertebral defects, anal atresia, tracheo-esophageal fistula with esophageal atresia, cardiac anomalies, renal anomalies, and limb anomalies). J Pediatr 2014;164:451–7.

37. Khincha PP, Savage SA. Genomic characterization of the inherited bone marrow failure syndromes. Semin Hematol 2013;50:333–47.

38. Agopian A, Marengo L, Mitchell LE. Descriptive epidemiology of nonsyndromic omphalocele in Texas, 1999–2004. Am J Med Genet A 2009;149A:2129–33.

39. Benjamin B, Wilson GN. Anomalies associated with gastroschisis and omphalocele: analysis of 2825 cases from the Texas Birth Defects Registry. J Pediatr Surg 2014;49:514–9.

40. Mac Bird T, Robbins JM, Druschel C, et al. Demographic and environmental risk factors for gastroschisis and omphalocele in the National Birth Defects Prevention Study. J Pediatr Surg 2009;44:1546–51.

41. Guo B, Lee S, Pakisma N. Polydactyly: a review. Bull Hosp Joint Dis 2013;71: 17–23.
42. Castilla E, Paz J, Mutchinick O, et al. Polydactyly: a genetic study in South America. Am J Hum Genet 1973;25:405–12.
43. Singer G, Thein S, Kraus T, et al. Ulnar polydactyly - an analysis of appearance and postoperative outcome. J Pediatr Surg 2014;49:474–6.
44. Manning M, Hudgins L. Array-based technology and recommendations for utilization in the medical genetics practice for detection of chromosomal abnormalities. Genet Med 2010;12:742–5.

Recognizable Syndromes in the Newborn Period

Anne Slavotinek, MB.BS, PhD*, Marwan Ali, MD

KEYWORDS

- Newborn period • Syndrome recognition • Dysmorphology • Birth defects

KEY POINTS

- Many syndromes have a different presentation in the newborn period compared with childhood or adult life, and recognition early in life is frequently based on a characteristic pattern of dysmorphic features and/or malformations that can vary from the classic presentation seen in childhood.
- Early recognition of syndromes is increasingly important, as for many of them there are professional guidelines for treatment and surveillance.
- Genetic testing with next-generation sequencing will increasingly be performed for diagnosis in the newborn period and will expand our understanding of the clinical variability within syndromes.

INTRODUCTION

The primary goals of the assessment of an infant with congenital anomalies in the neonatal period are to establish a diagnosis, identify associated abnormalities, develop a management plan, and assess the natural history and prognosis. The correct diagnosis enables parents and clinicians to obtain accurate information, plan for appropriate surveillance, determine recurrence risks and access support and advocacy groups. Standard tools for the diagnostic assessment in the newborn period include a pregnancy history, birth history and family history, physical examination, and investigations to delineate the presence of additional anomalies, including cranial ultrasound, chest radiograph, echocardiogram, abdominal or renal ultrasound, skeletal survey, and ophthalmologic examination. If the baby is stable, more detailed imaging or invasive testing, such as magnetic resonance imaging (MRI) scan of the brain or other relevant regions, can be considered.

Disclosures: none.
Division of Genetics, Department of Pediatrics, University of California, San Francisco, 1550 4th Street, Room RH384D, San Francisco, CA 94143-2711, USA
* Corresponding author.
E-mail address: slavotia@ucsf.edu

Clin Perinatol 42 (2015) 263–280
http://dx.doi.org/10.1016/j.clp.2015.02.003
0095-5108/15/$ – see front matter © 2015 Elsevier Inc. All rights reserved.
perinatology.theclinics.com

Chromosome testing with array comparative genomic hybridization (aCGH) is the standard of care in the investigation of many infants with multiple congenital anomalies, birth defects, or neurologic signs. Chromosomal aneuploidies and chromosomal deletions and duplications are identified in an estimated 7.5% of infants with multiple congenital anomalies. A growing number of infants also undergo gene panel sequencing or genomic testing with exome sequencing. Despite the increased testing options now available, an accurate knowledge of the presentation of syndromes in the neonatal period is often needed to obtain the correct diagnosis.

One of the most important initial decisions is whether an infant's presentation is syndromic, as opposed to an isolated birth defect or sequence that is less likely to be associated with additional malformations or an easily discernible underlying genetic cause. A syndrome can be defined as a set of developmental anomalies or pattern of defects occurring together in a recognizable and consistent pattern that is caused by a single cause.[1] Many syndromes are associated with dysmorphic features and a recognizable facial gestalt that enables a clinical diagnosis. Imaging or other investigations to determine the extent of phenotypic involvement and chromosomal, biochemical, and/or molecular genetic testing are usually performed to confirm the syndrome diagnosis. It is important to be aware that, just as the appearance and physiology of typically developing infants alters with time, the manifestations of syndromes can be specific to different developmental time periods. In the neonatal period, syndromes may either be more straightforward or more difficult to recognize. It is vital for clinicians to be aware of these differences, so that an age-appropriate differential diagnosis is considered at the baby's bedside.

This review describes a selection of the syndromes most frequently encountered in the newborn period, with an emphasis on the physical findings that present shortly after birth. The authors have focused on syndromes that are frequently encountered and that differ significantly in presentation in the newborn period compared with later in childhood, and on syndromes that are frequently encountered and for which early recognition is helpful because it prompts surveillance or more timely treatment. Space limitations have prevented the coverage of many conditions, and the craniosynostoses and disorders of sexual development that may present in the neonatal period are not included.

TEXT

Table 1 provides a summary of common syndromes that are recognizable in the newborn period based on cardinal symptoms and signs. Syndromes with causative genes have been grouped into body systems; syndromes caused by chromosome aberrations, metabolic conditions, and conditions with multifactorial or an unknown cause are listed separately. Genetic confirmation should be performed for those conditions for which it is available (**Table 2**), and it is important to remember that many chromosomal abnormalities can be phenocopies of Mendelian genetic syndromes. In the following text, the authors discuss selected conditions that have specific neonatal presentations, listing clinical features and reasons that an early diagnosis may be helpful.

CRANIOFACIAL SYNDROMES

The diagnosis of Van der Woude syndrome (MIM 119300) is a good example of the utility of a thorough examination, as the small lip pits that are pathognomonic for this condition in association with cleft lip/palate (CL/P) can sometimes be missed

(**Fig. 1**). Achieving a diagnosis in the neonatal period is important because of the autosomal dominant inheritance of this condition, which can result in a recurrence risk that is increased compared with the risks for isolated CL/P.[2] The lip pits can be surgically removed and, thus, may be less apparent at later ages.

Stickler Syndrome

Stickler syndrome (MIM 108300) classically presents with Pierre-Robin sequence (cleft soft palate with micrognathia) in the neonatal period. The diagnosis may be missed, as the ocular findings comprising vitreoretinopathy and retinal detachment, deafness, epiphyseal dysplasia, and degenerative joint disease may all be later manifestations.[3,4] A facial gestalt can aid recognition of Stickler syndrome in the newborn period and childhood, with infants demonstrating relatively prominent eyes and a flat facial profile with a hypoplastic midface and a short and anteverted nose, in addition to micrognathia (**Fig. 2**).[4] Stickler syndrome should also be considered in neonates with significant refractive errors, astigmatism, cataracts, and abnormal anterior chamber drainage that can predispose to glaucoma.[5] It is vital to distinguish Stickler syndrome from isolated Pierre-Robin sequence, as monitoring for the eye complications, such as retinal detachment, and prophylactic or early treatment can preserve vision. In addition, a cardiac assessment for complications, such as mitral valve prolapse, should be undertaken.

Stickler syndrome is an autosomal dominant condition with great variability, even within families; thus, a very careful family history may be an important diagnostic clue.[3] The condition is genetically heterogeneous, although most patients have mutations in the Collagen, Type II, Alpha-1 (*COL2A1*), Collagen, Type XI, Alpha-1 (*COL11A1*), and Collagen, Type XI, Alpha-2 (*COL11A2*) genes. A panel approach to genetic testing is frequently used (see **Table 2**).

SYNDROMES WITH HYPOTONIA
Prader-Willi Syndrome

Many infants present with hypotonia and feeding difficulties in the newborn period, and Prader-Willi syndrome [PWS; MIM 176270] should be considered in the differential diagnosis. PWS has an incidence of 1 in 10,000 to 1 in 15,000 individuals and a prevalence of up to 10% in a small series of infants with hypotonia.[6] The neonatal presentation of PWS includes central hypotonia that is frequently severe, leading to lethargy and feeding difficulties, with a weak suck and failure to thrive.[7] Dysmorphic features, such as bitemporal narrowing, almond-shaped palpebral fissures, and a thin upper lip, may also aid recognition in the newborn period.[7] Central sleep apnea has been described and may be ameliorated by oxygen therapy.[8] It is important to note that the classic features of truncal obesity and voracious appetite that develop later in childhood are absent in the neonatal period. Other features that are absent or less apparent in the newborn period include learning and behavioral differences, small hands and feet and short stature.[9,10]

PWS is caused by a variety of genetic mechanisms including paternal deletions at chromosome 15q11–15q13 (75% of patients), maternal uniparental disomy for this chromosome region (24% of patients) and imprinting defects (1% of patients). Diagnosis can be accomplished by determining methylation status of the small nuclear ribonucleoprotein polypeptide N gene (*SNRPN*; 99% yield). As therapy with growth hormone has been shown to be efficacious in normalizing the body habitus and lean body mass,[11] a timely diagnosis can help to prevent the complication of morbid obesity.

Table 1
Summary of selected syndromes that are recognizable in the newborn period: presentation

Syndromes	Characteristic Diagnostic Features	Differences in Presentation from Other Age Groups	Importance of Neonatal Diagnosis
Craniofacial Syndromes			
Van der Woude syndrome	CL/P, lip pits	No	Recurrence risk high
Stickler syndrome	Facial gestalt, Pierre-Robin sequence	Different dysmorphism	Screen for complications
Syndromes with Hypotonia			
Spinal muscular atrophy	Hypotonia	Severe in newborn	Appropriate care
Myotonic dystrophy	Respiratory difficulties	Severe in newborn	Screen for complications
Prader-Willi syndrome	Facial gestalt, hypotonia, FTT	FTT, no obesity	Early treatment
Cardiac Syndromes			
Noonan syndrome	Facial gestalt, cardiac defects, hypotonia, FTT	Different dysmorphism	Surveillance
Kabuki syndrome	Facial gestalt, cardiac defects, hypotonia	Different dysmorphism	Surveillance
Neonatal Marfan syndrome	Arachnodactyly, thin habitus; aortic dilatation	Different dysmorphism	Treatment of cardiac lesions
Gastrointestinal Syndromes			
Beckwith-Wiedemann	Macroglossia, macrosomia, abdominal wall defect	Severe in newborn	Screen for complications
Renal Syndromes			
WAGR	Wilms tumor, aniridia, genitourinary anomalies	No	Screen for complications
Skeletal Syndromes			
Achondroplasia	Facial gestalt, short limbs, short trunk	No	Screen for complications
Osteogenesis imperfecta	Multiple fractures, short stature, osteopenia	No	Early treatment
Syndromes with Skin Findings			
Incontinentia pigmenti	Multi-stage rash	Severe in newborn	Severe in newborn

Other Syndromes			
CHARGE syndrome	Coloboma, choanal atresia, heart defects	No	Screen for complications
Cornelia de Lange syndrome	Facial gestalt, limb defects	No	Screen for complications
Aneuploidy Syndromes			
Trisomy 21/18/13	See text	No	Screen for complications
Turner syndrome	Facial gestalt, cardiac defects, renal anomalies	Different dysmorphism	Screen for complications
Trisomy 8 mosaicism	Orthopedic manifestations	No	Screen for complications
Microdeletion Syndromes			
22q11 deletion syndrome	Outflow tract abnormalities, CP, hypocalcemia	Different dysmorphism	Screen for complications
William syndrome	Pulmonary stenosis, hypercalcemia, FTT	Different dysmorphism	Screen for complications
Smith-Magenis syndrome	Facial gestalt, cardiac manifestations	Different dysmorphism	Screen for complications
Metabolic Syndromes			
Smith-Lemli-Opitz syndrome	Facial gestalt, microcephaly, 2/3 syndactyly	No	Early treatment
Zellweger syndrome	Facial gestalt, hypotonia, liver disease, renal cysts	Different dysmorphism	Early treatment
Congenital adrenal hyperplasia	Ambiguous genitalia, salt wasting	No	Early treatment
Multifactorial/Environmental			
VATER/VACTERL	TEF, anal atresia, vertebral anomalies	No	Relatively good prognosis
Goldenhar syndrome	Facial asymmetry, microtia, epibulbar dermoids	No	Recurrence risk low
Infant of a diabetic mother	Macrosomia, sacral agenesis, multiple anomalies	—	Relatively good prognosis
Fetal alcohol syndrome	Facial gestalt, withdrawal syndrome	No	Screen for complications

Abbreviations: CHARGE, Coloboma-heart defects-atresia choanae-retardation of growth and development-genital defect-ear anomalies and/or deafness; CP, cleft palate; FTT, failure to thrive; NGS, next-generation sequencing; TEF, trachea-esophageal fistula; VATER/VACTERL, vertebral defects-anal atresia-cardiac anomalies-trachea-esophageal fistula-renal anomalies-limb defects; WAGR, Wilms tumor-aniridia-genitourinary anomalies-mental retardation.

Table 2
Summary of selected syndromes that are recognizable in the newborn period: inheritance and genetics

Syndromes	Inheritance	Genetic Cause	Testing Modalities
Craniofacial			
Van der Woude syndrome	Autosomal dominant	IRF6 mutations	Sanger sequencing
Stickler syndrome	Autosomal dominant	COL2A1, COL11A1, COL11A2 mutations	Panel/NGS approach
Central Nervous System			
Spinal muscular atrophy	Autosomal recessive	SMN1 deletion/gene conversion; other genes	Deletion testing
Myotonic dystrophy	Autosomal dominant	DMPK trinucleotide repeat expansion	PCR/Southern blotting
Prader-Willi syndrome	Majority sporadic	Imprinting defect at chromosome 15q11	Methylation assay
Cardiac			
Noonan syndrome	Autosomal dominant	PNPT11 mutations; other genes	Panel/NGS approach
Kabuki syndrome	Autosomal dominant	KMT2D mutations	Sanger sequencing
Neonatal Marfan syndrome	Autosomal dominant	FBN1 mutations	Sanger sequencing
Gastrointestinal			
Beckwith-Wiedemann syndrome	Sporadic; autosomal dominant	Imprinting defect at chromosome 11p15	Methylation assay
Renal			
WAGR	Autosomal dominant	WT1/PAX6 deletions	aCGH
Skeletal			
Achondroplasia	Autosomal dominant	FGFR3 mutation	Sanger sequencing
Osteogenesis imperfecta	Autosomal dominant/recessive	COL1A1 and COL1A2 mutations; other genes	Panel/NGS approach
Skin			
Incontinentia pigmenti	X-linked dominant	IKBKG gene deletion/mutations	Deletion testing; Sanger sequencing

Other			
CHARGE syndrome	Autosomal dominant	*CHD7* mutations; other genes	Sanger sequencing
Cornelia de Lange syndrome	Autosomal dominant	*NIPBL* mutations; other genes	Panel/NGS approach
Aneuploidy Syndromes			
Trisomy 21/18/13	Majority sporadic	Trisomy 21/18/13	Karyotype
Turner syndrome	Sporadic	XO chromosome complement	Karyotype
Trisomy 8 mosaicism	Sporadic	Trisomy 8	Karyotype
Microdeletion Syndromes			
22q11 deletion syndrome	Autosomal dominant	22q11.2 microdeletion	aCGH
Williams syndrome	Autosomal dominant	7q11.23 microdeletion	aCGH
Smith-Magenis syndrome	Autosomal dominant	17p11.2 microdeletion	aCGH
Metabolic Syndromes			
Smith-Lemli-Opitz syndrome	Autosomal recessive	*DHCR7* mutations	Sanger sequencing
Zellweger syndrome	Autosomal recessive	*PEX* gene mutations	Panel/NGS approach
Congenital adrenal hyperplasia	Autosomal recessive	*CYP21A2* mutations; other genes	Sanger sequencing
Multifactorial/Environmental			
VATER/VACTERL	Sporadic	Not known	—
Goldenhar syndrome	Sporadic	Not known	—
Infant of a diabetic mother	Environmental exposure	NA	—
Fetal alcohol syndrome	Environmental exposure	NA	—

Abbreviations: CHARGE, coloboma-heart defects-atresia choanae-retardation of growth and development-genital defect-ear anomalies and/or deafness; NGS, next-generation sequencing; PCR, polymerase chain reaction; VATER/VACTERL, vertebral defects-anal atresia-cardiac anomalies-trachea-esophageal fistula-renal anomalies-limb defects; WAGR, Wilms tumor-aniridia-genitourinary anomalies-mental retardation.

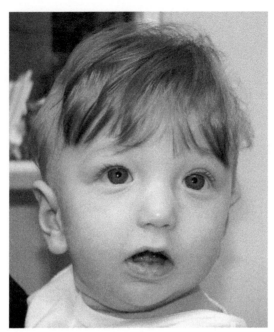

Fig. 1. Lip pits in Van der Woude syndrome. Frontal view of 13-month-old boy with a clinical diagnosis of Van der Woude syndrome, showing bilateral pits of the lower lip.

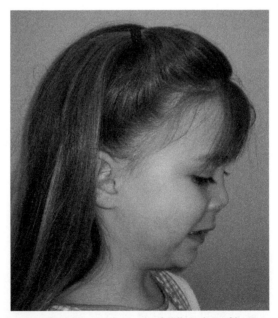

Fig. 2. Facial appearance of Stickler syndrome in childhood. Profile view of a 5-year-old girl with a clinical diagnosis of Stickler syndrome, showing midface hypoplasia, small and ante-verted nares, and micrognathia.

Myotonic Dystrophy Type I

Myotonic dystrophy type 1 (MD1; MIM 160900) can manifest with a severe presentation in the neonatal period (congenital MD1), with hypotonia, respiratory difficulties, facial diplegia, talipes, joint contractures, and weak facial muscles resulting in a tented upper lip.[12] Other diagnostically useful findings include polyhydramnios and reduced fetal movements during pregnancy.[13] The condition can be critical, and death can result from respiratory insufficiency or cardiac failure.[13] In contrast to MD1 with a later onset in childhood, the pathognomonic finding of myotonia and the characteristic electromyogram abnormalities are absent,[14] making molecular genetic testing helpful for establishing the diagnosis.

Congenital MD1 is caused by an expanded CTG repeat in the dystrophia myotonica protein kinase (*DMPK*) gene, typically resulting from the unstable expansion of a large, maternally inherited allele.[12] As mothers may be more mildly affected, maternal history and physical examination for evidence of myotonia should be performed. It is critical to recognize this condition in the newborn period for appropriate management of the infant's care as well as for maternal health management and recurrence risk/family planning.

CARDIAC SYNDROMES
Noonan Syndrome and Disorders of the Ras Mitogen-Activated Protein Kinase (RasMAPK) Pathway

Clinicians may be alerted to the possibility of Noonan syndrome (NS; MIM 163950) or related disorders of the RasMAPK pathway (such as cardiofaciocutaneous syndrome, MIM 115151, or Costello syndrome, MIM 218040) in pregnancy because of polyhydramnios, increased nuchal translucency, and hydrops fetalis.[15] After delivery, many of the characteristic dysmorphic findings of NS are apparent; the facial appearance may be most obvious at this time, comprising a tall forehead with coarse facial features, ptosis with thick, droopy eyelids, hypertelorism with striking blue or blue-green irises, epicanthic folds, low-set and posteriorly rotated ears with thickened helices and a deeply grooved philtrum with high, and wide peaks to the vermillion border of the upper lip.[16] The neck may be short, with a low posterior hairline and excess nuchal skinfolds. Birth length and weight are typically normal in contrast to short stature and microcephaly that can develop in childhood.[16] Other findings that are frequent in neonates and serve as diagnostic indicators include cardiac defects, including neonatal hypertrophic cardiomyopathy[17], pulmonic stenosis and septal defects, and disordered lymphatic development that can manifest as lymphatic dysplasia,[18] lymphedema involving the dorsal surfaces of the hands and feet, and effusions.[19] Infants can also have marked hypotonia, joint hyperextensibility, and ulerythema ophryogenes (inflammatory keratotic facial papules).[20] Cryptorchidism may be a useful diagnostic finding in boys. Finally, infants with NS often have feeding difficulties and failure to thrive that improve in early childhood.

NS shows high genetic heterogeneity (ie, many different genes can cause NS and related disorders) (see **Table 2**), and testing with RasMAPK gene panels or exome sequencing is frequently used in preference to single gene testing. Early diagnosis can facilitate screening for other physical manifestations, monitoring for potential complications, such as prolonged bleeding caused by clotting factor deficiencies, and ensure that appropriate educational services and support are available.

Neonatal Marfan Syndrome

Neonatal Marfan syndrome is a severe but rare condition that is diagnosable on examination in the neonatal period based on the phenotypic findings of dolichocephaly, micrognathia, striking arachnodactyly with thin hands and feet, and loose and redundant skin. Cardiac abnormalities are almost universal and can include aortic dilatation and valvular insufficiency that can lead to early mortality.[21] Other neonatal findings include lens dislocation, rocker bottom feet, joint hypermobility of the fingers and toes, hypotonia, and pulmonary emphysema.[22,23] The later clinical manifestations contrast to children with fibrillin-1 (*FBN1*) mutations who present in childhood, in whom there may be no findings in the neonatal period.[24]

A phenotype genotype correlation has been proposed for *FBN1* mutations in Marfan syndrome, with mutations in exons 24 to 32 of the *FBN1* gene causing the neonatal phenotype[22]; but exceptions have been noted.[25] Recently, a related but novel syndrome with prematurity and accelerated linear growth compared with weight, a progerioid appearance, and congenital lipodystrophy resulting from mutations in the penultimate exon of *FBN1* was recognized.[26,27]

Coloboma, Heart Defects, Atresia of the Choanae, Retarded Growth and Development, Genital Abnormalities, and Ear Anomalies Syndrome

CHARGE is an acronym for coloboma, heart defects, atresia of the choanae, retarded growth and development, genital abnormalities, and ear anomalies. CHARGE syndrome (MIM 214800) should be considered in the newborn period whenever a combination of any of the aforementioned features is present. The aural malformations are particularly characteristic, with asymmetric, small, low-set ears that have overfolded or severely hypoplastic helices. CHARGE syndrome is an autosomal dominant condition that demonstrates extreme phenotypic heterogeneity; other clinical aids for recognition include microphthalmia, cranial nerve dysfunction with unilateral or bilateral facial palsy, cleft palate, and characteristic inner malformations including hypoplasia of the semicircular canals and Mondini malformation.[28] It is important to accurately diagnose CHARGE syndrome, as morbidity and mortality are high, with intellectual impairment that can be severe. The main causative gene, chromodomain helicase DNA-binding protein 7 (*CHD7*), demonstrates loss of function in an estimated 50% to 70% of individuals with the condition.[29] Recently, semaphorin 3A (*SEMA3A*) has been suggested to modify the function of *CHD7*; but mutations in this gene have so far been predominantly found in individuals with Kallmann syndrome rather than CHARGE syndrome and have accounted for less than 10% of *CHD7*-negative patients.[30]

GASTROINTESTINAL SYNDROMES
Beckwith-Wiedemann Syndrome

The cardinal features of Beckwith-Wiedemann syndrome (BWS; MIM 130650), including neonatal macrosomia, macroglossia, abdominal wall defects, and hypoglycemia, are most obvious in the newborn period. Other characteristic findings include ear lobe creases and ear pits of the posterior helix, intra-abdominal visceromegaly including nephromegaly, hemihyperplasia, and renal and cardiac defects.[31] The newborn facial appearance can also be characteristic, with nevus flammeus, infraorbital creases, and midface hypoplasia in addition to the macroglossia. BWS can be considered antenatally because of polyhydramnios and fetal overgrowth, and delivery can be premature. The incidence of BWS is estimated at 1 in 10,340 live births,[32] and the diagnosis should be readily considered and investigated in view of the cancer predisposition conferred by this syndrome.[33] Monitoring for malignancies, such as Wilms tumor and hepatoblastoma, should start immediately after clinical diagnosis, as aggressive tumors have been described in the neonatal period.[32,34]

BWS is caused by epigenomic and genomic alterations on chromosome 11p15 that are found in up to 80% of affected individuals, including maternal microdeletions of imprinting centers 1 and 2 and paternal uniparental disomy and microduplications.[31] A link between BWS and assisted reproductive technologies was proposed, but this has not been confirmed in all studies.[35,36]

SYNDROMES WITH SKIN FINDINGS
Incontinentia Pigmenti

Incontinentia pigmenti (IP; MIM 308300) is a rare but highly diagnosable skin condition that most frequently commences in the neonatal period with blisters along the lines of Blaschko on the limbs and trunk, progressing through verrucous lesions, streaky lines of hyperpigmentation, and pale, atrophic streaks in childhood to adult life.[37,38] Neurologic complications include cognitive differences, seizures and microcephaly, and cerebral infarcts; brain atrophy and abnormalities of the corpus callosum have been noted on brain imaging.[39] Dental findings include hypodontia and microdontia; sparse hair, nail dystrophy, and retinal lesions may also be observed. The diagnosis is important to recognize in the newborn period, as the skin lesions may be less pronounced and harder to diagnose with certainty in childhood and adult life. IP is caused by loss-of-function mutations in the X-linked dominant inhibitor of kappa B kinase gamma (*IKBKG*) gene; a recurrent intragenic deletion involving exons 4 to 10 of *IKBKG* is found in most affected individuals.[38]

Goltz Syndrome

Goltz syndrome, also known as focal dermal hypoplasia (MIM 305600), can be diagnosed by skin lesions comprising patchy dermal hypoplasia, hyperpigmentation and hypopigmentation, fat herniation, and papillomas that manifest along Blaschko's lines and that are usually accompanied by digital (oligodactyly, ectrodactyly, syndactyly), ocular (microphthalmia, coloboma, cataracts), and dental abnormalities.[40] This condition is an X-linked dominant disorder caused by mutations in the Porcupine, Drosophila, Homolog-of (*PORCN*) gene that was considered fatal in boys and diagnosable only in males with mosaicism, Klinefelter syndrome, or a hypoplastic mutation.[41,42] The classic dermatologic findings can be present in the newborn period and confirmed on skin biopsy or mutation analysis, thus enabling a diagnosis and monitoring for other complications.

ANEUPLOIDY SYNDROMES
Trisomy 21: Down Syndrome

Although rarely missed, the diagnosis of trisomy 21 is important to achieve in the neonatal period, as specific management guidelines for health complications are available.[43,44] Infants with Down syndrome have a characteristic appearance that is familiar to many, with a flat facial profile, brachycephaly, excess skin at the back of the neck, upslanting palpebral fissures with epicanthic folds, small ears with overfolding of the upper helix, diminished middle phalanges of the fifth fingers, single transverse palmar creases, and a wide sandal gap between the first and second toes. These infants also have brachycephaly, mild microcephaly, late closure of fontanelles, Brushfield spots and peripheral iris hypoplasia, a small nose with a low nasal bridge, and a short hard palate. Joint hyperextensibility, an absent Moro reflex, and a dysplastic pelvis on radiographs are all frequent. The overall appearance is that of a hypotonic infant with an open mouth and a protruding tongue.

Infants with Down syndrome have a 50% incidence of congenital heart disease (CHD), with atrioventricular septal defect, ventricular septal defect, atrial septal defect, patent ductus arteriosus, overriding aorta, tetralogy of Fallot, and an aberrant subclavian artery among the commonly encountered lesions. Pulmonary hypoplasia may cause breathing difficulties independently from CHD. Duodenal stenosis/atresia and Hirschsprung disease are also seen. All individuals with Down syndrome have delayed growth, and measurements should be plotted on specific Down syndrome growth charts. These children are at risk for hearing loss that is exacerbated by serous otitis media and for cataracts, strabismus, nystagmus, and myopia.

Investigations should include a chest radiograph, electrocardiography, and echocardiography within the first month of life. A complete blood count should be performed to rule out hyperviscosity syndrome and transient myeloproliferative disorder, which has a 10- to 30-fold greater incidence in individuals with Down syndrome, as compared with the general population.[45] Transient megakaryocytic leukemia can be found in 10% of newborns with Down syndrome caused by specific mutations of Gata-binding protein 1 (GATA1). Newborns must also be screened for hypothyroidism, and all infants should be referred to early intervention services.

Ninety-five percent of individuals with Down syndrome have 3 free copies of chromosome 21 resulting from meiotic non-disjunction; but 3% to 4% of cases are caused by unbalanced translocations involving chromosome 21, and 1% are caused by mosaicism, making this one of the chromosomal conditions whereby a karyotype, rather than aCGH is indicated.

Trisomy 18 and Trisomy 13

These aneuploidies are important to diagnose promptly because of the likelihood of reduced survival, which can influence medical and surgical management decisions.[46] In trisomy 18, the 3 most common neonatal findings are clenched hands with overlapping fingers, rocker bottom feet, and low-set or malformed ears.[47] A newborn with trisomy 18 will typically be small for gestational age, with a prominent occiput, and a short sternum. Other major clinical features include hypertonia, anteroposterior elongation of the skull with a prominent occiput, micrognathia, CHD, a narrow chest with a short sternum, renal anomalies, and partial syndactyly of the toes with hypoplastic nails.[48] In trisomy 13, presentation is notoriously variable; one study found ear anomalies, CL/P, and heart disease to be the most common manifestations.[49] However, postaxial polydactyly and the appearance associated with holoprosencephaly, including microcephaly, microphthalmia, and hypotelorism, have also been considered hallmarks of this condition. Other physical findings in newborns with trisomy 13 include cutis aplasia of the scalp (may be confused with lacerations), omphalocele, genital abnormalities (including cryptorchidism and micropenis), cystic kidneys, and capillary hemangiomata.[50]

In most patients with trisomy 18 and 13, a full copy of the extra chromosome is present. However, mosaicism and translocations can occur; a karyotype is, therefore, recommended over aCGH.

MICRODELETION SYNDROMES
22q11 Deletion Syndrome

The 22q11.2 deletion syndrome (also known as diGeorge syndrome [MIM 188400] and velocardiofacial syndrome [MIM 192430]) is the most common microdeletion syndrome, with an incidence of 1 in 4000 births.[51,52] The 22q11.2 deletion syndrome is often diagnosed in the newborn period because of characteristic malformations, as the commonly recognized facial appearance is not always present. The malformations associated with 22q11 deletions include submucous cleft palate, bifid uvula and conotruncal heart defects, with right-sided aortic arch, tetralogy of Fallot, aberrant left subclavian artery and ventricular septal defect, neonatal hypocalcemia caused by hypoparathyroidism, and abnormal T-cell function caused by thymic hypoplasia. In infancy, the only notable dysmorphic features may be atypical ears, an anteverted nose, and microretrognathia. Later in childhood, the narrow palpebral fissures, prominent nose, squared nasal root and narrow alar base, and malar hypoplasia become more obvious, in addition to hypernasal speech and speech delay. Other common findings in infancy include hypotonia and microcephaly.

Recommended investigations include an electrocardiogram and echocardiogram; ionized calcium level; baseline immune profile; renal sonogram and cardiology, ear, nose and throat, and audiology and immunology consultations. The typical 3 megabase microdeletion at 22q11.2 contains an estimated 60 genes and is found in 90% of cases.[51] The deletion is caused by non-allelic homologous recombination between low-copy number repeats.[51] The diagnosis can be made by fluorescence in-situ hybridization (FISH) or aCGH.

Williams Syndrome

In the newborn period, the diagnosis of Williams syndrome (also known as Williams-Beuren syndrome; MIM 194050) can be suggested by a cardiologist following detection of the classic cardiac lesions of supravalvular aortic stenosis, peripheral pulmonary artery stenosis, pulmonic valvular stenosis, and supravalvular pulmonic stenosis. Persistent hypercalcemia is an additional sign that is diagnostically useful early in life. In contrast to the presentation in early childhood, the characteristic dysmorphic features of periorbital puffiness and full lips may be harder to recognize in the neonatal period, or the dysmorphic features may be non-specific. These newborns also manifest joint hypermobility and soft lax skin.[53] Renal anomalies, including nephrocalcinosis, asymmetry in kidney size, small solitary or pelvic kidney, bladder diverticulae, urethral stenosis, and vesicoureteral reflux, are also common.[54] Williams syndrome is caused by a deletion at 7q11.23, causing hemizygosity for the elastin gene[55] that is detectable either by FISH or aCGH.

METABOLIC SYNDROMES
Smith-Lemli-Opitz Syndrome

The phenotype of Smith-Lemli-Opitz (SLO) syndrome can be noticeable in the newborn period because of associated malformations, including cleft palate, cardiac defects with atrioventricular septal defects and total anomalous pulmonary venous drainage, hypospadias and cryptorchidism, postaxial polydactyly, and short thumbs.[56] The facial appearance may also be suggestive because of microcephaly, ptosis, a depressed nasal bridge, and a short and anteverted nares with micrognathia. Particularly pathognomonic is Y-shaped syndactyly of the second and third toes.[56] Although rare, recognition of SLO is critical because the biochemical pathway is well understood and multiple treatment options with cholesterol, statins, antioxidants, and gene therapy exist, although data from randomized controlled trials documenting improvement after therapeutic modalities are scarce.[57]

SLO syndrome is an autosomal recessive condition caused by deficiency of the enzyme 7-dehydrocholesterol reductase, leading to low cholesterol and elevated serum levels of 7- and 8-dehydrocholesterol that can be assayed to establish the diagnosis.[58] Genetic testing for 7-dehydro cholesterol reductase (*DHCR7*) gene mutations is also clinically available.

SYNDROME OF UNKNOWN CAUSE
Vertebral Defects, Anorectal Malformations, Cardiac Defects, Tracheoesophageal Fistula, Esophageal Atresia, Renal Anomalies, and Limb Deformities

VATER/VACTERL association (vertebral defects, anorectal malformations, cardiac defects, tracheoesophageal fistula, esophageal atresia, renal anomalies, and limb deformities) is a non-random association that has been well established. Prevalence has been estimated at 1 in 10,000 to 1 in 40,000.[59] The characteristic pattern of anomalies aids recognition in the newborn period; the diagnosis is important, as VATER/VACTERL is a sporadic condition and generally without implications for abnormal growth or developmental progress.[59,60] aCGH is frequently performed because the differential diagnosis may be broad; but the cause of this condition is unknown, and the mainstay of management is surgical with long-term care related to the underlying malformations.

Hemifacial Microsomia

Hemifacial microsomia (also known as Goldenhar syndrome, oculoauriculovertebral dysplasia, and craniofacial microsomia; MIM 164210) is diagnosed at birth in around two-thirds of cases, with the most frequent phenotypic findings comprising microtia, facial asymmetry or hemifacial microsomia, and ear tags.[61] It is important to consider this diagnosis because of the clinical variability and high prevalence (69.5%) of malformations in other organ syndromes, including cardiac defects.[61] The pathogenesis has been hypothesized to include both environmental (for example, maternal diabetes) and genetic factors but remains unknown in almost all cases.

SUMMARY/DISCUSSION

The authors provide brief descriptions for some of the most common syndromes that present in the newborn period, outlining the differences between presentations in the newborn period and those at later ages for selected conditions. Phenotypes may be more severe (for example, neonatal Marfan syndrome, congenital myotonic dystrophy, and IP) or less fully developed (for example, Stickler syndrome). Early recognition is important for specific surveillance (for example, BWS and Stickler syndrome) or for starting treatment (for example, SLO). Many syndromes can be recognized from a typical pattern of malformations in the newborn period (for example, 22q11 deletion syndrome and VATER/VACTERL).

Most of these conditions have cardinal manifestations and natural histories that were defined long in advance of current clinical practices. However, the growing availability of information continues to refine management; efforts to remain abreast of changes in the literature are increasingly important. Finally, the landscape of genetic testing has changed dramatically with the introduction of next-generation sequencing technologies, such as whole-exome or whole-genome sequencing; it is likely that these methodologies will be increasingly used in the newborn period.[62] Exome sequencing has resulted in an expansion of the clinical features connected with the phenotype for many different disorders; although less applicable to the common syndromes described earlier, it is likely that this test will substantially influence how clinicians approach syndrome diagnosis in the newborn period for rarer diseases in the future.

Best Practices

What is the current practice?

Many syndromes have a different presentation in the neonatal period compared with later in life. Most children with multiple anomalies undergo tests, such as cranial ultrasound, chest radiograph, echocardiogram, abdominal or renal ultrasound, skeletal survey, and ophthalmology examination, to define the extent of their anomalies. If the baby is stable, more detailed imaging or invasive testing, such as MRI of the brain or other relevant regions, can be considered. Chromosome testing with array comparative genomic hybridization is also commonly performed as an initial screening test.

Best practice/guideline/care path objectives

What changes in current practice are likely to improve outcomes? The introduction of next-generation sequencing technologies (for example, exome sequencing) is likely to increase diagnostic yield in the neonatal period.

Summary statement

It is important for clinicians to be aware that the presentation of common syndromes can vary with age. It is likely that exome sequencing will be increasingly used in diagnostic investigations in the newborn period in the future.

REFERENCES

1. Slavotinek A, Wynshaw-Boris A, Biesecker L. Dysmorphology. In: Kliegman R, Stanton B, St Geme J, editors. Nelson textbook of pediatrics. 19th edition. Philadelphia: Elsevier Inc; 2011. Chapter 108. p. 122–32.
2. Rizos M, Spyropoulos MN. Van der Woude syndrome: a review. Cardinal signs, epidemiology, associated features, differential diagnosis, expressivity, genetic counselling and treatment. Eur J Orthod 2004;26(1):17–24.
3. Lansford M. Focus on the physical assessment of the infant with Stickler syndrome. Adv Neonatal Care 2008;8(6):308–14.
4. Antunes RB, Alonso N, Paula RG. Importance of early diagnosis of Stickler syndrome in newborns. J Plast Reconstr Aesthet Surg 2012;65(8):1029–34.
5. Snead MP, McNinch AM, Poulson AV, et al. Stickler syndrome, ocular-only variants and a key diagnostic role for the ophthalmologist. Eye (Lond) 2011; 25(11):1389–400.
6. Tuysuz B, Kartal N, Erener-Ercan T, et al. Prevalence of Prader-Willi syndrome among infants with hypotonia. J Pediatr 2014;164(5):1064–7.
7. Cassidy SB, Schwartz S, Miller JL, et al. Prader-Willi syndrome. Genet Med 2012; 14(1):10–26.
8. Cohen M, Hamilton J, Narang I. Clinically important age-related differences in sleep related disordered breathing in infants and children with Prader-Willi syndrome. PLoS One 2014;9(6):e101012.
9. Miller SP, Riley P, Shevell MI. The neonatal presentation of Prader-Willi syndrome revisited. J Pediatr 1999;134(2):226–8.
10. Chen CJ, Hsu ML, Yuh YS, et al. Early diagnosis of Prader-Willi syndrome in a newborn. Acta Paediatr Taiwan 2004;45(2):108–10.
11. Bridges N. What is the value of growth hormone therapy in Prader Willi syndrome? Arch Dis Child 2014;99(2):166–70.
12. Echenne B, Bassez G. Congenital and infantile myotonic dystrophy. Handb Clin Neurol 2013;113:1387–93.

13. Kamsteeg EJ, Kress W, Catalli C, et al. Best practice guidelines and recommendations on the molecular diagnosis of myotonic dystrophy types 1 and 2. Eur J Hum Genet 2012;20(12):1203–8.

14. Meola G. Clinical aspects, molecular pathomechanisms and management of myotonic dystrophies. Acta Myol 2013;32(3):154–65.

15. Gargano G, Guidotti I, Balestri E, et al. Hydrops fetalis in a preterm newborn heterozygous for the c.4A>G SHOC2 mutation. Am J Med Genet A 2014;164A(4): 1015–20.

16. Allanson JE, Roberts AE. Noonan syndrome. In: Pagon RA, Adam MP, Ardinger HH, et al, editors. GeneReviews® [Internet]. Seattle (WA): University of Washington, Seattle; 2001. p. 1993–2014.

17. Sana ME, Spitaleri A, Spiliotopoulos D, et al. Identification of a novel de novo deletion in RAF1 associated with biventricular hypertrophy in Noonan syndrome. Am J Med Genet A 2014;164(8):2069–73.

18. Mathur D, Somashekar S, Navarrete C, et al. Twin infant with lymphatic dysplasia diagnosed with Noonan syndrome by molecular genetic testing. Fetal Pediatr Pathol 2014;33(4):253–7.

19. Katz VL, Kort B, Watson WJ. Progression of nonimmune hydrops in a fetus with Noonan syndrome. Am J Perinatol 1993;10(6):417–8.

20. Li K, Ann Thomas M, Haber RM. Ulerythema ophryogenes, a rarely reported cutaneous manifestation of Noonan syndrome: case report and review of the literature. J Cutan Med Surg 2013;17(3):212–8.

21. Robinson PN, Booms P, Katzke S, et al. Mutations of FBN1 and genotype-phenotype correlations in Marfan syndrome and related fibrillinopathies. Hum Mutat 2002;20(3):153–61.

22. Elçioglu NH, Akalin F, Elçioglu M, et al. Neonatal Marfan syndrome caused by an exon 25 mutation of the fibrillin-1 gene. Genet Couns 2004;15(2): 219–25.

23. Tekin M, Cengiz FB, Ayberkin E, et al. Familial neonatal Marfan syndrome due to parental mosaicism of a missense mutation in the FBN1 gene. Am J Med Genet A 2007;143A(8):875–80.

24. Stheneur C, Tubach F, Jouneaux M, et al. Study of phenotype evolution during childhood in Marfan syndrome to improve clinical recognition. Genet Med 2014;16(3):246–50.

25. Sípek A Jr, Grodecká L, Baxová A, et al. Novel FBN1 gene mutation and maternal germinal mosaicism as the cause of neonatal form of Marfan syndrome. Am J Med Genet A 2014;164A(6):1559–64.

26. Takenouchi T, Hida M, Sakamoto Y, et al. Severe congenital lipodystrophy and a progeroid appearance: mutation in the penultimate exon of FBN1 causing a recognizable phenotype. Am J Med Genet A 2013;161A(12):3057–62.

27. Jacquinet A, Verloes A, Callewaert B, et al. Neonatal progeroid variant of Marfan syndrome with congenital lipodystrophy results from mutations at the 3' end of FBN1 gene. Eur J Med Genet 2014;57(5):230–4.

28. Lalani SR, Hefner MA, Belmont JW, et al. CHARGE syndrome. In: Pagon RA, Adam MP, Ardinger HH, et al, editors. GeneReviews® [Internet]. Seattle (WA): University of Washington, Seattle; 2006. p. 1993–2014.

29. Janssen N, Bergman JE, Swertz MA, et al. Mutation update on the CHD7 gene involved in CHARGE syndrome. Hum Mutat 2012;33(8):1149–60.

30. Schulz Y, Wehner P, Opitz L, et al. CHD7, the gene mutated in CHARGE syndrome, regulates genes involved in neural crest cell guidance. Hum Genet 2014;133(8):997–1009.

31. Choufani S, Shuman C, Weksberg R. Molecular findings in Beckwith-Wiedemann syndrome. Am J Med Genet C Semin Med Genet 2013;163C(2):131–40.
32. Mussa A, Ferrero GB, Ceoloni B, et al. Neonatal hepatoblastoma in a newborn with severe phenotype of Beckwith-Wiedemann syndrome. Eur J Pediatr 2011; 170(11):1407–11.
33. Spivey PS, Bradshaw WT. Recognition and management of the infant with Beckwith-Wiedemann syndrome. Adv Neonatal Care 2009;9(6):279–84.
34. Smith AC, Shuman C, Chitayat D, et al. Severe presentation of Beckwith-Wiedemann syndrome associated with high levels of constitutional paternal uniparental disomy for chromosome 11p15. Am J Med Genet A 2007;143A(24): 3010–5.
35. Uyar A, Seli E. The impact of assisted reproductive technologies on genomic imprinting and imprinting disorders. Curr Opin Obstet Gynecol 2014;26(3): 210–21.
36. Scheuerle AE, Ursini MV. Incontinentia Pigmenti. In: Pagon RA, Adam MP, Ardinger HH, et al, editors. GeneReviews® [Internet]. Seattle (WA): University of Washington; 1993-2015.[1999; updated 2015].
37. Bodemer C. Incontinentia pigmenti and hypomelanosis of Ito. Handb Clin Neurol 2013;111:341–7.
38. Pizzamiglio MR, Piccardi L, Bianchini F, et al. Incontinentia pigmenti: learning disabilities are a fundamental hallmark of the disease. PLoS One 2014;9(1): e87771.
39. Miller SP, Riley P, Shevell MI. Systematic review of central nervous system anomalies in incontinentia pigmenti. Orphanet J Rare Dis 2013;8:25.
40. Sutton VR, Van den Veyver IB. Focal dermal hypoplasia. In: Pagon RA, Adam MP, Ardinger HH, et al, editors. GeneReviews® [Internet]. Seattle (WA): University of Washington, Seattle; 2008. p. 1993–2014.
41. Lombardi MP, Bulk S, Celli J, et al. Mutation update for the PORCN gene. Hum Mutat 2011;32(7):723–8.
42. Brady PD, Van Esch H, Fieremans N, et al. Expanding the phenotypic spectrum of PORCN variants in two males with syndromic microphthalmia. Eur J Hum Genet 2014. http://dx.doi.org/10.1038/ejhg.2014.
43. Carey JC. Health supervision and anticipatory guidance for children with genetic disorders (including specific recommendations for trisomy 21, trisomy 18, and neurofibromatosis I). Pediatr Clin North Am 1992;39(1):25–53.
44. Roizen NJ, Patterson D. Down's syndrome. Lancet 2003;361(9365):1281–9.
45. Roberts I, Alford K, Hall G, et al. GATA1-mutant clones are frequent and often unsuspected in babies with Down syndrome: identification of a population at risk of leukemia. Blood 2013;122(24):3908–17.
46. Niedrist D, Riegel M, Achermann J, et al. Survival with trisomy 18–data from Switzerland. Am J Med Genet A 2006;140(9):952–9.
47. Lin HY, Lin SP, Chen YJ, et al. Clinical characteristics and survival of trisomy 18 in a medical center in Taipei, 1988-2004. Am J Med Genet A 2006;140(9):945–51.
48. Taylor AI. Autosomal trisomy syndromes: a detailed study of 27 cases of Edwards' syndrome and 27 cases of Patau's syndrome. J Med Genet 1968;5: 227–41.
49. Griffith CB, Vance GH, Weaver DD. Phenotypic variability in trisomy 13 mosaicism: two new patients and literature review. Am J Med Genet A 2009;149A(6): 1346–58.
50. Hodes ME, Cole J, Palmer CG, et al. Clinical experience with trisomies 18 and 13. J Med Genet 1978;15:48–60.

51. Swerdlow AJ, Schoemaker MJ, Higgins CD, et al. Mortality risks in patients with constitutional autosomal chromosome deletions in Britain: a cohort study. Hum Genet 2008;123(2):215–24.
52. Michaelovsky E, Frisch A, Carmel M, et al. Genotype-phenotype correlation in 22q11.2 deletion syndrome. BMC Med Genet 2012;13:122.
53. Pober BR. Williams-Beuren syndrome. N Engl J Med 2010;362(3):239–52.
54. Pober BR, Lacro RV, Rice C, et al. Renal findings in 40 individuals with Williams syndrome. Am J Med Genet 1993;46(3):271–4.
55. Ewart AK, Morris CA, Atkinson D, et al. Hemizygosity at the elastin locus in a developmental disorder, Williams syndrome. Nat Genet 1993;5(1):11–6.
56. Nowaczyk MJ. Smith-Lemli-Opitz syndrome. In: Pagon RA, Adam MP, Ardinger HH, et al, editors. GeneReviews® [Internet]. Seattle (WA): University of Washington, Seattle; 1998. p. 1993–2014.
57. Svoboda MD, Christie JM, Eroglu Y, et al. Treatment of Smith-Lemli-Opitz syndrome and other sterol disorders. Am J Med Genet C Semin Med Genet 2012; 160C(4):285–94.
58. Haas D, Haege G, Hoffmann GF, et al. Prenatal presentation and diagnostic evaluation of suspected Smith-Lemli-Opitz (RSH) syndrome. Am J Med Genet A 2013;161A(5):1008–111.
59. Solomon BD. VACTERL/VATER association. Orphanet J Rare Dis 2011;6:56.
60. Winberg J, Gustavsson P, Papadogiannakis N, et al. Mutation screening and array comparative genomic hybridization using a 180K oligonucleotide array in VACTERL association. PLoS One 2014;9(1):e85313.
61. Barisic I, Odak L, Loane M, et al. Prevalence, prenatal diagnosis and clinical features of oculo-auriculo-vertebral spectrum: a registry-based study in Europe. Eur J Hum Genet 2014;22(8):1026–33.
62. Saunders CJ, Miller NA, Soden SE, et al. Rapid whole-genome sequencing for genetic disease diagnosis in neonatal intensive care units. Sci Transl Med 2012;4(154):154.

Congenital Limb Deficiency Disorders

William R. Wilcox, MD, PhD[a],*, Colleen P. Coulter, PT, DPT, PhD, PCS[b],
Michael L. Schmitz, MD[c]

KEYWORDS

- Limb deficiency • Split-hand • Split-foot • Ectrodactyly • Hemimelia • Phocomelia

KEY POINTS

- Congenital limb deficiencies are common birth defects, occurring in 1 in 2000 neonates.
- The presence of a limb deficiency should prompt a thorough examination for other skeletal and nonskeletal anomalies, a 3-generation pedigree, assessment of teratogenic exposures during the pregnancy, and often examination of the parents.
- Consultation with a medical geneticist should be sought especially for longitudinal deficiencies.
- Genetic testing is available and helpful for management and genetic counseling in many cases.
- Most families should be promptly referred to a specialized limb deficiency center for ongoing management.
- With appropriate specialized care, most children with isolated limb deficiencies are able to lead productive lives with excellent function.

INTRODUCTION

The limb deficiency disorders (LDDs) are a broad group of congenital anomalies featuring significant hypoplasia or aplasia of one or more bones of the limbs. LDDs of all types occur in approximately 1 in 1300 to 2000 births.[1–6] LDDs can occur in isolation or associated with other anomalies. The nomenclature of limb deficiencies is often confusing with many historical terms that are imprecise (**Table 1**). An international standard nomenclature was adopted in 1989, permitting a more precise description of the specific bones that are hypoplastic or absent in each case.[7–10] The standard nomenclature divides limb deficiencies into 2 basic types, longitudinal and transverse. Longitudinal deficiencies are

Disclosures: None.
[a] Department of Human Genetics, Emory University, 615 Michael Street, Whitehead 305H, Atlanta, GA 30322, USA; [b] Orthotics and Prosthetics Department, Children's Healthcare of Atlanta, 5445 Meridian Mark Road, Suite 200, Atlanta, GA 30342, USA; [c] Children's Orthopaedics of Atlanta, Children's Healthcare of Atlanta, 5445 Meridian Mark Road, Suite 250, Atlanta, GA 30342, USA
* Corresponding author.
E-mail address: william.wilcox@emory.edu

Clin Perinatol 42 (2015) 281–300
http://dx.doi.org/10.1016/j.clp.2015.02.004   **perinatology.theclinics.com**

Table 1
Descriptive terms for limb deficiencies

Standard terminology	
Transverse deficiency	Absence of limb elements distal to a specified level across the long axis of the limb, eg, the loss of the left distal forearm and hand (see **Fig. 1A**)
Longitudinal deficiency	Aplasia or hypoplasia of a bone along the long axis of the limb, eg, left radial and thumb aplasia (see **Fig. 1B**)
Historical terminology	
Amelia	Absence of one or more limbs
Ectrodactyly	Absent digit or digits (often used interchangeably with split-hand/foot)
Hemimelia	Absence or significant hypoplasia of the lower part of one or more limbs (fibular, radial, tibial, or ulnar hemimelia)
Oligodactyly	Fewer than 5 digits
Peromelia	Malformation of one or more limbs
Phocomelia	Absence of the proximal limbs with some preservation of the distal elements (seal limb or flipper-like
Split-hand, split-foot	Absent digit or digits producing a cleft appearance

Data from Prosthetics and orthotics - limb deficiencies- Part 1: Method of describing limb deficiencies present at birth. ISO 8548-1:1989. International Standards Organization; 1989. Available at: http://www.iso.org.

along the long axis of the limb, such as absence of the radius. In contrast, a transverse deficiency is across the long axis of the limb, such as an amputation of the foot (**Fig. 1**, see **Table 1**). It is common to refer to transverse deficiencies as preaxial (radial and tibial side), postaxial (ulnar and fibular side), and central.[6]

The LDDs have traditionally been placed in the skeletal dysostosis group (early developmental disorders that are fixed at birth), as opposed to the skeletal dysplasias (disorders with ongoing abnormalities of skeletal development). However, disorders that have features of both have made this distinction less useful.[11] There is no classification system for the LDDs that is useful for the practicing clinician; only the better-defined LDDs are listed in the International Nosology of Genetic Skeletal Disorders,[11] a catalog of skeletal disorders.

Limb development in tetrapods is complex, involving numerous interconnected regulatory circuits including the wingless family (WNTs), bone morphogenic proteins (BMPs), fibroblast growth factors, hedgehog proteins, homeobox and other transcription factors, and retinoic acid. Despite intense study for decades, many essential components remain to be discovered.[12–14]

Studying the genetics of human limb malformations and dysplasias has led to new understandings of limb development; this has been especially true for the brachydactylies[15] and skeletal dysplasias (reviewed by Krakow elsewhere in this issue). As in the brachydactylies and skeletal dysplasias, the molecular pathways identified to date in the LDDs are diverse; some were predicted based on animal studies, whereas others were unexpected until the defect in humans was identified. Examples of the variety of pathways involved in the LDDs include chromatid adhesion in Roberts SC phocomelia (268300 [numbers in parentheses in this review correspond to Online Mendelian Inheritance in Man (OMIM; www.ncbi.nlm.nih.gov/omim) numbers]); cell adhesion in the ectodermal dysplasia, ectrodactyly, and macular dystrophy syndrome (225280); transcription factors in synpolydactyly 1 (186000), split-hand/foot malformation with

A

Left upper limb, transverse
Radius: partial, distal 1/3
Ulna: partial, distal 1/3
Carpus: total
Ray: 1-5 total

B

Left upper limb, longitudinal
Radius: Total
Carpus: Partial
Ray: 1 total

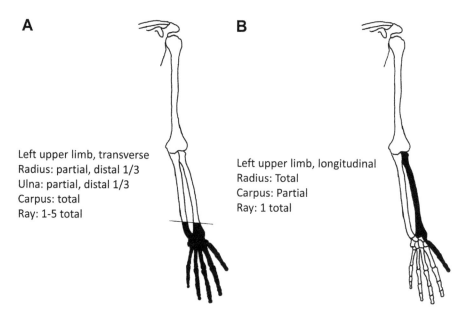

Fig. 1. Examples using the standard nomenclature for limb deficiencies. (*A*) Transverse loss of the left distal forearm and hand. (*B*) Longitudinal left radial and thumb aplasia.

sensorineural hearing loss (220600), VACTERLX (314390), Okihiro syndrome (607323), deficiency of long bones with mirror-image polydactyly (119800), Holt-Oram syndrome (142900), IVIC syndrome (147750), and the ulnar-mammary and allelic syndromes (181450); Rho and Rac signaling in the Adams-Oliver syndrome (100300); semaphorin signaling in CHARGE association (214800); retinoic acid signaling in radiohumeral fusions with other skeletal and craniofacial anomalies (614416); abnormal Gli3 signaling in orofacial digital syndrome type IV (258860); pyrimidine biosynthesis in Miller syndrome (263750); DNA repair in Fanconi anemia (227650), Baller-Gerold and allelic syndromes (218600); ribosomal biogenesis in Diamond-Blackfan anemia (105650); RNA processing in TAR (274000) and Nager acrofacial dysostosis (154400); Wnt signaling in the Goltz-Gorlin syndrome (305600), Robinow syndrome (268310), and some cases with fibular and ulnar aplasia (228930, 276820); sonic hedgehog (Shh) signaling in acheiropody (200500), syndactyly type IV (186200), and Werner mesomelic dysplasia (188770); BMP signaling in acromesomelic dysplasia with genital anomalies (609441), ophthalmoacromelic syndrome (206920), and Grebe and allelic syndromes (200700); protein ubiquitination, tumor suppressor, and Wnt signaling in some cases of split-hand/foot malformation type 1 (183600); and a tumor suppressor in limb-mammary and allelic split-hand/foot syndromes (603543).

There are more than 120 clinical LDDs in OMIM (there are sometimes several OMIM entries per clinical entity, one for each genetic defect identified, eg, 16 entries for Fanconi anemia; the authors count these as one clinical entity). The molecular basis is known for less than 40% of the disorders listed in OMIM. Even for many of the disorders for which a genetic defect is known, there is evidence for genetic locus heterogeneity, with genes remaining to be discovered (split-hand/foot [183600][16] is one example). Some disorders with known genetic defects form an allelic series, such as for mutations in *GDF5* (Grebe [200700], Hunter-Thompson [201250], and Du Pan [228900] syndromes) and *TP63* (limb-mammary [603543], ectrodactyly with ectodermal dysplasia and cleft lip/palate [EEC] [604292], acrodermatoungual-lacrimal-tooth syndrome [ADULT] [103285], and split-hand/foot [605289] syndromes). Many of the disorders with unknown genetic causes overlap in their clinical features and may represent allelic conditions (eg, femoral hypoplasia with and without abnormal facies [134780]; tibial aplasia/hypoplasia with and without polydactyly [188770, 275220]; and split-hand/foot with varying combinations of brachydactyly, tri-phalangeal thumbs, and nail dysplasia [106990, 190680, 106995, 106900]). The heterogeneity of the LDDs is more extensive than the number of OMIM entries might suggest, as many cases do not fit well into any described syndrome.

DIAGNOSTIC EVALUATION

When a congenital limb deficiency is identified, the child should have a thorough evaluation beginning with a physical examination looking for other anomalies of the limbs, face, spine, nipples, genitals, and anus (**Fig. 2**). A 3-generation pedigree should be taken, including any history of pregnancy losses, congenital anomalies, and consanguinity. Unsuspected consanguinity can be common when parents are from rural areas with small populations. A pregnancy history should include drug use, medications, chorionic villus sampling, diabetes, and high fevers during the first trimester. In the case of a transverse deficiency, placental pathology for identification of amniotic bands may be helpful and radiography helps define the extent of the bony deficiencies.

Longitudinal deficiencies can be isolated but are often part of a syndrome or chromosome anomaly. Radiography of the affected and contralateral limbs should be taken, but frequently, a skeletal survey is required to detect abnormalities of the spine and distinguish symmetric limb deficiencies from a skeletal dysplasia. If there are neurologic abnormalities, a brain MRI is indicated. The parents should be examined for limb anomalies, keeping in mind that they may be subtle (eg, a child with radial

Congenital limb deficiency

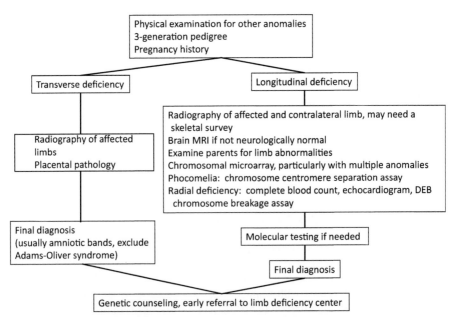

Fig. 2. Strategy for the evaluation of congenital limb deficiencies. DEB, diepoxybutane.

and thumb hypoplasia may have a parent with only mild thumb hypoplasia or a triphalangeal thumb). If multiple anomalies are present, a chromosomal microarray to look for copy number variants is indicated. The many syndromes associated with specific anomalies are discussed in the relevant section later in the article. Molecular testing of a single gene, if the phenotype is clear and there is no genetic locus heterogeneity, or a panel of genes can help make a final diagnosis and permit informed genetic counseling and subsequent prenatal testing, if indicated.

SPECIFIC LIMB DEFICIENCIES
Transverse Deficiencies

Transverse deficiencies are the most common of the limb deficiencies, mostly often caused by the early amnion rupture disruption sequence, also referred to as amniotic bands (**Fig. 3**).[6,17,18] The risk for transverse deficiencies, especially of the central digits in the hand, is increased with chorionic villus sampling, particularly when performed before 10 weeks of gestation,[19,20] as well as failed abortions with the use of misoprostol.[21] There may be no history of rupture or leakage of amniotic fluid, but fibrous cords of amnion can often be found constricting hypoplastic limbs. Good placental pathology is indicated for any newborn with a transverse limb deficiency. The damage from an amniotic band can range from constriction of a limb to hypoplasia of digits with syndactyly, rudimentary digits, and absence of the limb distally from the site of the in utero amputation. Amniotic bands can also cause disruptions at other sites, such as the face and body wall. Typically, the transverse deficiencies are not symmetric.

Care must be taken to distinguish disruptions due to amniotic bands from Adams-Oliver syndrome (100300, 614219, 614814), which may be inherited in an autosomal

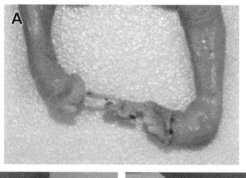
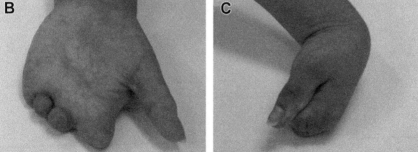

Fig. 3. Transverse deficiency. (A) Amniotic band of fibrous tissue extending between the feet in a fetal autopsy. (B, C) Transverse deficiency of digits 2 to 5. Despite the loss of digits, the child still is able to form grasp.

dominant (AD) or autosomal recessive (AR) manner and has asymmetric terminal transverse limb defect–associated aplasia cutis congenita and frequently congenital heart disease.

Longitudinal Deficiencies

Longitudinal deficiencies can involve 1 limb or may be symmetric, with often some significant differences in severity between the sides. Although 1 bone may be predominantly involved, there are many conditions with hypoplasia/aplasia of several bones. In addition to variation in manifestations between different limbs in a given person, there is significant variability between affected individuals in a family, with some in AD pedigrees showing at most subtle limb abnormalities. For some of the severe disorders with AD inheritance, most cases are due to *de novo* mutations.

The longitudinal deficiencies have been divided into groups depending on which bone is predominantly involved (radius, ulna, humerus, tibula, fibula, femur, or multiple) and a separate group for disorders with split-hand/foot. Although each disorder is listed only once, some could easily be included in more than one category. Because some of the mesomelic dysplasias are restricted in the extent of their skeletal involvement, they could also be categorized as limb deficiencies and have been included.

Although most longitudinal deficiencies are genetic or sporadic (perhaps also due to new AD mutations), some longitudinal deficiencies are teratogenic in origin. The most notorious teratogenic agent was thalidomide, which caused a variety of limb anomalies, including phocomelia, where there is aplasia of the proximal limb structures producing so-called flipper-like or seal-like residual limbs.[21] Maternal hyperthermia is associated with oromandibular-limb hypogenesis as well as Poland anomaly (hypoplasia of the pectoralis major) that may also have hypoplasia of the ipsilateral upper extremity.[22] Maternal cigarette smoking increases the risk for longitudinal deficiencies, particularly preaxial deficiencies of the lower extremity.[23] Congenital varicella can result in limb hypoplasia.[24] Poor control of maternal diabetes during the first trimester can cause longitudinal deficiencies, sacral agenesis with lower extremity hypoplasia, and a variety of other skeletal and nonskeletal anomalies.[25,26] Radial ray deficiencies are increased with valproic acid use along with other limb and visceral abnormalities.[21]

Radial deficiency

Radial deficiencies are the most common of the transverse limb deficiencies. They are commonly associated with other anomalies[2,27] (**Table 2**) and frequently have a known genetic cause. Radial deficiency is often associated with hypoplasia or aplasia of the thumb, absent scaphoid and trapezium, and bowing of the ulna (so-called radial club hand, **Fig. 4**). Isolated thumb hypoplasia or triphalangeal thumb is the mildest manifestation of a radial ray (preaxial) deficiency. The most frequently encountered of the disorders in **Table 2** are trisomy 18, Brachmann-de Lange syndrome, Fanconi anemia, Holt-Oram syndrome, thrombocytopenia absent radius (TAR), and the VACTERL association. Several disorders with radial deficiency have, or develop, hematalogic abnormalities (Diamond-Blackfan anemia, Fanconi anemia, TAR, and WT limb-blood syndrome). Concomitant cardiac and renal anomalies are also commonly found with radial ray deficiencies.

Ulnar deficiency

Ulnar deficiency is less common than radial deficiency (**Table 3**). Ulnar hypoplasia is often associated with radioulnar synostosis, absence of the postaxial digits (fourth and fifth fingers), and fibular deficiency. Many of the syndromes with ulnar deficiency also have mammary hypoplasia and/or Mullerian abnormalities.

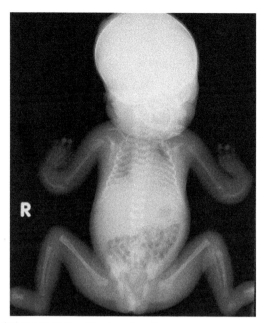

Fig. 4. Bilateral radial ray aplasia with ulnar bowing.

Humeral deficiency

Humeral deficiencies are seldom isolated and are usually occasional findings in deficiencies of the radius and/or ulna (see **Tables 2** and **3**). Humeral deficiencies, usually the entire limb, can also be seen with Poland anomaly (173800). Deficiency of the humerus may also occur with much more extensive limb deficiencies (see **Table 7**). SAMS syndrome (short stature, auditory canal atresia, mandibular hypoplasia, skeletal abnormalities; 602471) is an AR disorder with humeral hypoplasia and humeroscapular synostosis. AD omodysplasia (164745) has shortening of the humeri, whereas the AR form (258315) also has shortening of the femora.

Tibial deficiency

Tibial deficiencies are often associated with equinovarus deformities, and there may be fibular hypoplasia/aplasia of the fibula as well (**Table 4**). In contrast to preaxial radial ray deficiencies whereby hypoplasia/aplasia of the thumb is common, tibial deficiencies are frequently associated with polydactyly of the feet (**Fig. 5**).

Fibular deficiency

Fibular deficiency is often found with ipsilateral tibial bowing and shortening (**Fig. 6**, **Table 5**). It frequently occurs with ulnar deficiency (see **Table 3**) and postaxial loss of digits in the foot.

Femoral deficiency

Deficiency of the proximal femur (proximal femoral focal deficiency, **Fig. 7**) is one of the most common longitudinal deficiencies of the lower extremity.[3] It can be unilateral or bilateral, and there can be an associated fibular deficiency. When isolated, it seems to be sporadic. There is a known association with dysmorphic facies (small nose, micrognathia, and cleft palate) called the femoral hypoplasia-unusual facies syndrome (134780). Aside from these 2 disorders, femoral deficiency is usually found with other limb deficiencies.

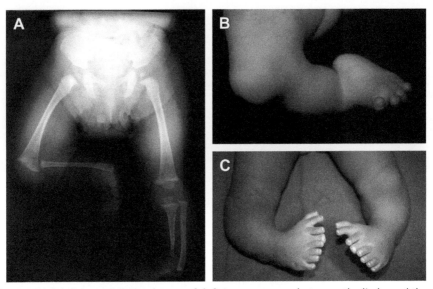

Fig. 5. Tibial deficiency. (*A*) The degree of deficiency may vary between the limbs and there can be (*B*) aplasia of the hallux or (*C*) mirror-image polydactyly.

Split-hand/split-foot malformations

A longitudinal deficiency of the central digits often involving the associated carpal/tarsal bones leads to a split-hand (**Fig. 8**A) or split-foot appearance, which was pejoratively referred to in the historical literature as a "lobster-claw" deformity (**Table 6**). Ectrodactyly, although imprecise, is often used interchangeably (and is part of many of the syndrome names) with split-hand/foot. The most severe form of split-hand/foot is monodactyly, where the hand or foot has but a single digit. In many cases of split-hand/foot, there is syndactyly and hypoplasia of some of the remaining digits (see **Fig. 8**B). The variability between the different limbs in a patient can be striking, as it is between family members in dominant kindreds. Split-hand/foot can be caused by single gene mutations; chromosomal rearrangements, some of which affect distant regulatory elements; and possibly digenic inheritance (mutations at more than 1 locus are required

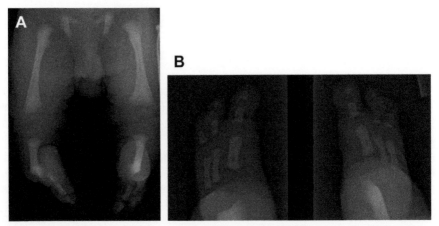

Fig. 6. Fibular deficiency. (*A*) Bilateral fibular deficiency with tibial bowing and (*B*) aplasia of the fourth and fifth toes.

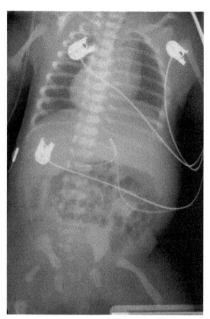

Fig. 7. Femoral deficiency. Note the severe proximal deficiency of one femur and shortening and bowing of the other.

to produce a phenotype).[16] Split-hand/foot may be isolated, or there may be deficiency of the adjacent long bones of the limbs. Split-hand/foot is part of a large group of syndromes, some with overlapping features. The most common of these is EEC.

Multiple Limb Deficiencies

There are several defined syndromes with multiple limb deficiencies, but the clinician must keep in mind that additional deficiencies, especially of adjacent bones, can be occasional findings in several of the syndromes listed in **Tables 2–7**. Some syndromes, such as Roberts, CHARGE, and Brachmann-de Lange, can have a range of single and multiple limb anomalies. Many of the syndromes in **Table 7** have bilateral, symmetric upper and lower extremity involvement and are usually classified with the mesomelic dysplasias. Roberts syndrome (SC phocomelia, pseudothalidomide) (**Fig. 9**) is one of the most common of the multiple limb deficiency syndromes and an important AR disorder to diagnose by a chromosome centromere separation assay or molecular testing.

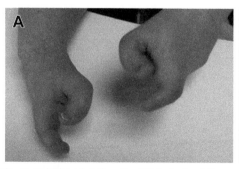
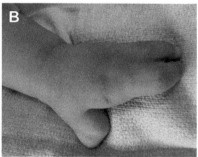

Fig. 8. Split-hand deformity. (*A*) Aplasia of the central digits and incurving of the 2 remaining digits and (*B*) syndactyly of the postaxial digits with thumb hypoplasia.

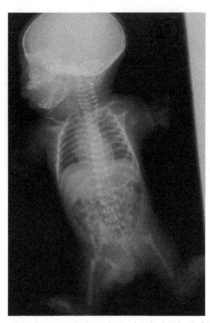

Fig. 9. Roberts syndrome (SC phocomelia) with multiple limb deficiencies.

MANAGEMENT

The management of a patient with an LDD requires a multidisciplinary effort during the entire life span. Genetic counseling should be provided to all families, particularly those with longitudinal deficiencies. As patients approach reproductive age, a review of the genetic aspects of the particular LDD is important. Overall management depends on the specific diagnosis and whether there are other nonlimb anomalies. For example, a child with Fanconi anemia (227650) should be followed up by hematology, Holt-Oram syndrome (142900) by cardiology, and so on.

Although some children with syndromes or chromosomal anomalies may have poor cognitive function, most children with an LDD should be immediately referred to a specialized LDD clinic, which has expertise in orthopedics, prosthetics, and occupational and physical therapy. LDD clinics have experience with the long-term emotional and physical adjustments patients and their families must make and can put the families in touch with others with a similar LDD.[28]

Resources for patients and a list of specialized LDD clinics can be found on the Web site of The Association of Children's Prosthetic-Orthotic Clinics (www.acpoc.org/). The management of each patient is individualized and adjusted according to the needs and developmental stage of the child.[8] Orthopedic and prosthetic care is continuing to evolve and is beyond the scope of this review. However, with care in a specialized center, most children with isolated limb deficiencies can lead productive lives with excellent function.[29]

FUTURE DIRECTIONS

The genetic bases for many of the LDDs are unknown, largely because they are often sporadic or family sizes are small. Although some LDDs may be caused by environmental exposures, the interaction of multiple genes, or a combination of factors, many are likely due to *de novo* genetic mutations. Genomic sequencing now makes it possible to approach these disorders in a research setting. Knowing the specific causes of the LDDs will bring new insight into the mechanisms of limb development and permit more informed genetic counseling.

SUMMARY

Congenital limb deficiencies are common birth defects that may be associated with other anomalies or occur in isolation. A multidisciplinary evaluation and management strategy tailored to the particular patient is required for the best outcomes and accurate genetic counseling. In most cases, early evaluation by a medical geneticist and referral to a limb deficiency team are essential components of optimal management.

Table 2
Selected syndromes with radial ray deficiencies

Syndrome	Syndrome OMIM[a]	Inheritance	Other Features
Atrioventricular septal defect with blepharophimosis and anal and radial defects	600123	?AR	Ulnar hypoplasia, congenital heart disease, blepharophimosis, micrognathia, malformed ears, anal anomalies
Baller-Gerold syndrome	218600	AR	Craniosynostosis
Brachmann-de Lange syndrome	122470 300590	AD XLD	Intrauterine growth retardation, microcephaly, intellectual disability, dysmorphic facies (synophrys, long eyelashes, small nose), may have other limb deficiencies
Diamond-Blackfan anemia	105650	AD	Hypoplastic anemia, short stature
Fanconi anemia	227650	AR	Short stature, hypoplastic anemia, renal anomalies
	300514	X-linked	May also have features of VACTERL
Goldenhar syndrome (oculoauriculovertebral spectrum)	141400	AD	Microtia, malar hypoplasia, epibulbar dermoid, vertebral and renal anomalies
Holt-Oram syndrome	142900	AD	Congenital heart disease (atrial and ventricular septal defects)
IVIC syndrome	147750	AD	Hearing loss, ocular movement abnormalities, imperforate anus, retrovaginal fistula
Nager acrofacial dysostosis	154400	AD	Hearing loss, malar hypoplasia
Oculo-otoradial syndrome	147750	AD	Strabismus, hearing loss
Okihiro syndrome (acroreno-ocular syndrome)	607323	AD	Allelic and similar to IVIC syndrome but may also have renal, vertebral, and other limb and ocular anomalies

(continued on next page)

Table 2
(continued)

Syndrome	Syndrome OMIM[a]	Inheritance	Other Features
Radial aplasia, X-linked	312190	X-linked	Hydrocephalus, hypospadius, imperforate anus
Radial hypoplasia, triphalangeal thumbs, hypospadius, and maxillary distema	179250	AD	Triphalangeal thumbs, hypospadius, anterior maxillary diastema
Radial ray deficiency, X-linked	300378	X-linked	Ulnar hypoplasia, absent patellae, congenital heart disease, Dandy-Walker malformation
Radial ray hypoplasia with choanal atresia	179270	AD	Choanal stenosis/atresia
Radiohumeral fusions with other skeletal and craniofacial anomalies	614416	AR	Radiohumeral fusion, oligodactyly, advanced osseous maturation, craniosynostosis
Radius, aplasia of, with cleft lip/palate	179400	?AD	Cleft lip/palate
Rapadilino syndrome	266280	AR	Patellar hypoplasia, joint dislocations, infantile diarrhea, short stature
Richieri-Costa-Pereira syndrome	268305	AR	Robin sequence, cleft mandible, hallux hypoplasia, may have ulnar, tibial, fibular hypoplasia
Robinow syndrome	268310 180700	AR AD	Ulnar hypoplasia, hemivertebrae, brachydactyly, hypertelorism, hypoplastic genitalia
Smith-Lemli-Opitz syndrome	270400	AR	Small for gestational age, failure to thrive, intellectual disability, microcephaly, dysmorphic facies, 2–3 toe syndactyly, genital anomalies, congenital heart disease
Thrombocytopenia absent radius	274000	AR	Thumb is present, thrombocytopenia
Trisomy 18			Intrauterine growth retardation, dysmorphic facies (low-set, abnormal ears, micrognathia), clenched hands with overlapping fingers, congenital heart disease, renal anomalies
VACTERL association	192350	Sporadic	Nonrandom association of anomalies, including vertebral anomalies, anal atresia, cardiovascular anomalies, tracheoesophageal fistula, esophageal atresia, renal anomalies, preaxial limb anomalies
WT limb-blood syndrome	194350	AD	Radioulnar synostosis, hypoplastic anemia

Abbreviations: AD, autosomal dominant; AR, autosomal recessive; XLD, X-linked dominant.
 [a] If there is more than one clinical OMIM number, the first one is listed here.

Table 3
Selected syndromes with ulnar ray deficiencies

Syndrome	Syndrome OMIM[a]	Inheritance	Other Features
Acromesomelic dysplasia with genital anomalies	609441	AR	Fibular hypoplasia, severe brachydactyly, Mullerian abnormalities
Femur-fibula-ulna syndrome	228200	Sporadic	Hypoplasia/aplasia of the femur, fibula
Fibuloulnar aplasia with renal anomalies	228940	AR	Fibular aplasia, renal anomalies, micrognathia, congenital heart disease
Fuhrmann syndrome	228930	AR	Fibular hypoplasia/aplasia; polydactyly, syndactyly, and oligodactyly; nail dysplasia
Mayer-Rokitansky-Kuster-Hauser syndrome	277000	AD (female limited)	Mullerian and urinary anomalies
Miller syndrome (postaxial acrofacial dysostosis)	263750	AR	Malar hypoplasia, cleft lip and/or palate, micrognathia, absent fifth toes, may have radial hypoplasia
Ulna and fibula, absence of, with severe limb deficiency	276820	AR	Hypoplasia of femur and fibula, oligodactyly, Mullerian defects
Ulnar agenesis and endocardial fibroelastosis	276822	?AR	Endocardial fibroelastosis, oligodactyly
Ulnar/fibular ray defect and brachydactyly	608571	AD	Fibular hypoplasia/aplasia, brachydactyly, midface hypoplasia
Ulnar hypoplasia	191440	AD	—
Ulnar hypoplasia with mental retardation	276821	AR	Anonychia, intellectual disability
Ulnar-mammary syndrome	181450	AD	Axillary apocrine and breast hypoplasia, genital anomalies and pubertal delay in males
Ulnar ray dysgenesis with postaxial polydactyly and renal cystic dysplasia	604380	?AR	Oligodactyly, polydactyly, dysplastic kidneys
Mesomelic dysplasia, Reinhardt-Pfeiffer type	191400	AD	Fibular hypoplasia
Weyers ulnar ray/oligodactyly syndrome	602418	AD	Single central incisor, fibular hypoplasia/aplasia, oligodactyly, renal, splenic, and cardiac anomalies

Abbreviations: AD, autosomal dominant; AR, autosomal recessive.
[a] If there is more than one clinical OMIM number, the first one is listed here.

Table 4
Selected syndromes with tibial deficiencies

Syndrome	Syndrome OMIM[a]	Inheritance	Other Features
Acromelic frontonasal dysostosis	603671	AD	Preaxial polydactyly, frontonasal dysostosis, cleft lip/palate, brain malformations
Brachyphalangy, polydactyly, and tibial aplasia/hypoplasia	609945	Sporadic	Brachydactyly, foot preaxial polysyndactyly, genitourinary anomalies, dysmorphic facies, anonychia
Clubfoot, congenital, with or without deficiency of long bones and/or mirror-image polydactyly	119800	AD	Preaxial polydactyly, equinovarus deformity
Mesomelic dysplasia, Savarirayan type	605274	AR	Fibular hypoplasia/aplasia
Orofacial digital syndrome type IV	258860	AR	Preaxial and postaxial polydactyly, dysmorphic features, tongue hamartoma, cystic kidneys, deafness
Tibia, hypoplasia of, with polydactyly (includes Werner mesomelic dysplasia)	188770	AD	Polydactyly, radioulnar synostosis
Tibial hemimelia	275220	AR, AD	

Abbreviations: AD, autosomal dominant; AR, autosomal recessive.
[a] If there is more than one clinical OMIM number, the first one is listed here.

Table 5
Selected syndromes with fibular deficiencies

Syndrome	Syndrome OMIM[a]	Inheritance	Other Features
Acrodysplasia with ossification abnormalities, short stature and fibular hypoplasia	603740	AR	Brachydactyly, short stature
Acrofrontofacionasal dysostosis	201180	AR	Postaxial polysyndactyly, hypertelorism, cleft lip/palate, cleft nose, intellectual disability
Camptodactyly syndrome, Guadalajara, type I	211910	AR	Intrauterine growth retardation, camptodactyly, blepharophimosis, broad nasal bridge, pectus carinatum/excavatum
Craniosynostosis with fibular aplasia	218550	AR	Craniosynostosis
Du Pan syndrome	228900	AR	Brachydactyly, short stature
Fibular aplasia, tibial campomelia and oligosyndactyly	246570	?AD	Tibial hypoplasia, oligosyndactyly to absent hands and/or feet, congenital heart disease
Santos syndrome	613005	AD, ?AR	Oligodactyly, brachydactyly, preaxial polydactyly, nail hypoplasia/anonychia

Abbreviations: AD, autosomal dominant; AR, autosomal recessive.
[a] If there is more than one clinical OMIM number, the first one is listed here.

Table 6
Selected syndromes with split-hand/foot malformations

Syndrome	Syndrome OMIM[a]	Inheritance	Other Features
Acrocardiofacial syndrome	600460	AR	Cleft lip/palate, congenital heart disease, genital anomalies, intellectual disability
Acrodermatoungual-lacrimal-tooth (ADULT) syndrome	103285	AD	Nail dysplasia, mammary hypoplasia, lacrimal duct atresia, hypodontia, alopecia
Acrorenal	102520	?AD	Preaxial polydactyly, renal malformation
Anonychia-ectrodactyly	106900	AD	Anonychia of some digits
Anonychia-onychodystrophy with brachydactyly type B and ectrodactyly	106990	AD	Brachydactyly, nail dysplasia/anonychia
Brachydactyly-ectrodactyly with fibular aplasia or hypoplasia	113310	AD	Fibular hypoplasia
Ectrodactyly-cleft palate syndrome	129830	AD	Cleft palate (without cleft lip)
Ectrodactyly and ectodermal dysplasia without cleft lip/palate	129810	AD	Ectodermal dysplasia (hypotrichosis, abnormal teeth)
Ectrodactyly, ectodermal dysplasia and cleft lip/palate (EEC) syndrome	129900	AD	Polydactyly, ectodermal dysplasia (hypotrichosis, oligodontia), cleft lip/palate, genitourinary anomalies
Ectrodactyly of lower limbs, congenital heart disease, and micrognathia	601348	Sporadic	Congenital heart disease, micrognathia
Ectodermal dysplasia, ectrodactyly, and macular dystrophy syndrome	225280	AR	Ectodermal dysplasia, macular dystrophy
Facioauriculoradial dysplasia	171480	AD	Radial, ulnar hypoplasia, ear deformities, hearing loss, sinus arrhythmia
Femur, unilateral bifid, with monodactylous ectrodactyly	228250	AR	Ulnar, tibial hypoplasia, bifid distal femur, may have monodactyly, vertebral anomalies, congenital heart disease
Goltz-Gorlin syndrome	305600	X-linked (male lethal)	Atrophy and linear pigmentation of the skin, osteopathia striata, eye anomalies, dental hypoplasia

(continued on next page)

	Syndrome		
Syndrome	**OMIM[a]**	**Inheritance**	**Other Features**
Hypomelia with Mullerian duct anomalies (limb-uterus syndrome)	146160	AD	Split-hand, radial and ulnar hypoplasia, postaxial polydactyly, Mullerian anomalies
Limb-mammary syndrome	603543	AD	Mammary hypoplasia/aplasia
Microphthalmia syndrome 8	601349	?	Microcephaly, microphthalmia, cleft lip/palate, congenital heart disease
Odontotrichomelic syndrome	273400	AR	Ectodermal dysplasia, malformed ears, mammary hypoplasia, hypogonadism
Opthalmoacromelic syndrome	206920	AR	Tibial, fibular hypoplasia, polydactyly, oligodactyly, hemivertebrae, micro/anopthalmia, renal anomalies
Split-foot deformity with mandibulofacial dysostosis	183700	AD	Robin sequence, abnormal ears, hearing loss
Split-hand with congenital nystagmus, fundal changes and cataracts (Karsh-Neugebauer) syndrome	183800	AD	May have monodactyly, nystagmus, cataracts
Split-hand with obstructive uropathy, spina bifida and diaphragmatic defects	183802	AD	Spina bifida, renal anomalies, diaphragmatic defect
Split-hand/foot malformation	183600 225300 313350	AD AR X-linked	
Split-hand/foot malformation 1 with sensorineural hearing loss	220600	AR	Sensorineural hearing loss, may have dysmorphic facies, abnormal ears
Split-hand/foot malformation with long-bone deficiency 1	119100	AD ?	Tibial, distal femoral hypoplasia, may be bifurcated
Split-hand/foot malformation with long-bone deficiency 2	610685	?	Tibial hypoplasia
Split-hand/foot malformation with long-bone deficiency 3	612576	AD	Tibial hypoplasia, bifid distal femur
Split-hand/foot with hypodontia	183500	?AD	Hypodontia (may be part of EEC spectrum)
Split-hand/foot with micrognathia	246560	AD	Micrognathia
Triphalangeal thumbs with brachyectrodactyly	190680	AD	Brachydactyly, nail dysplasia
Ulnar hypoplasia with lobster-claw deformity of feet	314360	X-linked	Ulnar hypoplasia, split-foot, may have split-hand

Abbreviations: AD, autosomal dominant; AR, autosomal recessive.

[a] If there is more than one clinical OMIM number, the first one is listed here.

Table 7
Selected syndromes with multiple limb deficiencies

Syndrome	Syndrome OMIM[a]	Inheritance	Anomalies
Acheiropody	200500	AR	Hypoplasia/aplasia of the radius, ulna, tibia, fibula, distal humerus, aplasia of hands and feet
Acromesomelic dysplasia, Hunter-Thompson type	201250	AR	Hypoplastic ulna, tibia, fibula, small fingers and toes
Amelia, autosomal recessive	601360	AR	All limbs absent, may have defects in other organs
Anonychia-onchodystrophy with hypoplasia or absence of distal phalanges (Cooks syndrome)	106995	AD	Triphalangeal thumb, hypoplasia/aplasia of distal phalanges, nail dysplasia or anonychia
Aprosencephaly	207770	AR	Oligodactyly, radiohumeral fusion, brain and craniofacial malformations
Brachial amelia, cleft lip, holoprosencephaly	601357	Sporadic	Upper limb amelia, femoral, fibular hypoplasia, oligodactyly, cleft lip, holoprosencephaly, omphalocele, congenital heart disease
CHARGE syndrome	214800	AD	Ocular coloboma, congenital heart disease, choanal atresia, retarded growth and development, genital anomalies, ear anomalies and deafness; can have a variety of limb deficiencies
Faciocardiomelic dysplasia	227270	AR	Radial, ulnar, tibial, fibular, digital hypoplasia; micrognathia; microglossia; microstomia; congenital heart disease
Grebe dysplasia	200700	AR	Radial, ulnar, tibial, fibular hypoplasia; small fingers and toes; polydactyly
Hanhart syndrome (hypoglossia-hypodactylia)	103300	Sporadic	Variable hypoplasia/aplasia of any segment, hypoglossia, hypoplastic mandible
Laryngeal atresia, encephalocele, limb deformities	601732	AR	Radial, ulnar, tibial hypoplasia, oligodactyly, laryngeal atresia, encephalocele, renal anomalies
Mesomelic dysplasia, Kantaputra type	156232	AD	Ulna > radial, fibula > tibia hypoplasia
Mesomelic dysplasia, Langer type	249700	AR	Radial, ulnar, fibula > tibia hypoplasia, micrognathia
Microgastria-limb reduction defects association	156810	Sporadic	Hypoplasia of the upper limb, microgastria, hypoplastic lungs, genitourinary anomalies
Nievergelt mesomelic dysplasia	163400	AD	Hypoplasia of the radius, ulna, tibia, fibula

(continued on next page)

Syndrome	Syndrome OMIM[a]	Inheritance	Anomalies
Orofacial digital syndrome type 10	165590	AD	Radial and fibular hypoplasia, oligodactyly, preaxial polydactyly, dysmorphic facies, oral frenula
Roberts syndrome (SC phocomelia)	268300	AR	Humeral, radial, ulnar, femoral, tibial, fibular hypoplasia/aplasia. Upper extremities more severely affected than lower, may have tetraphocomelia, oligosyndactyly. Cleft lip/palate, congenital heart disease, microcephaly, intellectual disability
Rodriguez acrofacial dysostosis	201170	AR	Radial, ulnar, humeral, fibular hypoplasia/aplasia to phocomelia, oligodactyly, micrognathia, microtia, brain, cardiac, and lung malformations
Skeletal defects, genital hypoplasia, mental retardation	612447	AR	Hypoplasia of all segments, hypoplastic clavicle and scapula, oligodactyly, genital hypoplasia, microcephaly, dysmorphic facies, intellectual disability
Tetramelic monodactyly	187510	AD	Only fifth digit present
Tukel syndrome	609428	AR	Postaxial oligosyndactyly, opthalmoplegia

Table 7
(continued)

Abbreviations: AD, autosomal dominant; AR, autosomal recessive.
[a] If there is more than one clinical OMIM number, the first one is listed here.

ACKNOWLEDGMENTS

The authors thank the International Skeletal Dysplasia Registry (http://ortho.ucla.edu/body.cfm?id=279) and Dr Allan Peljovich for some of the images in the figures.

REFERENCES

1. Evans JA, Vitez M, Czeizel A. Congenital abnormalities associated with limb deficiency defects: a population study based on cases from the Hungarian Congenital Malformation Registry (1975-1984). Am J Med Genet 1994;49(1):52–66.
2. Froster UG, Baird PA. Upper limb deficiencies and associated malformations: a population-based study. Am J Med Genet 1992;44(6):767–81.
3. Froster UG, Baird PA. Congenital defects of lower limbs and associated malformations: a population based study. Am J Med Genet 1993;45(1):60–4.
4. Froster-Iskenius UG, Baird PA. Limb reduction defects in over one million consecutive livebirths. Teratology 1989;39(2):127–35.

5. Koskimies E, Lindfors N, Gissler M, et al. Congenital upper limb deficiencies and associated malformations in Finland: a population-based study. J Hand Surg Am 2011;36(6):1058–65.

6. Gold NB, Westgate MN, Holmes LB. Anatomic and etiological classification of congenital limb deficiencies. Am J Med Genet A 2011;155A(6):1225–35.

7. Prosthetics and orthotics - Limb deficiencies - Part 1: Method of describing limb deficiencies present at birth. ISO 8548-1:1989. International Standards Organization; 1989. Available at: http://www.iso.org.

8. Smith DG, Michael JW, Bowker JH, American Academy of Orthopaedic Surgeons. Atlas of amputations and limb deficiencies: surgical, prosthetic, and rehabilitation principles. 3rd edition. Rosemont (IL): American Academy of Orthopaedic Surgeons; 2004.

9. Day HJ. The ISO/ISPO classification of congenital limb deficiency. Prosthet Orthot Int 1991;15(2):67–9.

10. Kay HW, Day HJ, Henkel HL, et al. The proposed international terminology for the classification of congenital limb deficiencies. Dev Med Child Neurol Suppl 1975;(34):1–12.

11. Warman ML, Cormier-Daire V, Hall C, et al. Nosology and classification of genetic skeletal disorders: 2010 revision. Am J Med Genet A 2011;155A(5):943–68.

12. Rabinowitz AH, Vokes SA. Integration of the transcriptional networks regulating limb morphogenesis. Dev Biol 2012;368(2):165–80.

13. Towers M, Tickle C. Generation of pattern and form in the developing limb. Int J Dev Biol 2009;53(5–6):805–12.

14. Zeller R, Lopez-Rios J, Zuniga A. Vertebrate limb bud development: moving towards integrative analysis of organogenesis. Nat Rev Genet 2009;10(12):845–58.

15. Stricker S, Mundlos S. Mechanisms of digit formation: human malformation syndromes tell the story. Dev Dyn 2011;240(5):990–1004.

16. Gurrieri F, Everman DB. Clinical, genetic, and molecular aspects of split-hand/foot malformation: an update. Am J Med Genet A 2013;161A(11):2860–72.

17. Froster UG, Baird PA. Amniotic band sequence and limb defects: data from a population-based study. Am J Med Genet 1993;46(5):497–500.

18. Graham JM. Smith's recognizable patterns of human deformation. 3rd edition. Philadelphia: Saunders/Elsevier; 2007.

19. Brumback BA, Cook RJ, Ryan LM. A meta-analysis of case-control and cohort studies with interval-censored exposure data: application to chorionic villus sampling. Biostatistics 2000;1(2):203–17.

20. Golden CM, Ryan LM, Holmes LB. Chorionic villus sampling: a distinctive teratogenic effect on fingers? Birth Defects Res A Clin Mol Teratol 2003;67(8):557–62.

21. Holmes LB. Teratogen-induced limb defects. Am J Med Genet 2002;112(3):297–303.

22. Graham JM Jr, Edwards MJ, Edwards MJ. Teratogen update: gestational effects of maternal hyperthermia due to febrile illnesses and resultant patterns of defects in humans. Teratology 1998;58(5):209–21.

23. Caspers KM, Romitti PA, Lin S, et al. Maternal periconceptional exposure to cigarette smoking and congenital limb deficiencies. Paediatr Perinat Epidemiol 2013;27(6):509–20.

24. Smith CK, Arvin AM. Varicella in the fetus and newborn. Semin Fetal Neonatal Med 2009;14(4):209–17.

25. Garne E, Loane M, Dolk H, et al. Spectrum of congenital anomalies in pregnancies with pregestational diabetes. Birth Defects Res A Clin Mol Teratol 2012; 94(3):134–40.

26. Correa A, Gilboa SM, Besser LM, et al. Diabetes mellitus and birth defects. Am J Obstet Gynecol 2008;199:237.e1–9.

27. Pakkasjarvi N, Koskimies E, Ritvanen A, et al. Characteristics and associated anomalies in radial ray deficiencies in Finland–a population-based study. Am J Med Genet A 2013;161A(2):261–7.

28. Kerr SM, McIntosh JB. Coping when a child has a disability: exploring the impact of parent-to-parent support. Child Care Health Dev 2000;26(4):309–22.

29. Michielsen A, Van Wijk I, Ketelaar M. Participation and quality of life in children and adolescents with congenital limb deficiencies: a narrative review. Prosthet Orthot Int 2010;34(4):351–61.

Skeletal Dysplasias

Deborah Krakow, MD[a,b,c,*]

KEYWORDS

- Osteochondrodysplasias • Skeletal dysplasias • Nonassortive mating
- Achondroplasia • Type II collagenopathies • Osteogenesis imperfecta

KEY POINTS

- Approximately 5% of children with congenital birth defects have skeletal dysplasias.
- Lethality usually results from small chest, pulmonary hypoplasia, and respiratory compromise.
- Diagnosis is made based on clinical and radiographic findings, including molecular diagnosis when possible.
- Nonlethal skeletal dysplasias are associated with short stature, but overall affected individuals are cognitively normal and have a good quality of life.

The skeletal dysplasias or osteochondrodysplasias are a heritable group of more than 450 well-delineated disorders that affect primarily bone and cartilage, but also can have significant effects on muscle, tendons, and ligaments.[1] By definition, skeletal dysplasias are heritable diseases that have generalized abnormalities in cartilage and bone, whereas dysostoses are genetic disorders characterized by abnormalities in a single or group of bones.[2] Over time, the distinction between these disorders has become blurred, as the field has recognized that there is radiographic, clinical, and molecular overlap. Recent advances in genetic technologies have identified the molecular basis in more than 350 of these disorders, providing us with the opportunity to translate research findings into clinical service. Understanding the genes that

Disclosures: None.

D. Krakow is supported by NIH grants RO1 AR066124, the March of Dimes Birth Defects Foundation, the Joseph Drown Foundation and the Orthopedic Institute for Children/Orthopedic Hospital Research Center. Support was also provided by NIH/National Center for Advancing Translational Science (NCATS) UCLA CTSI Grant Number UL1TR000124.

[a] Department of Orthopaedic Surgery, David Geffen School of Medicine at UCLA, BSRB/OHRC 615 Charles E. Young Drive South, Room 410, Los Angeles, CA 90095, USA; [b] Department of Human Genetics, David Geffen School of Medicine at UCLA, BSRB/OHRC 615 Charles E. Young Drive South, Room 410, Los Angeles, CA 90095, USA; [c] Department of Obstetrics and Gynecology, David Geffen School of Medicine at UCLA, BSRB/OHRC 615 Charles E. Young Drive South, Room 410, Los Angeles, CA 90095, USA
* Department of Orthopaedic Surgery, David Geffen School of Medicine at UCLA, BSRB/OHRC 615 Charles E. Young Drive South, Room 410, Los Angeles, CA 90095.
E-mail address: dkrakow@mednet.ucla.edu

Clin Perinatol 42 (2015) 301–319
http://dx.doi.org/10.1016/j.clp.2015.03.003
0095-5108/15/$ – see front matter © 2015 Elsevier Inc. All rights reserved.

produce these disorders allows us to delineate the extent of spectrum of disease associated with a particular disorder, provides diagnostic service for families at risk for recurrence based on mode of inheritance, as well as furthering our understanding of pathways involved in the development and maintenance of the skeleton.

EMBRYOLOGY

The skeleton forms under 2 distinct processes; endochondral and membranous ossification. Endochondral ossification is responsible for the formation of most of the mammalian appendicular skeleton and it involves a sequence of carefully orchestrated developmental processes. These include embryonic limb bud initiation and its outgrowth from lateral plate mesoderm, specification of mesenchymal cells for the future limb elements, mesenchymal condensations triggering cartilage differentiation, ossification of developing bones, and, finally, their proper growth and maturation in the postnatal period.[3,4] Membraneous ossification is the developmental event in which condensing mesenchymal cells progress almost directly to bone cells. The bones of the skull, lateral clavicle, and pubis form via mesenchymal ossification. Postnatally, growth continues through the cartilage growth plate in which resting chondrocytes proliferate, undergo hypertrophy, then apoptosis, becoming the growing scaffold of bone.[5] Multiple molecular mechanisms (genes) underlie skeleton formation and perturbations to these highly orchestrated processes can lead to skeletal dysplasias.[6]

GENETICS

Best Practices

Determine the diagnosis either through clinical, radiographic, and molecular testing to determine the mode of inheritance and recurrence risk.

Be aware of nonassortive mating in the short-stature community and that outcomes for children with compound heterozygosity for autosomal disorders can be guarded and variable.

The skeletal dysplasias are inherited in an autosomal-recessive, autosomal-dominant, X-linked recessive, X-linked dominant, and Y-linked manner.[1] Appreciation of the mode of inheritance is important because it imparts information to families regarding future recurrences. Family history, including parental and familial heights and growth patterns, should be obtained from the parents of any affected child to determine if there are similarly affected siblings, or other family members, which can lead to a diagnosis or establish the mode of inheritance. There are several X-linked skeletal disorders that recur in male family members and carrier females are either unaffected or only mildly affected (eg, X-linked spondyloepiphyseal tarda).[7] **Table 1** lists some of these more commonly seen disorders seen in the neonatal period with their respective inheritance pattern. The Nosology and Classification of Genetic Skeletal Disorders[1] and Online Mendelian Inheritance in Man (OMIM:www.omim.org/) are sources that include information on these disorders and include data on their patterns of inheritance. There are some uncommonly seen patterns of inheritance in the skeletal dysplasias. These include somatic mosaicism, in which one of the parents is mildly affected and their offspring is more severely affected.[8] Evaluation of the parents should be considered if there is any question that one of the parents could have a mild skeletal disorder. Gonadal mosaicism is characterized by familial recurrence of

Table 1
Well delineated disorders seen in the neonatal period

Group or Name of the Disorder	Mode of Inheritance	Gene Symbol
Fibroblast growth factor receptor 3 (FGFR3) disorders		
Thanatophoric dysplasia	AD	FGFR3
Achonodroplasia	AD	FGFR3
Hypochondroplasia	AD	FGFR3
Severe achondroplasia with developmental delay and acanthosis nigricans (SADDAN)	AD	FGFR3
Type II collagen disorders		
Achondrogenesis II	AD	COL2A1
Hypochondrogenesis	AD	COL2A1
Spondyloepiphyseal dysplasia congenita (SEDC)	AD	COL2A1
Kniest dysplasia	AD	COL2A1
Type X1 collagen disorders		
Fibrochondrogenesis	AR	COL11A1
Fibrochondrogenesis	AD	COL11A1, COL11A2
Otospondylomegaepiphyseal dysplasia (OSMED)	AR	COL11A2
Sulfation disorders		
Achondrogenesis IB	AR	SLC26A2
Atelosteogenesis II	AR	SLC26A2
Diastrophic dysplasia	AR	SLC26A2
Chondrodysplasia with congenital joint dislocations	AR	CHST3
Perlecan disorders		
Dyssegmental dysplasia	AR	PLC
Dyssegmental dysplasia, Silverman-Handmaker type	AR	PLC
Dyssegmental dysplasia, Rolland Desbuquois type	AR	PLC
Filamin disorders and similar disorders		
Otopalatodigital syndrome I and II	XLD	FLNA
Osteodysplasty, Melnick-Needles	XLD	FLNA
Atelosteogenesis types I and III	AD	FLNB
Larsen syndrome	AD	FLNB
Spondylo-carpal-tarsal dysplasia	AR	FLNB
Serpentine fibula-polycystic kidney syndrome	AD	NOTCH2
TRPV4 disorders		
Metatropic dysplasia	AD	TRPV4
Short-rib dysplasias (with and without polydactyly)		
Chondroectodermal dysplasia (Ellis-van Creveld [EVC])	AR	EVC1, EVC2
Short-rib polydactyly syndrome I, II, III, and IV including asphyxiating thoracic dystrophy	AR	DYNC2H1 IFT80 NEK WDR35 WDR19 WDR34
Thoracolaryngeal dysplasia	AD	Unknown

(continued on next page)

Table 1
(continued)

Group or Name of the Disorder	Mode of Inheritance	Gene Symbol
Metaphyseal dysplasias		
Cartilage-hair hypoplasia	AR	RMRP
Metaphyseal dysplasia, Jansen type	AD	PTHR1
Spondylo-epi-(meta)-physeal dysplasia (SEMD)		
SEMD, short limb abnormal calcification type	AR	DDR2
Severe spondylodysplastic dysplasias		
Achondrogenesis 1A	AR	GMAP210
Schneckenbecken dysplasia	AR	SLC35D1
Opsismodysplasia	AR	INPPL1
Acromesomelic disorders		
Acromesomelic dysplasia, type Maroteaux	AR	NPR2
Mesomelic and rhizo-mesomelic dysplasias		
Langer type (homozygous dyschondrosteosis)	Pseudo-AR/XLD	SHOX
Omodysplasia	AR	GPC6
Robinow syndrome, recessive	AR	ROR2
Robinow syndrome, dominant	AD	WNT5
Bent bone dysplasias		
Campomelic dysplasia	AD	SOX9
Stuve-Wiedemann dysplasia	AR	LIFR
Bent bone dysplasia FGFR2 type	AD	FGFR2
Slender bone dysplasias		
Microcephalic osteodysplastic primordial dwarfism (MOPD1)	AR	RNU4ATAC
Microcephalic osteodysplastic primordial dwarfism (MOPD2)	AR	PCNT
Osteocraniostenosis		FAM111A
Dysplasias with multiple joint dislocations		
Desbuquois dysplasia	AR	CANT1, XYLT1
Pseudodiatrophic dysplasia	AR	Unknown
Chondrodysplasia punctata group (CDP)		
CDP, X-linked dominant	XLD	EBP
Conradi-Hunermann type (CDPX2)	XLR	ARSE
brachytelephalangic type (CDPX1)	XLD	NSDHL
Congenital hemidysplasia with ichthyosiform erythroderma and limb defects (CHILD) syndrome	XLD	EBP
Greenberg dysplasia	AR	LBR
Rhizomelic CDP type 1	AR	PEX7
Rhizomelic CDP type 2	AR	DHPAT
Rhizomelic CDP type 3	AR	AGPS
Neonatal osteosclerotic dysplasias		
Bloomstrand dysplasia	AR	PTHR1
Desmosterolosis	AR	DHCR24
Caffey disease (infantile)	AD	COL1A1
Raine dysplasia	AR	FAM20C

(continued on next page)

Group or Name of the Disorder	Mode of Inheritance	Gene Symbol
Table 1 (*continued*)		
Increased bone density group		
Osteopetrosis (severe neonatal or infantile forms)	AR	TCIRG1
Osteopetrosis (severe neonatal or infantile forms)	AR	CLCN7
Dysosteosclerosis	AR	SLC29A3
Lenz-Majewski hyperostotic dysplasia	SP	PTDSS1
Osteogenesis imperfecta and decreased bone density group		
Osteogenesis imperfecta (OI), moderate, severe, and perinatal lethal	AD	COL1A1, COL1A2 IFITM5
OI, moderate, severe, and perinatal lethal	AR	CRTAP P3H1 PPBI FKBP10 HSP47 SP7 WNT1 TMEM33B
Bruck syndrome		PLOD2 FKBP10
Osteoporosis-pseudoglioma syndrome	AR	LRP5
Cole-Carpenter dysplasia	SP	SEC24D, P4HB, CRTAP
Abnormal mineralization group		
Hypophosphatasia, perinatal and infantile forms	AR	ALPL

a known dominant disorder resultant from one parent carrying heterozygosity for a mutation in one of the cell lineages that comprise the pool of progenitor germ cells and the parent is clinically unaffected.[9] This is a rare occurrence, but influences counseling of all dominant disorders because if a newborn is diagnosed with an autosomal-dominant disorder, counseling should include a less than 1% recurrence risk based on gonadal mosaicism.

In the short-stature community, it is common to see nonassortive mating, meaning that both parents have skeletal dysplasias. Under these circumstances, it is common to evaluate pregnancies at risk for differing outcomes. In cases in which one parent has a recessively inherited skeletal disorder and the other parent has a dominantly inherited skeletal disorder, the fetus is at 50% risk for only the dominantly inherited disorder. Whether carrying the recessive allele for another skeletal disorder influences adult height or skeletal complications is unknown, although the concept of genetic load and disease could be applicable in this situation. More commonly, couples are seen in whom both have the same autosomal-dominant disorder, or have 2 different autosomal-dominant disorders. In either scenario, the fetuses or newborns are at 25% risk for inheriting both dominant conditions. Compound heterozygosity has been seen for achondroplasia-achondroplasia,[10] achondroplasia-hypochondroplasia (non-FGFR3 [fibroblast growth factor receptor 3]),[11] achondroplasia-spondyloepiphyseal congenita[12–14] pseudoachondroplasia-achondroplasia,[15,16] pseudoachondroplasia-spondyloepiphyseal dysplasia,[17] achondroplasia-osteogenesis imperfecta (OI) mild type,[11] Leri-Weil dyschondrosteosis-achondroplasia,[18] pseudoachondroplasia-OI severe type, achondroplasia-OI[19] severe type (Deborah Krakow, MD, personal communication, 2013), and achondroplasia-acromicric dysplasia (Deborah Krakow, MD, personal communication, 2013). The outcomes for these infants are based on the severity of each individual skeletal disorder. Many of these children have guarded prognoses based on respiratory insufficiency due to restrictive lung disease and die within the first year of life. For longer-term survivors, issues of severe cervical canal stenosis, foramen magnum stenosis with spinal cord compression, cervical spine instabilities, abnormalities of the brainstem, hydrocephalous, brain dysgenesis (FGFR3 compound heterozygosity), seizures, poor feeding with gastrointestinal reflux, apnea, joint hypermobility, truncal hypermobility, scoliosis, fixed angle kyphosis, fractures, and orthopedic complications have been reported, but the body of literature remains small.

Information regarding the severity and natural history of an individual disorder is critical for the family and providers. There is no large single source summarizing the findings, and in some cases is dependent on the private mutations that each parent carries. If possible, it is important to establish that the child carries 2 deleterious mutations if the genes for the disorders are known, assuring the caretakers and family that the child indeed has 2 autosomal-dominant disorders. If the child survives the neonatal period, then care should be individualized based on each organ system abnormality and its severity.

The explosion in molecular genetics has allowed for gene identification in more than two-thirds of the skeletal dysplasias. This technical advancement has allowed for more precise diagnosis and physicians and health care providers can direct their care based on the established natural history of each disorder. When a disorder is diagnosed based on family history, clinical or radiographic data, clinical gene testing is performed by many laboratories (GeneTests: https://www.genetests.org/), as well as through skeletal dysplasia gene panels offered by many diagnostic laboratories. The historical approach of clinical diagnosis through physical evaluation and radiographic review then directed molecular testing has now in many centers been supplanted by use of skeletal dysplasia panels that are somewhat unbiased to clinical findings. The limitations to this approach include delay in diagnosis, cost, and potential nondiagnosis, because panels may not be comprehensive for all skeletal disorders. However, the benefits include molecular diagnosis in a group of disorders that are rare and often difficult to diagnose, and for some of these disorders there are multiple potential responsible genes (locus heterogeneity), allowing for diagnosis not based on a serial testing approach. As advancing technology evolves, and the cost and the precision of newer gene sequencing approaches improves, it should become available to a larger portion of the population.

Molecular diagnosis can be important particularly for disorders associated with both allelic and locus heterogeneity. For some disorders, the type and location of the mutation within the disease-producing gene (protein) can impart long-term natural history information (eg, nonsense or loss of protein mutations can lead to a different severity of disease relative to missense mutations). This is well illustrated in OI; nonsense or nonstop mutations in the genes that encode type I collagen, *COL1A1* and *COL1A2*, cause the mildest form of the disease,[20] whereas missense mutations in the same genes produce more severe progressive deforming forms of OI.[21] Further complicating counseling is that approximately 90% of cases of OI result from mutations in type I collagen; however, most of the remaining 10% result from mutations in recessively inherited genes that are primarily involved in the processing and trafficking of type I collagen.[22] These recessively inherited forms of OI illustrate the explosion in our molecular understanding of a single osteochondrodysplasia.[23] Although immediate care of a neonate with OI is similar regardless of the molecular basis, the familial recurrence risk and long-term natural history differs based on the underlying genetic basis of disease. For example, severe progressing OI is typically associated with normal intelligence, whereas the same radiographic form of OI due to homozygosity for *Wintless 1 (WNT 1)* mutations are associated with subnormal intelligence.[24,25]

PRENATAL DIAGNOSIS OF OSTEOCHONDRODYSPLASIAS

> Ideally, the diagnosis of the skeletal dysplasia should be made in the prenatal period to improve implementation of a plan of management.
> Discussion should ensue with families before and immediately after delivery regarding management of disorders associated with high incidences of lethality.

Rapid advances in both imaging modalities and the aforementioned molecular diagnostics have improved our ability to recognize osteochondrodysplasias in the prenatal period.[26,27] For those families with a parent affected by an autosomal-dominant disorder, either molecular diagnostics via invasive techniques or by ultrasound imaging can aid in predicting whether the fetus will be similarly affected (**Fig. 1**). For at-risk families based on a previously affected child with an autosomal-recessive disorder, the same above-mentioned approach can be used. However, affected neonates with skeletal dysplasias are often the first affected children in their respective families.

Many pregnant women are offered an array of noninvasive tests to determine if their fetuses are at risk for genetic disorders.[28,29] These molecular screening panels are for autosomal-recessive and X-linked disorders, including skeletal dysplasias such as diastrophic dysplasia; however, many genes and mutations that can cause skeletal

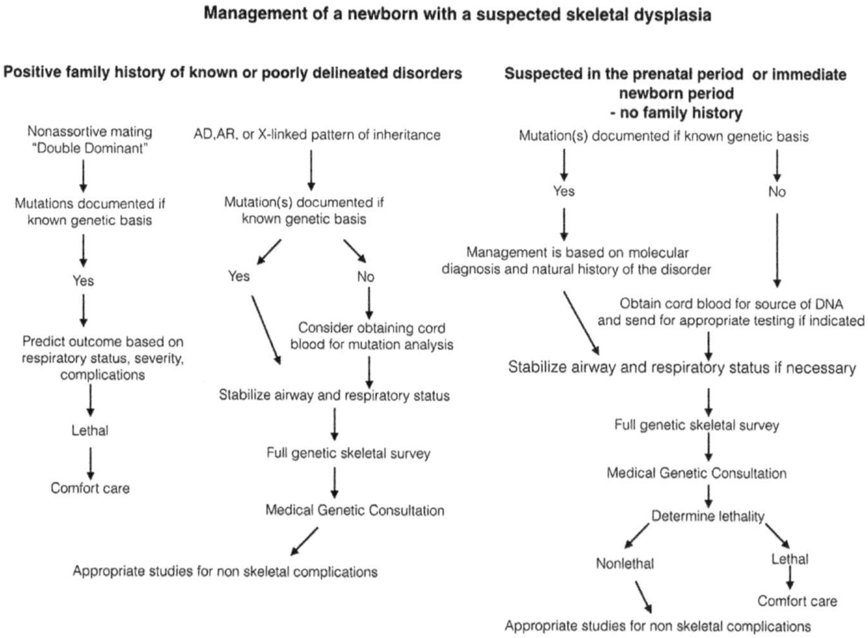

Fig. 1. Scheme of management in newborns with a skeletal dysplasia.

dysplasias are presently not included in these panels. Usually if one parent screens positive for a disorder, then the other parent is screened, determining a baseline risk for a disorder. First trimester ultrasound analysis, usually used to identify aneuploidy, is also affective in identifying severe, usually lethal skeletal dysplasias, including OI, thanatophoric dysplasia, and the short-rib polydactyly syndromes, as some examples.[30–32] If a neonate with a skeletal disorder was noted to have abnormal ultrasound findings in the first trimester, including a small crown-rump length for gestational age and increased nuchal fold thickness, the likelihood is that the fetus has a severe, probable lethal skeletal dysplasia.

Many prenatal skeletal dysplasias are diagnosed in the late second trimester when many pregnant women are screened by ultrasound for congenital anomalies.[33] The advantages to early detection (with and without a precise diagnosis) allows for preparation before delivery. This includes discussion of active resuscitation, proper assembly of consultants, collection of appropriate material for molecular diagnosis from cord blood, and smoother transition for the fetus from the prenatal to neonatal period. This is particularly important if the neonate is predicted to have a severe, but nonlethal skeletal disorder.

Experience has informed us that many skeletal disorders are not diagnosed in the late second trimester, but either in the third trimester or at birth. These disorders tend to be milder, with a less profound effect on the skeleton, including the thorax; thus, severe respiratory compromise is not usually encountered. Achondroplasia, spondyloepiphyseal dysplasia congenita (SEDC), and nonlethal forms of OI are frequency first encountered in the newborn period. Many parents are distraught if the suggestion of a skeletal dysplasia is made at birth, and question if "something" was missed at second trimester ultrasound evaluation. It is helpful to explain that for the milder skeletal disorders, long-bone measurements are frequently on the normal growth curves at 20 weeks, and fall off occurs in the third trimester, because in most of these disorders the defect is in endochondral ossification (not condensation or other earlier-occurring processes), which is a process that is most active in the third trimester.[34]

Beyond ultrasound and enhanced carrier screening panels, noninvasive prenatal testing from maternal blood for Mendelian disorders may soon be a clinical reality. Screening for cell-free fetal DNA in maternal blood during the first trimester of gestation is used for the detection of aneuploidy, including disorders of copy number variations.[35] Reports of de novo FGFR3 mutations (thanatophoric dysplasia) from the fetal cell-free DNA fraction in maternal blood illustrates that this technology has the future potential to diagnose de novo autosomal-dominant skeletal disorders.[36]

DEFINING LETHALITY

> Lethality should ideally be determined in the prenatal period based on ultrasound parameter and/or by molecular diagnosis.
> Infants with skeletal dysplasias with small chests and need for aggressive ventilation are likely to have a lethal skeletal dysplasia and counseling of families is necessary.

If a newborn has been diagnosed with a known lethal disorder in the fetal period, then treating physicians should offer comfort care for the newborn, but not aggressive management. Defining lethality in the prenatal period can be accomplished by

2 means: molecular diagnosis of a known lethal disorder and precise diagnosis by ultrasound or chest size abnormalities seen by ultrasound that correlate with lethality. If the chest-to-abdominal circumference ratio is less than 0.7, the heart-to-chest circumference is greater than 50%, or the abdomen-to-femur length ratio is less than 0.16, these objective measures are highly correlated with lethality. However, these measurements can be dependent on gestational age and may not apply to the infant[27] with significant prematurity and a skeletal dysplasia; the presenting disorder may be a known lethal disorder, but the aforementioned criteria may not quite have been reached, or conversely a severely affected child may survive for a prolonged period of time. When lethality is suspected based only on prenatal ultrasound measurements, it is important to counsel parents that although a lethal condition is suspected, only at birth will a true assessment of lethality be possible.

Postnatally, similar criteria can apply to management of a newborn. If clinical and radiographic findings and/or molecular findings indicate a known lethal diagnosis, then supportive care is indicated. Some of the more difficult clinical management scenarios result from the clinical spectrum of disease that is associated with individual gene defects. This is particularly true for the disorders listed in the categories in **Table 1**. For example, in type II collagen disorders, hypochondrogenesis diagnosed by radiographic criteria is often associated with lethality due to a small chest and respiratory compromise, yet some of these infants survive the neonatal period and then are categorized as severe spondyloepiphyseal dysplasia congenita.[37] Thus, for each group of skeletal dysplasias, clinical judgment must be used to determine the severity of the skeletal disorder and whether aggressive management is indicated. If highly aggressive ventilation is necessary because of severe respiratory insufficiency, particularly due to a small chest, respiratory failure and lethality commonly occurs.[38] For all newborns who die of complications from skeletal disorders, radiographs and a source of DNA should be obtained, and families should be offered autopsy. Collection of postmortem material aids in final diagnosis, which helps to provide parents emotional closure and determine recurrence risk for families through clinical molecular diagnosis or research participation (**Box 1**).

The approach to the initial evaluation of a newborn with a suspected skeletal dysplasia is outlined in **Fig. 1**. If the newborn is known to have a uniformly lethal disorder, then supportive care is indicated. Similarly, if the diagnosis is known before delivery, then management is predicated on the knowledge regarding the natural history of the disorder.

Newborns with recognized skeletal disorders present in the newborn period with disproportion. Dependent on the skeletal disorder, there are some common findings: relative macrocephaly, narrow chest appearance relative to the abdomen, rhizomelia (short upper portion extremity), mesomelia (short midportion extremity), and frequently brachydactyly (short hands, including phalanges). Frequently the face is normal but there are numerous disorders associated with a flat nasal bridge, frontal bossing,

---

Box 1
Approach to the initial evaluation of a neonate with a skeletal dysplasia

Newborns should be evaluated by clinical examination and radiographs.

Initial care should be highly focused on respiratory status.

Close attention should be paid to the status of the trachea/larynx.

Awareness of the high incidence of cervical abnormalities in the skeletal dysplasias should be communicated to all caregivers.

and midface hypoplasia, and include many of the lethal skeletal disorders, achondroplasia, campomelic dysplasia, chondrodysplasia punctate (all forms), type II collagen disorders, Larsen syndrome, and the mucopolysaccharidoses (most forms). Disorders with micrognathia include some of the following disorders: type II collagen disorders, acrofacial dysostoses, Robinow syndrome, and, again, many of the lethal skeletal dysplasias. Attention must be paid to the Robin-Pierre sequence (small mandible and posterior cleft palate) associated with these disorders. Few of these newborns are delivered by ex utero intrapartum treatment (EXIT) procedures because of the mandibular abnormality and safety of the airway,[39] but some of these children require postdelivery intubation and subsequent tracheostomies until definitive surgery for jaw retraction or time, awaiting facial growth. If the newborn has Pierre-Robin sequence, timing of the repair of the cleft palate should be deferred to the craniofacial surgery team or plastic surgeons[40] (see the article by Robin and Hamm elsewhere in this issue).

Care should be taken regarding the trachea in the skeletal dysplasias. The trachea is composed of 15 to 20 incomplete C-shaped tracheal rings that contain cartilage that reinforces the front and sides of the trachea to protect and maintain the airway.[41] Pediatricians, neonatologists, and anesthesiologists should be informed that many skeletal disorders have been associated with tracheal anatomic changes complicating respiratory status, intubation, and any manipulations. The abnormalities include tracheal agenesis, congenital stenosis, premature cartilage calcifications, short trachea, and tracheomalacia, as well as disorders associated with tracheoesophageal fistulas.[42] Caretakers should be aware of this when caring for newborns with skeletal abnormalities, and can affect prognosis in many of the nonlethal skeletal disorders.

DIAGNOSIS OF A SKELETAL DYSPLASIA

How does one make the diagnosis of a skeletal dysplasia? If the diagnosis has been determined in the prenatal period or based on family history, then laboratory testing or radiographs should be obtained to confirm the clinical or molecular diagnosis. If the skeletal dysplasia is undiagnosed or unexpected, then a similar approach should be taken. Once the newborn is stable, a thorough physical examination should be undertaken. Key measurements include head circumference, birth weight, birth length, chest circumference if it appears small, and palm and middle finger lengths. Carefully delineation of any dysmorphic facial features should be performed and include evaluation of the fontanels, nasal bridge, midface, philtrum, mandible, palate, and ears. Frequently, the neck will appear short, and if the chest is small, the nipples may appear widely spaced. In many disorders, the hands will appear small, and the fingers will appear to have wide spaces between them because they are short. Attention should be paid to the proportion of the upper and mid sections of the arm. In most newborns, they appear subjectively one to one, and in skeletal disorders, there is frequently subjective disproportion. Rhizomelia is common in achondroplasia and spondyloepiphyseal dysplasia congenita, 2 of the commonly seen nonlethal disorders. Very significant mesomelia relative to the rhizomelic segment suggests a group of specific disorders: the mesomelic dysplasias. Frequently, when there is rhizomelia and mesomelia, there are increased skin creases and skin folds due to the abnormal underlying bone length. A significantly curved long bone may appear substantially much shorter externally than by radiographs.

After clinical evaluation, it is critical to obtain complete anterior/posterior and lateral radiographs. This includes images of the skull, extremities (including hands and feet!), and the spine. Radiographic evaluation should start with overall assessment of epiphyseal ossification to determine if they are delayed or irregular for age, then there should be consideration for an epiphyseal dysplasia. If the metaphyses are widened, flared, or irregular, then the diagnosis of a metaphyseal chondrodysplasia should be entertained. If diaphyseal abnormalities are present, such as widening and/or cortical thickening, or marrow space expansion, then a diaphyseal dysplasia is implied. Combination of the aforementioned abnormalities helps categorize the disorder (eg, epimetaphyseal disorder). If the vertebral bodies are affected, then there is a spondylo-component present, further categorizing the disorder. Once the extent of radiographic abnormalities is determined and placed within a category (eg, spondylometaphyseal dysplasia), then radiographic textbooks can aid in refining the diagnosis.

Organ system abnormalities beyond the skeleton are occasionally seen and can be clues to diagnosis. Congenital heart defects are commonly seen in the skeletal ciliopathies (chondroectodermal dysplasia, asphyxiating thoracic dysplasia, short-rib polydactyly syndromes), abnormal formed genitalia in the skeletal ciliopathies, campomelic dysplasia, omodysplasia, Robinow dysplasia, Antley-Bixler syndrome, and severe disorders of cholesterol metabolism.[43–48] Immune deficiency and Hirschsprung disease are seen in metaphyseal chondrodysplasia, McKusick type (cartilage-hair hypoplasia).[49,50]

COMMONLY SEEN DISORDERS
Achondroplasia Group

Radiographs and molecular testing can differentiate severe achondroplasia from thanatophoric dysplasia, particularly if there is respiratory compromise.

Caregivers should be aware of the need to evaluate the foramen magnum in the first few months of life, and special attention should be paid to rapidly increasing head size and bulging anterior fontanel.

This group of disorders all result from heterozygosity for activation mutations in the gene that encodes FGFR3.[51] This group of disorders includes thanatophoric dysplasia, achondroplasia, hypochondroplasia, and the very rare severe achondroplasia with developmental delay and acanthosis nigricans. Thanatophoric dysplasia is almost uniformly lethal without aggressive management. Radiographic findings include macrocephaly with narrow skull base, long narrow trunk with handlebar clavicles, flat vertebral bodies, small flared iliac bones with very narrow sacrosciatic notches, and generalized micromelia (illustrated in **Fig. 2**A).

Achondroplasia is by far the most common form of nonlethal skeletal dysplasia. Most cases present at birth, although some children are diagnosed in early infancy. Newborns present with relative macrocephaly; frontal bossing; and rhizomelia, mesomelia, and acromelia, with a splaying of the fingers between digits and 3 and 4 (known as the "trident" deformity). Radiographic findings include a large skull with short, flat vertebral bodies; short, narrow sciatic notch with flat acetabular roof; short, thick tubular bones; and flared metaphyses (see **Fig. 2**B). In the newborn period, most of the children are stable; however, neurologic complications, including brainstem compression due to a tight foramen magnum, can lead to hydrocephalous, sleep apnea, and increased incidence of sudden infant death in addition to long-term neurologic sequelae.[52] These complications usually present in the first few months of life and frequently present with rapidly increasing head size, bulging anterior fontanel, irritability, sweating, increased head extension when asleep, increased deep tendon

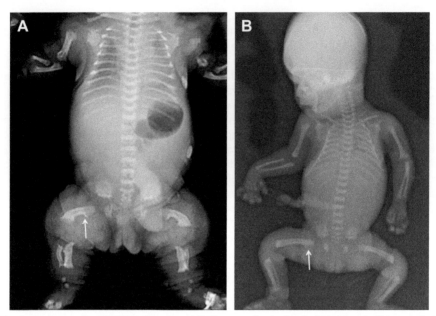

Fig. 2. Radiographs of FGFR3 disorders. (*A*) Thanatophoric dysplasia in the newborn period. Note the small chest, severe rhizo-mesomelia, curved femora with proximal fade-out, and distal irregularities. (*B*) Thirty-two–week fetus with achondroplasia. Note the relatively mild narrowing of the chest, rhizomelia, and fade-out of the proximal femora (*arrow*).

reflexes, and clonus. Families should be counseled that formal evaluation of the foramen magnum should be obtained in the first few months of life under the supervision of a medical geneticist, neurosurgeon, or orthopedic surgeon; rarely is this indicated in the newborn period. There are published guidelines by the American Academy of Pediatrics on health supervision in children with achondroplasia.[53] Hypochondroplasia is usually a milder phenotypic presentation than achondroplasia and may not be detected in the newborn period.

TYPE II COLLAGENOPATHIES

> Caregivers should be aware of the high incidence of odontoid hypoplasia and cervical vertebrae 1 and 2 hypoplasia.
> Club feet can present in these disorders, and these children should be evaluated by pediatric orthopedic surgeons with experience in caring for children with skeletal dysplasias.

The type II collagenopathies are a heterogeneous group of disorders that all show some relationship to each other clinically and radiographically.[37] These disorders typically result from heterozygosity for mutations in the type II collagen gene, *COL2A1*. Achondrogenesis II and hypochondrogenesis are lethal disorders that present with large skulls, very small and short ribs, and almost lack of mineralization of most vertebral bodies. The pelvis has small iliac wings with absent ischia, pubic bones, and sacral elements. The extremities show severe rhizomelia and mesomelia with relative sparing of the hands (**Fig. 3**).

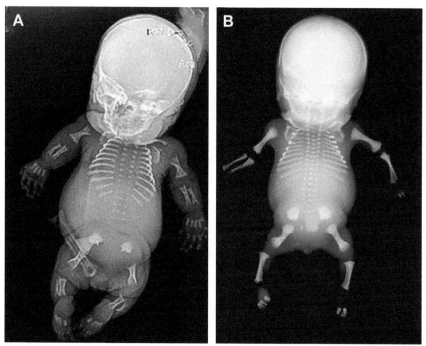

Fig. 3. Radiographs of type II collagen disorders. (*A*) Achondrogenesis II in the late second trimester. Note the severe rhizomelia and mesomelia with relative sparing of the hands, lack of ossification of the vertebral bodies, and absent ischia. (*B*) Hypochondrogenesis in the late second trimester. Vertebral bodies are underossified with dumbbell-shaped humeri and femora, and lack of ossification of the ischia.

Spondyloepiphyseal dysplasia is usually nonlethal, and clinical presentation includes a severely short-trunked, short-limbed infant with normal-appearing hands, feet, and skull. There may be micrognathia and a Pierre-Robin sequence, and attention should be paid to the upper cervical spine, which can be hypomineralized. Radiographic findings in the newborn period include short thorax with short ribs, pear-shaped or oval vertebral bodies, absent pubic ossification, short long bones, and unossified talus and calcaneus (which are typically ossified by approximately 24 weeks of gestation) (**Fig. 4** A and B).[54] Pediatricians should be aware that these children can have some respiratory issues based on small rib cage, feeding difficulties due to micrognathia and flat midface, and are at risk for recurrent ear infections. Families should be counseled that serial evaluation of the cervical spine by a team of specialists who can manage odontoid hypoplasia in childhood should be part of long-term care for these children (**Box 2**).

There are a large group of skeletal disorders that present with decreased bone density. The most common among these disorders is OI, or brittle bone disease, in which severe forms may present in the newborn period with fractures sustained in utero. This disorder has been classified in numerous forms: mild, moderate, severe, and perinatal forms. These classifications are used by clinicians to manage the complications and predict some of the natural history associated with the disorder, and are somewhat arbitrary.[55] In the past decade there has been enormous progress in unwinding the molecular genetics associated with OI.[56] Approximately 90% of the cases result from mutations in the genes that encode type I collagen, *COL1A1* and *COL1A2*. Most of the

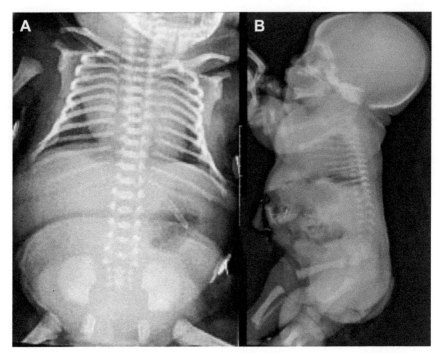

Fig. 4. Radiographs of SEDC in the newborn period. (*A*) Anteroposterior (AP) view of the chest showing bell-shaped chest with normal appearance of the rib ends, subjective platy-spondyly and lack of ossification of the pubis. (*B*) Lateral radiograph showing delayed ossification of the base of the skull, short ribs, and platyspondyly.

remaining cases result from gene mutations that are recessively inherited.[56] These recessively inherited cases usually present with severe forms of OI, some of them perinatal lethal.[57–59] They are extremely rare, and unless there is a family history consistent with autosomal-recessive inheritance (previously affected sibling or consanguinity), most OI cases result from dominantly or sporadically inherited mutations.

Newborns with OI present with relative macrocephaly, flat facies, short limbs, narrow thorax, and deformed and fractured extremities, with normal-appearing hands and feet. Radiographs show poor ossification of the skull, fractured ribs, undermineralized bone with fractures and, in very severe cases, femurs that are accordion in

---

Box 2
Osteogenesis imperfecta

Osteogenesis imperfecta (OI) can present with a broad phenotypic and genetic basis of disease; thus, molecular diagnosis can be helpful in predicting severity and recurrence risk.

Bisphosphonates can be used in the newborn period in severe cases of OI after consultation with medical genetics or another pediatric specialist experienced in the use of intravenous bisphosphonates.

Caregivers should be counseled on how to handle a newborn with OI.

Pediatric orthopedic surgeons should be consulted regarding the management of appendicular skeletal fractures.

appearance, diffuse osteopenia including the vertebrae, flattened acetabulae, and relatively normal-appearing hands and feet (**Fig. 5**). Similarly to the aforementioned skeletal dysplasias, there is a broad phenotypic spectrum in OI. The perinatal lethal form usually presents with a very small chest and deformed extremities. Care should be taken if a newborn with OI and in utero–occurring fractured ribs requires ventilator assistance. There is probable underlying pulmonary insufficiency due to a small chest, and ventilation may cause ongoing fractures in a probable lethal condition; thus, the degree and period of active intervention should be discussed with the family.

For those newborns who are stable, but present with fractures, orthopedic surgeons should evaluate the patient. In many instances, the treatment modality depends on the site of the fracture and degree of angulation at the site. Many of these fractures are managed by immobilization using strapping (eg, femoral fractures in the subtrochanteric region are managed by strapping of the thigh to abdomen), whereas fractures of the shaft of bones may be managed by casting.[60] In nonlethal but severe cases, consultation should be obtained from medical genetics or pediatric endocrinology for consideration of treatment with intravenous bisphosphonates while in the nursery. Studies have shown that early treatment with bisphosphonates decreases the number of subsequent fractures.[61,62] Individuals with OI also have fragile skin and blood vessels because type I collagen is an important component of connective tissue. Care in handling of these children should be discussed with staff.

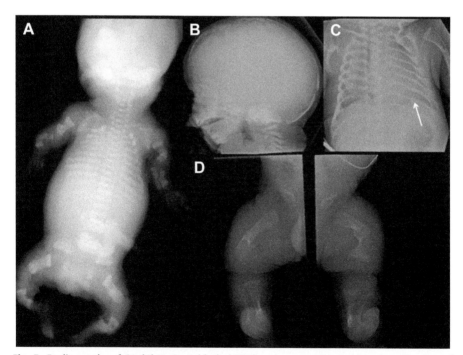

Fig. 5. Radiographs of OI. (*A*) Perinatal lethal OI showing complete undermineralization of the skeleton with crumbled appendicular bone due to recurrent fractures and poor healing. (*B*) Lateral skull of a newborn with OI. Note poor ossification of the calvarium, visualization of the anterior fontanel, and wormian bones. (*C*) AP view of the chest showing narrowness and rib fractures (*arrow*). (*D*) AP view of the lower extremities showing poorly modeled and undermineralized long bones, and crumbled appearance due to recurrent fractures.

LONG-TERM FOLLOW-UP

Children with skeletal disorders are best managed by a multidisciplinary approach that includes obstetricians (before delivery), pediatricians, neonatologists, medical geneticists, endocrinologists, neurosurgeons, otolaryngologists, and orthopedic surgeons. Subspeciality care should be directed toward the individual presenting issue. Families should be prepared for ongoing visits to supervise health management. For most children with nonlethal skeletal dysplasias, their quality of life is good. Families should be encouraged to seek out support from organizations dedicated to the well-being of individuals with forms of dwarfism that include Little People of America (www.lpaonline.org) and the Osteogenesis Imperfecta Foundation (www.oif.org). Pediatricians should be aware that these children with normal immune systems should receive standard doses of vaccines on routine schedules, as well as recognizing the potential for increased ear infections in disorders associated with midface hypoplasia, hearing loss due to increased infection and abnormalities of the stapes, as well as hydrocephalous in disorders associated with foramen magnum stenosis (achondroplasia, hypochondroplasia, diastrophic dysplasia, and metatropic dysplasia).

Best Practices

What is the current practice?

Best Practice/Guideline/Care Path Objective(s)

What changes in current practice are likely to improve outcomes?

1. Advances in molecular diagnosis through gene discovery will lead to improved counseling of families with affected children.

2. Knowing the precise diagnosis of type of skeletal dysplasia also will allow clinicians to tailor the treatment of children based on objective natural history data.

3. Improvement in imaging of the skeleton through MRI and computed tomography will aid in identifying children at risk for cervical vertebrae abnormalities.

Major Recommendations

1. In skeletal disorders it is important to identify those affected individuals with lethal disorders.

2. Evaluation of lethality is outlined in **Fig. 1**.

3. Children with skeletal dysplasias are ideally be managed by a multidisciplinary team.

4. Cervical vertebral abnormalities occur commonly in skeletal disorders and merits close evaluation by orthopedic and/or neurosurgeons in childhood.

Bibliographic Source(s)

Krakow D, Rimoin DL. The skeletal dysplasias. Genet Med 2010;12(6):327–41.

Krakow D, Lachman RS, Rimoin DL. Guidelines for the prenatal diagnosis of fetal skeletal dysplasias. Genet Med 2009;11(2):127–33.

Summary statement

Children with skeletal disorders are ideally cared for by a multidisciplinary approach that includes obstetricians (before delivery), pediatricians, neonatologists, medical geneticists, endocrinologists, neurosurgeons, otolaryngologists, and orthopedic surgeons. There are more than 450 skeletal disorders, some primarily affecting cartilage, some primarily bone, and some both. Knowledge of the precise diagnosis determined by clinical and radiographic data, confirmed by available molecular testing, provides clinicians with the basis to care for a newborn with a skeletal disorder.

REFERENCES

1. Warman ML, Cormier-Daire V, Hall C, et al. Nosology and classification of genetic skeletal disorders: 2010 revision. Am J Med Genet A 2011;155A(5):943–68.
2. Krakow D, Rimoin DL. The skeletal dysplasias. Genet Med 2010;12(6):327–41.
3. Provot S, Schipani E. Molecular mechanisms of endochondral bone development. Biochem Biophys Res Commun 2005;328(3):658–65.
4. Hall BK, Miyake T. All for one and one for all: condensations and the initiation of skeletal development. Bioessays 2000;22(2):138–47.
5. Ballock RT, O'Keefe RJ. The biology of the growth plate. J Bone Joint Surg Am 2003;85(4):715–26.
6. Kronenberg HM. Developmental regulation of the growth plate. Nature 2003; 423(6937):332–6.
7. Gedeon ÁK, Colley A, Jamieson R, et al. Identification of the gene (SEDL) causing X-linked spondyloepiphyseal dysplasia tarda. Nat Genet 1999;22(4):400–4.
8. Edwards MJ, Wenstrup RJ, Byers PH, et al. Recurrence of lethal osteogenesis imperfecta due to parental mosaicism for a mutation in the COL1A2 gene of type I collagen. The mosaic parent exhibits phenotypic features of a mild form of the disease. Hum Mutat 1992;1(1):47–54.
9. Cohn D, Starman B, Blumberg B, et al. Recurrence of lethal osteogenesis imperfecta due to parental mosaicism for a dominant mutation in a human type I collagen gene (COL1A1). Am J Hum Genet 1990;46(3):591.
10. Pauli RM, Conroy MM, Langer LO, et al. Homozygous achondroplasia with survival beyond infancy. Am J Med Genet 1983;16(4):459–73.
11. Flynn MA, Pauli RM. Double heterozygosity in bone growth disorders: four new observations and review. Am J Med Genet A 2003;121(3):193–208.
12. Young I, Ruggins N, Somers J, et al. Lethal skeletal dysplasia owing to double heterozygosity for achondroplasia and spondyloepiphyseal dysplasia congenita. J Med Genet 1992;29(11):831–3.
13. Günthard J, Fliegel C, Ohnacker H, et al. Lung hypoplasia and severe pulmonary hypertension in an infant with double heterozygosity for spondyloepiphyseal dysplasia congenita and achondroplasia. Clin Genet 1995;48(1):35–40.
14. Chitty LS, Tan AW, Nesbit DL, et al. Sonographic diagnosis of SEDC and double heterozygote of SEDC and achondroplasia—a report of six pregnancies. Prenat Diagn 2006;26(9):861–5.
15. Langer LO, Schaefer GB, Wadsworth DT. Patient with double heterozygosity for achondroplasia and pseudoachondroplasia, with comments on these conditions and the relationship between pseudoachondroplasia and multiple epiphyseal dysplasia, Fairbank type. Am J Med Genet 1993;47(5):772–81.
16. Woods C, Rogers J, Mayne V. Two sibs who are double heterozygotes for achondroplasia and pseudoachondroplastic dysplasia. J Med Genet 1994;31(7): 565–9.
17. Unger S, Korkko J, Krakow D, et al. Double heterozygosity for pseudoachondroplasia and spondyloepiphyseal dysplasia congenita. Am J Med Genet 2001; 104(2):140–6.
18. Ross JL, Bellus G, Scott CI, et al. Mesomelic and rhizomelic short stature: the phenotype of combined Leri-Weill dyschondrosteosis and achondroplasia or hypochondroplasia. Am J Med Genet A 2003;116(1):61–5.
19. Kitoh H, Oki T, Arao K, et al. Bone dysplasia in a child born to parents with osteogenesis imperfecta and pseudoachondroplasia. Am J Med Genet 1994;51(3): 187–90.

20. Cohn D, Apone S, Eyre D, et al. Substitution of cysteine for glycine within the carboxyl-terminal telopeptide of the alpha 1 chain of type I collagen produces mild osteogenesis imperfecta. J Biol Chem 1988;263(29):14605–7.
21. Marini JC, Forlino A, Cabral WA, et al. Consortium for osteogenesis imperfecta mutations in the helical domain of type I collagen: regions rich in lethal mutations align with collagen binding sites for integrins and proteoglycans. Hum Mutat 2007;28(3):209–21.
22. Byers PH, Pyott SM. Recessively inherited forms of osteogenesis imperfecta. Annu Rev Genet 2012;46:475–97.
23. Forlino A, Cabral WA, Barnes AM, et al. New perspectives on osteogenesis imperfecta. Nat Rev Endocrinol 2011;7(9):540–57.
24. Laine CM, Joeng KS, Campeau PM, et al. WNT1 mutations in early-onset osteoporosis and osteogenesis imperfecta. N Engl J Med 2013;368(19):1809–16.
25. Pyott SM, Tran TT, Leistritz DF, et al. WNT1 mutations in families affected by moderately severe and progressive recessive osteogenesis imperfecta. Am J Hum Genet 2013;92(4):590–7.
26. Krakow D, Alanay Y, Rimoin LP, et al. Evaluation of prenatal-onset osteochondrodysplasias by ultrasonography: a retrospective and prospective analysis. Am J Med Genet A 2008;146A(15):1917–24.
27. Krakow D, Lachman RS, Rimoin DL. Guidelines for the prenatal diagnosis of fetal skeletal dysplasias. Genet Med 2009;11(2):127–33.
28. Levenson D. New test could make carrier screening more accessible. Am J Med Genet A 2010;152(4):vii–viii.
29. Carmichael M. One hundred tests. Sci Am 2010;303(6):50.
30. Parilla BV, Leeth EA, Kambich MP, et al. Antenatal detection of skeletal dysplasias. J Ultrasound Med 2003;22(3):255–8.
31. Makrydimas G, Souka A, Skentou H, et al. Osteogenesis imperfecta and other skeletal dysplasias presenting with increased nuchal translucency in the first trimester. Am J Med Genet 2001;98(2):117–20.
32. Dugoff L, Thieme G, Hobbins J. First trimester prenatal diagnosis of chondroectodermal dysplasia (Ellis–van Creveld syndrome) with ultrasound. Ultrasound Obstet Gynecol 2001;17(1):86–8.
33. Schramm T, Gloning K, Minderer S, et al. Prenatal sonographic diagnosis of skeletal dysplasias. Ultrasound Obstet Gynecol 2009;34(2):160–70.
34. Krakow D, Williams J, Poehl M, et al. Use of three-dimensional ultrasound imaging in the diagnosis of prenatal-onset skeletal dysplasias. Ultrasound Obstet Gynecol 2003;21(5):467–72.
35. Fan HC, Blumenfeld YJ, Chitkara U, et al. Noninvasive diagnosis of fetal aneuploidy by shotgun sequencing DNA from maternal blood. Proc Natl Acad Sci U S A 2008;105(42):16266–71.
36. Saito H, Sekizawa A, Morimoto T, et al. Prenatal DNA diagnosis of a single-gene disorder from maternal plasma. Lancet 2000;356(9236):1170.
37. Kannu P, Bateman J, Savarirayan R. Clinical phenotypes associated with type II collagen mutations. J Paediatr Child Health 2012;48(2):E38–43.
38. Harding CO, Green CG, Perloff WH, et al. Respiratory complications in children with spondyloepiphyseal dysplasia congenita. Pediatr Pulmonol 1990;9(1):49–54.
39. Costello BJ, Edwards SP, Clemens M. Fetal diagnosis and treatment of craniomaxillofacial anomalies. J Oral Maxillofac Surg 2008;66(10):1985–95.
40. Schaefer RB, Gosain AK. Airway management in patients with isolated Pierre Robin sequence during the first year of life. J Craniofac Surg 2003;14(4):462–7.

41. Minnich DJ, Mathisen DJ. Anatomy of the trachea, carina, and bronchi. Thorac Surg Clin 2007;17(4):571–85.

42. Wells AL, Wells TR, Landing BH, et al. Short trachea, a hazard in tracheal intubation of neonates and infants: syndromal associations. Anesthesiology 1989;71(3): 367–73.

43. Mansour S, Hall C, Pembrey M, et al. A clinical and genetic study of campomelic dysplasia. J Med Genet 1995;32(6):415–20.

44. Kelley RI, Kratz LE, Glaser RL, et al. Abnormal sterol metabolism in a patient with Antley-Bixler syndrome and ambiguous genitalia. Am J Med Genet 2002;110(2): 95–102.

45. Patton M, Afzal A. Robinow syndrome. J Med Genet 2002;39(5):305–10.

46. Ho NC, Francomano CA, van Allen M. Jeune asphyxiating thoracic dystrophy and short-rib polydactyly type III (Verma-Naumoff) are variants of the same disorder. Am J Med Genet 2000;90(4):310–4.

47. Maroteaux P, Sauvegrain J, Chrispin A, et al. Omodysplasia. Am J Med Genet 1989;32(3):371–5.

48. Baujat G, Le Merrer M. Ellis-van Creveld syndrome. Orphanet J Rare Dis 2007; 2(6):27.

49. Lux SE, Johnston RB Jr, August CS, et al. Chronic neutropenia and abnormal cellular immunity in cartilage-hair hypoplasia. N Engl J Med 1970;282(5):231–6.

50. Mäkitie O, Kaitila I. Cartilage-hair hypoplasia—clinical manifestations in 108 Finnish patients. Eur J Pediatr 1993;152(3):211–7.

51. Vajo Z, Francomano CA, Wilkin DJ. The molecular and genetic basis of fibroblast growth factor receptor 3 disorders: the achondroplasia family of skeletal dysplasias, Muenke craniosynostosis, and Crouzon syndrome with acanthosis nigricans 1. Endocr Rev 2000;21(1):23–39.

52. Hecht JT, Butler IJ, Scott CI Jr. Long-term neurological sequelae in achondroplasia. Eur J Pediatr 1984;143(1):58–60.

53. Trotter TL, Hall JG. Health supervision for children with achondroplasia. Pediatrics 2005;116(3):771–83.

54. Unger S. A genetic approach to the diagnosis of skeletal dysplasia. Clin Orthop Relat Res 2002;(401):32–8.

55. Sillence D. Osteogenesis imperfecta: an expanding panorama of variants. Clin Orthop Relat Res 1981;(159):11–25.

56. Marini JC, Blissett AR. New genes in bone development: what's new in osteogenesis imperfecta. J Clin Endocrinol Metab 2013;98(8):3095–103.

57. Cabral WA, Chang W, Barnes AM, et al. Prolyl 3-hydroxylase 1 deficiency causes a recessive metabolic bone disorder resembling lethal/severe osteogenesis imperfecta. Nat Genet 2007;39(3):359–65.

58. Barnes AM, Chang W, Morello R, et al. Deficiency of cartilage-associated protein in recessive lethal osteogenesis imperfecta. N Engl J Med 2006;355(26): 2757–64.

59. Baldridge D, Schwarze U, Morello R, et al. CRTAP and LEPRE1 mutations in recessive osteogenesis imperfecta. Hum Mutat 2008;29(12):1435–42.

60. Kancherla R, Sankineani SR, Naranje S, et al. Birth-related femoral fracture in newborns: risk factors and management. J Child Orthop 2012;6(3):177–80.

61. Chien YH, Chu SY, Hsu CC, et al. Pamidronate treatment of severe osteogenesis imperfecta in a newborn infant. J Inherit Metab Dis 2002;25(7):593–5.

62. Cheung MS, Glorieux FH. Osteogenesis imperfecta: update on presentation and management. Rev Endocr Metab Disord 2008;9(2):153–60.

Newborn Craniofacial Malformations

Orofacial Clefting and Craniosynostosis

J. Austin Hamm, MD[a], Nathaniel H. Robin, MD[a,b,c],*

KEYWORDS

- Orofacial clefting • Craniosynostosis • Craniofacial malformations
- Genetic syndromes • Multidisciplinary clinics

KEY POINTS

- Craniofacial malformations are among the most common serious birth defects.
- Although most cases of orofacial clefting and craniosynostosis are isolated and sporadic, these abnormalities are associated with a wide range of genetic syndromes, and making the appropriate diagnosis can guide management and counseling.
- Absence of the premaxilla in patients with orofacial clefting may indicate an underlying brain malformation.
- Posterior positional plagiocephaly must be differentiated from craniosynostosis, as plagiocephaly responds to conservative management, and craniosynostosis requires surgical intervention.
- Patients with craniofacial malformation are best cared for in a multidisciplinary clinic that can coordinate the care delivered by a diverse team of providers.

INTRODUCTION

Craniofacial malformations, including orofacial clefting (OFC) and craniosynostosis (CS), are among the most common of birth defects. Most craniofacial malformations are sporadic, occurring with no family history, but they still may represent a genetically determined disorder. This determination is only one reason to make a correct genetic diagnosis (**Box 1**). Correct diagnosis can also aid in guiding management, assessing prognosis, and providing families with accurate genetic counseling and adequate access to appropriate support groups. The morbidity associated with these

The authors have no financial disclosures.

[a] Department of Genetics, The University of Alabama at Birmingham, 213 Kaul Human Genetics Building, 720 20th Street South, Birmingham, AL 35294, USA; [b] Department of Pediatrics, The University of Alabama at Birmingham, 1600 7th Avenue South, CPPI 310, Birmingham, AL 35233, USA; [c] Division of Otolaryngology, Department of Surgery, The University of Alabama at Birmingham, 563 Boshell Building, Birmingham, AL 35294, USA
* Corresponding author. Department of Genetics, The University of Alabama at Birmingham, 213 Kaul Human Genetics Building, 720 20th Street South, Birmingham, AL 35294.
E-mail address: nrobin@uab.edu

http://dx.doi.org/10.1016/j.clp.2015.02.005
perinatology.theclinics.com

Box 1
Reasons to make the diagnosis of a genetic syndrome

Benefits of making the diagnosis of a genetic syndrome

- Helps clarify the prognosis and anticipate complications
- Guides management, including use of or avoidance of specific therapies
- Can establish risk in other family members and future offspring
- Provides patients and their families with access to appropriate support groups
- Reduces cost by obviating need for unnecessary diagnostic tests or unhelpful therapies
- Provides families with a sense of closure

---

malformations is significant and includes disorders of feeding, hearing, speech, oral health, and psychosocial adjustment. Craniofacial defects present a formidable challenge to patients and their families and have a significant impact on the health care system. For example, expenditures by Medicaid[1] and private insurers[2] have been estimated to be 5 to 10 times higher for children with OFC compared with children without OFC during the first 5 years of life.

OROFACIAL CLEFTING
Epidemiology

OFC is the most common birth defect, occurring in about 1 in 600 newborns worldwide, although prevalence varies based on type of defect, gender, and ethnicity. In the United States alone, more than 7000 children are born with orofacial clefting each year according to the Centers for Disease Control.[3] The prevalence of cleft lip with or without cleft palate (CL±P) has geographic variation—from 3.4 to 22.9 per 10,000 births, with the highest prevalence among Asians and Latin Americans, the lowest among Africans, and an intermediate prevalence in European whites. Additionally, a recent survey of 13.5 million live US births found that the prevalence of CL±P among Amerindians is almost twice that of non-Hispanic whites.[4] In contrast, cleft palate only (CPO) is consistent across the world, with prevalence 1.3 to 25.3 per 10,000.[5] Studies of migrant populations in the United States[6,7] and the United Kingdom[8] suggest that the geographic variation of clefting incidence is more closely linked to genetic factors rather than environmental influences.

The ratio of boys to girls affected by CL±P is roughly 2:1, whereas with CPO, the there is a female predominance. Unilateral CL±P is the most common type of OFC and accounts for about one-third of cases. Isolated cleft lip and isolated CPO account for approximately 20% to 25% each, with the remaining cases being caused by bilateral CL±P, submucous clefts, interrupted clefts, bifid uvula, or other variations. Notably, CPO is roughly twice as likely to be associated with other anomalies or to be implicated as part of a recognized genetic syndrome than defects on the CL±P spectrum.[9]

Pathogenesis

The first distinction to be made when considering orofacial clefting is between CL±P and CPO, as these have classically been considered distinct entities.[10] Cleft lip (**Fig. 1**A) arises from the failure of fusion of the median nasal prominence with the premaxillary process at 42 days of gestation, and the defect often extends to the anterior hard palate, as the primary palate is also formed during this event. Failure of appropriate fusion may later result in the inability of the lateral palatine processes to unite

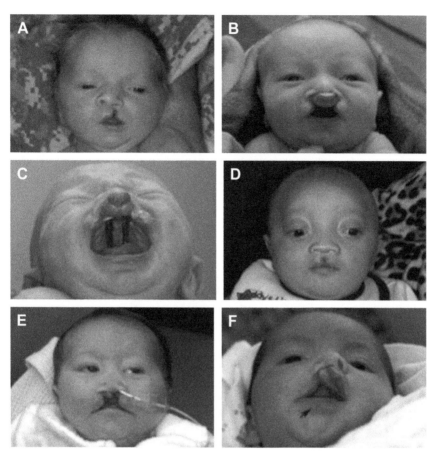

Fig. 1. Variations of CL±P. (*A*) Infant with unilateral cleft lip. (*B, C*) Infant with bilateral cleft lip and palate. (*D*) An infant with widely spaced eyes and median cleft lip that was also found to have a frontonasal encephalocele. (*E*) An infant with hypotelorism, median cleft lip with agenesis of the premaxilla, and holoprosencephaly. (*F*) An infant with unilateral cleft lip and palate and a lower lip pit (*arrow*), consistent with a diagnosis of Van der Woude syndrome. (*From* Evans K, Hing AV, Cunningham M. Avery's diseases of the newborn, 1331–1350. Philadelphia: Saunders; 2012; with permission.)

to form the soft palate at 63 days of gestation because of the increased intraoral space separating these 2 structures. Therefore, CL±P (see **Fig. 1**B and C) represents a spectrum of defects caused by the primary failure of the fusion between the nasal prominence and the premaxillary process. However, CPO arises from a different embryologic mechanism, as fusion of the palate normally occurs weeks after the lip is formed. This distinction is important for appropriate counseling, as parents with a child with cleft lip are at increased risk of having another child with CL±P, whereas parents with a child with CPO are similarly at risk for having another child with cleft palate without cleft lip. This distinction generally holds true regardless of whether the child is identified as having a genetic syndrome.

Although CL±P and CPO typically segregate as a result of different embryologic mechanisms, multiple families with mixed clefting (individuals with CL±P or CPO within the same family) have been described. Because of the high prevalence of OFC, some of these cases are likely owing to chance alone, but genetic associations have also been delineated, including *IRF6* mutations, which have been associated with mixed familial clefting in up to 9.1% of cases.[11,12] Notably, *IRF6* mutations also cause van der Woude syndrome (VWS), which is characterized by CL±P or CPO associated with lip pits and hypodontia (see **Fig 1F**).[13] VWS is the most common genetic syndrome associated with CL±P and is transmitted in an autosomal dominant fashion when associated with *IRF6* mutations. These mutations are incompletely penetrant for CL±P or CPO, but increase recurrence risk estimates for affected families to up to 50%, which is substantially higher than the empiric 3% to 5% risk of recurrence that is typical in siblings of a child with isolated OFC.

Syndromic Orofacial Clefting

VWS is only one of the more than 300 genetic syndromes that can manifest OFC.[14] Approximately 15% OFC are syndromic (12% of CL±P, 25% of CPO), meaning that they are associated with other findings. The remaining patients without other anomalies have isolated clefting, although this does not indicate that there is not a genetic component.

Select orofacial clefting syndromes

Deletion 22q11.2 syndrome (**Fig. 2**) is the most common genetic microdeletion syndrome. It is associated with a variety of congenital malformations, and up to 30% of patients have CPO, with additional patients showing submucous clefts or other structural palatal anomalies. Because of its clinical diversity, this syndrome has been variously identified as DiGeorge syndrome, velocardiofacial syndrome, and conotruncal anomaly-face syndrome, among others. Other congenital anomalies such as conotruncal heart defects and immune deficiency may also be present. Patients have a distinctive facial appearance that includes narrow palpebral fissures, malar hypoplasia, and small mouth with down-turned corners and small ears. Most

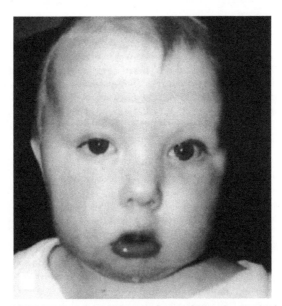

Fig. 2. A patient with 22q11.2 microdeletion syndrome shows short palpebral fissures, malar hypoplasia, squared nasal root, small mouth with downturned corners, and small ears. (*From* Turnpenny PD. Emery's elements of medical genetics. Philadelphia: Churchill Livingstone, an imprint of Elsevier Ltd; 2012; with permission.)

patients have learning disabilities and or behavioral problems, and up to one-third of patients have psychiatric disorders, including schizophrenia. Nearly all patients are affected with velopharyngeal insufficiency, regardless of whether a cleft is present, caused by neuromuscular weakness within these tissues. Pharyngeal abnormalities coupled with the neuropsychiatric conditions also associated with this disorder can lead to a distinctive hypernasal, pressured speech profile.

Stickler syndrome (**Fig. 3**) is characterized by CPO, severe myopia and retinal detachment, and early-onset arthritis. Stickler syndrome is the most common syndrome associated with the Pierre Robin sequence (PRS). In PRS, a cascade of developmental anomalies is initiated by micrognathia, which causes the tongue to be displaced posteriorly and superiorly resulting in obstruction that prevents the appropriate fusion of the palatine shelves and causes a U-shaped (rather than the typical V-shaped) cleft palate. About half of PRS is associated with an underlying genetic syndrome, with Stickler syndrome accounting for approximately half of these cases.

Importance of the premaxilla

A critical feature to assess on physical examination of a patient with OFC is the presence of the premaxillary segment, which is the tissue between the philtral columns above the upper lip. Absence or hypoplasia of this tissue is sometimes referred to as *median CL±P* and can be indicative of a more severe malformation, particularly holoprosencephaly (HPE) (see **Fig. 1**D and E). HPE is a major brain malformation that results from a failure of cerebral separation and is classified into alobar, semilobar, or lobar defects, in descending order of severity. HPE is often associated with major malformations of other organ systems and is commonly seen along with OFC in trisomy 13. However, about half of HPE cases are caused by a single gene defect, which may have significant implications for the patient's family. It is important to exclude this diagnosis in any child being evaluated for OFC.[9]

Nonsyndromic Clefting

Nonsyndromic clefting is classically viewed as a multifactorial trait that arises from interplay of genetic and environmental factors. The empiric recurrence risk for couples with a child with a nonsyndromic form of OFC is 3% to 5% compared with the general

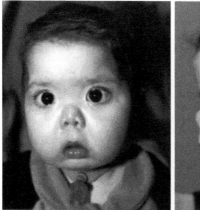
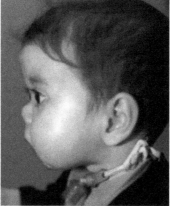

Fig. 3. A patient with typical features of Stickler syndrome, including a flat facial profile, prominent eyes, epicanthal folds, a low nasal bridge, a short nose, and a small chin. (*From* Graham JM. Smith's recognizable patterns of human deformation. Philadelphia: Elsevier; 2007. p. 124–9; with permission.)

population risk of about 0.1%. Currently, more than 20 single genes or cytogenetic loci are being studied for their role in nonsyndromic OFC,[15,16] including *IRF6*. A 2010 Danish study of nonsyndromic isolated CL±P and CPO found a recurrence risk of 3.5%, 0.8%, and 0.6% for first, second, and third degree relatives of patients with isolated OFC, respectively, with offspring of affected patients being most at risk. Another consideration is the recurrence risk of subepithelial defects of the orbicularis oris musculature, which some view as the mildest manifestation of CL±P defects. The recurrence risk of this subclinical defect has been estimated to be as high as 16.4% for first-degree relatives,[17] which suggests that in some cases of nonsyndromic CL±P, recurrence risk may approach levels typical of Mendelian patterns.

Environmental Factors

Environmental factors, including teratogen exposure, are also implicated in OFC. In a recent meta-analysis,[18] maternal factors associated with increased risk included tobacco or alcohol exposure, obesity, low blood zinc levels, fever during pregnancy, and stressful life events during the periconceptional period. Folic acid intake was identified as protective. Tobacco exposure and stressful life events had the strongest associations-, although a more recent article has questioned the role of maternal stress.[19] Food fortification programs with folic acid supplementation showed a protective effect in the United States,[20] although this protective effect has not been observed in similar programs in other countries.[21,22] A 2010 Cochrane review did not find a clear benefit[23] of folic acid supplementation, although more recent studies[24,25] have supported it. Furthermore, variations within the folate metabolism pathway[26] and the action of folic acid antagonists[27] have been associated with OFC.

CRANIOSYNOSTOSIS

CS is the premature fusion of one or more of the cranial sutures and usually comes to medical attention with the identification of an abnormal skull shape in the newborn period or early infancy. Severely affected patients may also have increased intracranial pressure, Chiari malformation, upper airway obstruction, or proptosis.[28] These complications are more common in syndromic cases. Diagnosis is often confirmed by a variety of radiologic techniques, including skull plain radiographs, cranial ultrasound scan, and 3-dimensional computed tomographic reconstruction, although assessing the shape of the skull on physical examination alone may be diagnostic in up to 98% of cases (**Fig. 4**).[29] The birth prevalence of congenital CS been estimated at 3 to 5 per 10,000 live births.[30–33]

PATHOGENESIS

Calvarial intramembranous bone formation begins with condensations of mesenchymal cells differentiating into osteoblasts after they have achieved a critical mass. Osteogenesis then proceeds in a centrifugal direction from multiple foci. As the osteogenic fronts encounter each other, they either merge into a single bone or form sutures. Cranial sutures represent joints between the flat calvarial bones separated by mesenchyme.[34] Further bone growth continues along these osteogenic fronts until the final closure of the major sutures in the third decade of life.[35] Well-orchestrated osteogenesis coupled with normal underlying brain growth lead to proper calvarial formation.

Primary and Secondary Craniosynostoses

CS is typically categorized as primary or secondary. Primary CS is caused by a defect in cranial suture osteogenesis, whereas in secondary CS the suture biology is normal.

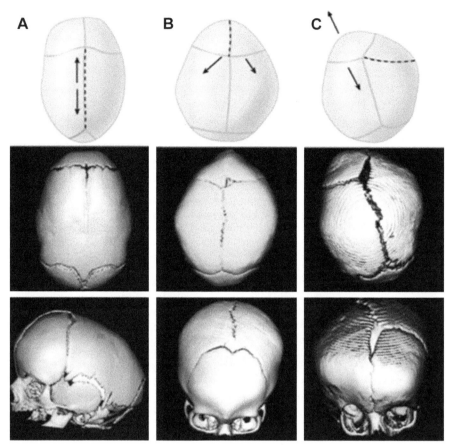

Fig. 4. Illustrations and 3-dimensional computed tomography reconstructions show (*A*) sagittal synostosis, (*B*) metopic synostosis, and (*C*) coronal synostosis. Arrows indicate direction of growth. (*From* Graham JM. Smith's recognizable patterns of human deformation. 3rd edition. Philadelphia: Elsevier; 2007. p. 173–9; with permission.)

The most common causes of secondary CS are insufficient brain growth and prolonged deformation. Primary CS typically results in an abnormal skull shape, as the underlying brain continues to grow but in an asymmetric fashion. Secondary CS caused by deficient brain growth typically demonstrates a normal, although microcephalic, head shape, possible ridging of the cranial sutures, and frequent neurodevelopmental deficits. This abnormal brain growth may be caused by central nervous system injury or to a primary developmental or genetic defect, such as Seckel syndrome, which is an autosomal recessive disorder characterized by microcephaly, a beaked nose, short stature, and neurodevelopmental delay (**Fig. 5**).[9] Additional causes of secondary CS include hyperthyroidism, hematologic abnormalities such as thalassemia, storage disorders, multiple teratogens,[36] and hypophosphatemic rickets.[37]

Isolated and Syndromic Craniosynostoses

Another key distinction is whether a patient has isolated CS or whether he has other findings that may indicate a syndromic diagnosis. Isolated craniosynostosis refers to

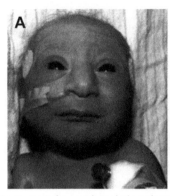
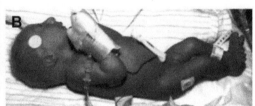

Fig. 5. An infant with Seckel syndrome has (*A*) microcephaly, prominent nose, and (*B*) low-set ears. (*From* Jones KL. Smith's recognizable patterns of human malformation. Philadelphia: Elsevier; 2013. p. 118–51 and; *Courtesy of* Dr MC Jones, MD, San Diego, CA; with permission.)

the presence of CS in the absence of other physical abnormalities; it is not meant to exclude a genetic component from having a role in pathogenesis of the condition. In a 2008 study of infants with CS, 84% had an isolated form of CS, 7% had multiple anomalies, and 9% had a recognized genetic syndrome. In nonsyndromic patients, sagittal synostosis was the most common (39%), followed by metopic (19%). Coronal and lambdoidal craniosyntostosis accounted for 17% each, with unilateral forms being most common. Eight percent had multiple suture types affected. White race, advanced maternal age, multiple gestation, male sex, and birth weight less than 1500 g or greater than 4000 g were associated with increased risk of isolated single-suture CS.[33] Increased risk associated with advance paternal age has also been reported.[38] Patients may also have CS of multiple sutures, sometimes referred to as *complex CS* with or without an underlying syndromic diagnosis. Clover leaf skull deformity, also known as *Kleeblattschädel* or *trilobed skull* (**Fig. 6**C), is a rare malformation characterized by a trilobar skull resulting from prenatal fusion of multiple sutures, most frequently the lambdoid and coronal sutures.[39] It is reported to occur as an isolated finding or as part of a genetic syndrome,[40] most commonly Pfeiffer syndrome.

Although dozens of syndromes have been associated with CS,[14] most syndromic cases are caused by a mutation in a fibroblast growth factor receptor (FGFR) gene or the *TWIST1* gene [33,41] and are listed in **Table 1**. FGFR-related craniosynostoses, also known as *acrocephalosyndactyly syndromes*, are autosomal dominant disorders caused by mutations in *FGFR1*, *FGFR2*, and *FGFR3* and are characterized by CS along with variable abnormalities of the extremities (see **Fig. 6**A, B, D, and E). *FGFR2* mutations can also be associated with isolated coronal synostosis. Saethre-Chotzen syndrome is phenotypically similar to this group but results from mutations in *TWIST1*.[42] Additional genes associated with isolated, complex, or syndromic CS include *ERF*[43] and *TCF12*,[44] and potentially others.[45]

Plagiocephaly

CS must be differentiated from deformational plagiocephaly, which does not involve premature fusion of the cranial sutures and therefore does not require surgical intervention. It is caused by a deformational force, most commonly intrauterine constraint or continual supine positioning of infants and is observed in 13% of singleton newborns[46] and up 19.7% of 4-month-olds. However, as the skull grows and children

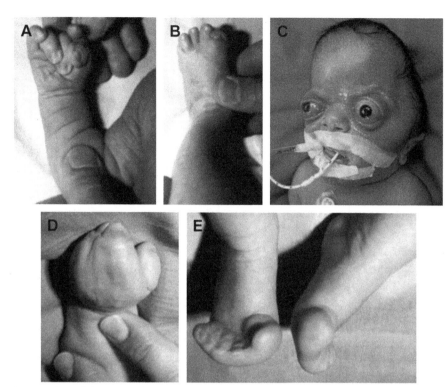

Fig. 6. Selected features of craniosynostosis syndromes. (*A*) Broad thumb and (*B*) broad great toe with medial deviation and cutaneous syndactyly, typical of Pfeiffer syndrome. (*C*) Clover leaf skull, seen in Pfeiffer syndrome type II. (*D*) Mitten and (*E*) sock malformations, which characterize the polysyndactyly of Apert syndrome. (*From [A, B, D, E]* Jones KL. Smith's recognizable patterns of human malformation. Philadelphia: Elsevier; 2013. p. 530–559; with permission; [*C*] Seruya M, Magge SN, Keating RF. Principles of neurological surgery. Philadelphia: Saunders; 2012. p. 137–55; with permission.)

develop more head control, prevalence decreases to 3.3% by 2 years of age.[47] After the American Academy of Pediatrics' recommendation in 1992 that infants be placed supine for sleep in efforts to decrease the incidence of sudden infant death syndrome,[48] there were multiple reports of increased incidence of deformational plagiocephaly, also known as *posterior positional plagiocephaly* (PPP).[49,50] The Back to Sleep campaign has been effective in lowering the incidence of sudden infant death syndrome, but routine supine positioning of infants has forced clinicians to become more adept at managing PPP, an important component of which is differentiating it from lambdoidal synostosis, which can be difficult.

Lamdoidal synostosis results in ipsilateral frontal bossing, whereas contralateral frontal bossing is observed in PPP. Additionally, the ipsilateral ear canal is displaced forward by deformational forces in PPP and pulled posteriorly in instances of labdoid synostosis (**Fig. 7**).[51] However, some studies have concluded that ear canal position is not a reliable diagnostic sign.[52,53] In contrast to CS, PPP is generally responsive to behavioral modification or physiotherapy in settings complicated by torticollis. Orthotic molding helmets may be indicated in refractory cases and are most effective when used at age 4 to 12 months. Surgery for deformational plagiocephaly is exceedingly rare but is the mainstay of therapy for CS.[54]

Table 1
Features of select craniosynostosis syndromes

Syndrome	Genes	Craniofacial	Extremities	Other
Apert	*FGFR2*	• Irregular craniosynostosis, especially coronal • Midface hypoplasia	• Osseus or cutaneous polysyndactly of fingers and toes, most commonly complete fusion of fingers 2–4. Occasional radiohumeral synostosis	• Mild cognitive impairment is common. • Often associated with other congenital anomalies, with up to 10% will having cardiac or genito urinary malformations
Beare Stevenson	*FGFR2*	• Craniosynostosis, cloverleaf skull • Midface hypoplasia	• Furrowed palms and soles	• Significant cognitive impairment • Cutis gyrata • Umbilical and genitourinary abnormalities
Crouzon	*FGFR2* *FGFR3*	• Craniosynostosis of coronal, sagittal, or lambdoidal sutures • Maxillary hypoplasia, shallow orbits with proptosis	• Normal	• Occasionally associated with other anomalies • Surgery may be deferred in mild cases • *FGFR3* is causative when associated with acanthosis nigricans
Jackson-Weiss	*FGFR2* *FGFR1(rare)*	• Craniosynostosis • Mandibular prognathism	• Broad and medially deviated halluces • Abnormal tarsals and metatarsals	• Normal intellect
Muenke	*FGFR3*	• Coronal craniosynostosis • Mild maxillary hypoplasia, downslanting palpebral fissures, and hypertelorism	• ± broad thumbs and halluces, ± carpal/tarsal fusion	• Variable expression with girls being more severely affected
Pfeiffer	*FGFR2* (69%) *FGFR1* (8%) *FGFR3* (3%) (Rocioli, 2013)	• Coronal ± sagittal craniosynostosis • Hypertelorism with proptosis • Cloverleaf skull in type 2	• Broad, medially deviated thumbs. ± partial syndactlyly • Variable radiohumeral synostosis	• Normal intelligence in type 1 • Types 2 and 3 have more severe malformations and poorer prognosis • Cloverleaf skull is pathomnemonic for type 2
Saethre-Chotzen	*TWIST1*	• Uni- or bicoronal synostosis • Hypertelorism, ptosis, maxillary hypoplasia	• Brachydactyly, ±2,3 finger or 3,4 toe syndactyly	• Normal intellect

Data from Jones KL, Jones MC, Del Campo M. Craniosynostosis syndromes. In: Jones KL, ed. Smith's recognizable patterns of human malformation. Philadelphia: Elsevier; 2013. p. 530–559; and refs.[41,42]

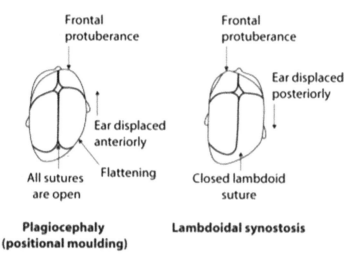

Frontal protuberance

Frontal protuberance

Ear displaced posteriorly

Ear displaced anteriorly

All sutures are open

Flattening

Closed lambdoid suture

Plagiocephaly (positional moulding)

Lambdoidal synostosis

Fig. 7. Differentiating labdoidal synostosis from posterior positional plagiocephaly. Note the ipsilateral frontal protuberance and posterior displacement of the ear in lambdoidal synostosis compared with the contralateral frontal protuberance and the anterior ear displacement in posterior positional plagiocephaly. (*From* Lissauer T. Illustrated textbook of paediatrics. Philadelphia: Elsevier Ltd; 2012. p. 181–99; with permission.)

Neurologic Function

Patients with isolated CS are a higher risk of neurodevelopmental dysfunction than the general population, although most have normal intelligence. A recent systematic review of neurodevelopmental outcomes in patients with single-suture craniosynostosis found that some studies did not detect a significant developmental delay in preoperative patients, although most studies reported affected patients being at increased risk for delay in the preoperative and postoperative periods. Additionally, affected patients tend to have a higher prevalence of learning, behavioral, and language problems.[55] Intelligence Quotient scores generally fall within the normal range, although a larger percentage of patients are in the below-average range and a smaller percentage in the above-average range compared with normal controls. Similarly, a 2006 study by Da Costa, and colleagues[56] found that 77% (10 of 13) of children and adolescents with syndromic CS developed normal intelligence, and some studies report an even higher prevalence of normal intelligence.[57]

TREATMENT

Craniofacial surgery is the mainstay of therapy for CS to correct the associated facial abnormalities and to treat impairment of regional cerebral blood flow caused by increased intracranial pressure and prevent its potentially negative developmental and neurologic sequelae. Although surgery offers the definitive treatment, other interventions such as airway support may be necessary in the newborn period, especially in instances of multisutural or syndromic cases.[51]

In the future, pharmacologic treatments may be available to patients with craniosynostosis. Characterization of the molecular pathways involved in the FGFR-related craniosynostosis syndromes has helped to identify multiple potential targets. A handful of approaches, including introduction of truncated FGFR receptors, use of specific interference RNA molecules, and targeting molecules within the FGF and transforming growth factor beta signaling pathways have furnished encouraging results.[58]

Furthermore, knowledge of the molecular pathways is advancing surgical care, such as the use of targeted therapy to help prevent premature resynostsois postoperatively.[59,60]

THE MULTIDISCIPLINARY CRANIOFACIAL CLINIC

The American Cleft Palate-Craniofacial Association offers guidelines for the optimal care for OFC and other craniofacial disorders, including CS.[61] Given the breadth of associated complications, these patients should be evaluated by a cleft craniofacial team, which includes the coordinated services of multiple health professionals. These teams are composed of numerous specialists—speech-language pathology, surgery, and orthodontics—and offer access to professionals in psychology, social work, psychiatry, audiology, genetics, dentistry, otolaryngology, and primary care.

Thorough evaluation in infancy is critically important because of the associated feeding problems and disorders of hearing and language development and risk of underlying genetic syndrome. However, it is also important to address the significant parental psychosocial burden of caring for a child with one of these disorders, as both OFC clefting[62,63] and CS[64,65] are associated with adverse psychosocial outcomes for the affected child and his or her parents. Additionally, the necessity of ongoing evaluation of the educational and psychological needs of the patient persists through childhood[66] into adolescence and adulthood.[67,68]

Best Practices

- Assessment of airway and feeding ability in patients with craniofacial malformations during the perinatal period is critical.

- Patients with craniofacial malformations should be cared for in a multidisciplinary clinic staffed professionals in speech-language pathology, surgery, and orthodontics with access to psychology, social work, psychiatry, audiology, genetics, dentistry, otolaryngology, and primary care providers.

- For children with craniofacial malformations, arriving at the correct genetic diagnosis can guide help guide management and is necessary to provide families with accurate recurrence risk and referral to appropriate support groups.

REFERENCES

1. Cassell CH, Meyer R, Daniels J. Health care expenditures among Medicaid enrolled children with and without orofacial clefts in North Carolina, 1995–2002. Birth Defects Res A Clin Mol Teratol 2008;82:785–94.
2. Boulet SL, Grosse SD, Honein MA, et al. Children with orofacial clefts: health-care use and costs among a privately insured population. Public Health Rep 2009;124:447–53.
3. The Center for Disease Control. Facts about cleft lip and cleft palate. Available at: http://www.cdc.gov/ncbddd/birthdefects/cleftlip.html. Accessed April 23, 2014.
4. Canfield MA, Mai CT, Wang Y, et al. The association between race/ethnicity and major birth defects in the United States, 1999–2007. Am J Public Health 2014; 104(9):e14–23.
5. Mossey PA, Modell B. Epidemiology of oral clefts 2012: an international perspective. Front Oral Biol 2012;16:1–18.
6. Croen LA, Shaw GM, Wasserman CR, et al. Racial and ethnic variations in the prevalence of orofacial clefts in California, 1983–1992. Am J Med Genet 1998;79:42–7.

7. Kirby R, Petrini J, Alter C. Collecting and interpreting birth defects surveillance data by hispanic ethnicity: a comparative study. The Hispanic Ethnicity Birth Defects Workgroup. Teratology 2000;61:21–7.
8. Leck I, Lancashire RJ. Birth prevalence of malformations in members of different ethnic groups and in the offspring of matings between them, in Birmingham, England. J Epidemiol Community Health 1995;49:171–9.
9. Robin NH. Medical genetics: its application to speech, hearing, and craniofacial disorders. San Diego (CA): Plural Publishing, Inc; 2008.
10. Fogh-Anderson P. Inheritance of harelip and cleft palate. Copenhagen (Denmark): Munksgaard; 1942.
11. Salahshourifar I, Wan Sulaiman WA, Halim AS, et al. Mutation screening of IRF6 among families with non-syndromic oral clefts and identification of two novel variants: review of the literature. Eur J Med Genet 2012;55:389–93.
12. Rutledge KD, Barger C, Grant JH, et al. IRF6 mutations in mixed isolated familial clefting. Am J Med Genet A 2010;152A:3107–9.
13. Van der W. Syndrome. In: Jones KL, Jones MC, Del Campo M, editors. Smith's recognizable patterns of human malformation. Philadelphia: Elsevier; 2013. p. 318–9.
14. Hennekam RCM. Gorlin's syndromes of the head and neck. New York: Oxford University Press; 2010.
15. Mangold E, Ludwig KU, Nothen MM. Breakthroughs in the genetics of orofacial clefting. Trends Mol Med 2011;17:725–33.
16. Dixon MJ, Marazita ML, Beaty TH, et al. Cleft lip and palate: understanding genetic and environmental influences. Nat Rev Genet 2011;12:167–78.
17. Klotz CM, Wang X, Desensi RS, et al. Revisiting the recurrence risk of nonsyndromic cleft lip with or without cleft palate. Am J Med Genet A 2010;152A: 2697–702.
18. Molina-Solana R, Yanez-Vico RM, Iglesias-Linares A, et al. Current concepts on the effect of environmental factors on cleft lip and palate. Int J Oral Maxillofac Surg 2013;42:177–84.
19. Carmichael SL, Ma C, Tinker S, et al. Maternal stressors and social support as risks for delivering babies with structural birth defects. Paediatr Perinat Epidemiol 2014;28:338–44.
20. Yazdy MM, Honein MA, Xing J. Reduction in orofacial clefts following folic acid fortification of the U.S. grain supply. Birth Defects Res A Clin Mol Teratol 2007; 79:16–23.
21. Ray JG, Meier C, Vermeulen MJ, et al. Association between folic acid food fortification and congenital orofacial clefts. J Pediatr 2003;143:805–7.
22. Lopez-Camelo JS, Castilla EE, Orioli IM, INAGEMP, ECLAMC. Folic acid flour fortification: impact on the frequencies of 52 congenital anomaly types in three South American countries. Am J Med Genet A 2010;152A:2444–58.
23. De-Regil LM, Fernandez-Gaxiola AC, Dowswell T, et al. Effects and safety of periconceptional folate supplementation for preventing birth defects. Cochrane Database Syst Rev 2010;(10):CD007950.
24. Kelly D, O'Dowd T, Reulbach U. Use of folic acid supplements and risk of cleft lip and palate in infants: a population-based cohort study. Br J Gen Pract 2012;62:e466–72.
25. Li S, Chao A, Li Z, et al. Folic acid use and nonsyndromic orofacial clefts in China: a prospective cohort study. Epidemiology 2012;23:423–32.
26. Blanton SH, Henry RR, Yuan Q, et al. Folate pathway and nonsyndromic cleft lip and palate. Birth Defects Res A Clin Mol Teratol 2011;91:50–60.
27. Hernandez-Diaz S, Werler MM, Walker AM, et al. Folic acid antagonists during pregnancy and the risk of birth defects. N Engl J Med 2000;343:1608–14.

28. Tamburrini G, Caldarelli M, Massimi L, et al. Complex craniosynostoses: a review of the prominent clinical features and the related management strategies. Childs Nerv Syst 2012;28:1511–23.
29. Fearon JA, Singh DJ, Beals SP, et al. The diagnosis and treatment of single-sutural synostoses: are computed tomographic scans necessary? Plast Reconstr Surg 2007;120:1327–31.
30. French LR, Jackson IT, Melton LJ 3rd. A population-based study of craniosynostosis. J Clin Epidemiol 1990;43:69–73.
31. Lajeunie E, Le Merrer M, Bonaiti-Pellie C, et al. Genetic study of nonsyndromic coronal craniosynostosis. Am J Med Genet 1995;55:500–4.
32. Cohen MM Jr. Craniofacial disorders caused by mutations in homeobox genes MSX1 and MSX2. J Craniofac Genet Dev Biol 2000;20:19–25.
33. Boulet SL, Rasmussen SA, Honein MA. A population-based study of craniosynostosis in metropolitan Atlanta, 1989–2003. Am J Med Genet A 2008;146A: 984–91.
34. Lana-Elola E, Rice R, Grigoriadis AE, et al. Cell fate specification during calvarial bone and suture development. Dev Biol 2007;311:335–46.
35. Non-syndromic Craniosynostosis. In: Guyuron B, editor. Plastic surgery indications and practice. Edinburgh, TX: Saunders/Elsevier; 2009. p. 389–404.
36. Cohen MM Jr. Etiopathogenesis of craniosynostosis. Neurosurg Clin N Am 1991; 2:507–13.
37. Pivnick EK, Kerr NC, Kaufman RA, et al. Rickets secondary to phosphate depletion. A sequela of antacid use in infancy. Clin Pediatr 1995;34:73–8.
38. Barik M, Bajpai M, Das RR, et al. Study of environmental and genetic factors in children with craniosynostosis: a case-control study. J Pediatr Neurosci 2013;8: 89–92.
39. Manjila S, Chim H, Eisele S, et al. History of the Kleeblattschadel deformity: origin of concepts and evolution of management in the past 50 years. Neurosurg Focus 2010;29:E7.
40. Sloan GM, Wells KC, Raffel C, et al. Surgical treatment of craniosynostosis: outcome analysis of 250 consecutive patients. Pediatrics 1997;100:E2.
41. Roscioli T, Elakis G, Cox TC, et al. Genotype and clinical care correlations in craniosynostosis: findings from a cohort of 630 Australian and New Zealand patients. Am J Med Genet C Semin Med Genet 2013;163C:259–70.
42. Robin NH, Falk MJ, Haldeman-Englert CR. FGFR-Related Craniosynostosis Syndromes. 1998 Oct 20 [Updated 2011 Jun 7]. In: Pagon RA, Adam MP, Ardinger HH, et al, editors. GeneReviews® [Internet]. Seattle, WA: University of Washington; 1993–2015. Available at: http://www.ncbi.nlm.nih.gov/books/NBK1455/. Accessed February 23, 2015.
43. Twigg SR, Vorgia E, McGowan SJ, et al. Reduced dosage of ERF causes complex craniosynostosis in humans and mice and links ERK1/2 signaling to regulation of osteogenesis. Nat Genet 2013;45:308–13.
44. Sharma VP, Fenwick AL, Brockop MS, et al. Mutations in TCF12, encoding a basic helix-loop-helix partner of TWIST1, are a frequent cause of coronal craniosynostosis. Nat Genet 2013;45:304–7.
45. Justice CM, Yagnik G, Kim Y, et al. A genome-wide association study identifies susceptibility loci for nonsyndromic sagittal craniosynostosis near BMP2 and within BBS9. Nat Genet 2012;44:1360–4.
46. Peitsch WK, Keefer CH, LaBrie RA, et al. Incidence of cranial asymmetry in healthy newborns. Pediatrics 2002;110:e72.

47. Hutchison BL, Stewart AW, de Chalain T, et al. Serial developmental assessments in infants with deformational plagiocephaly. J Paediatr Child Health 2012;48: 274-8.
48. American academy of pediatrics AAP Task force on infant positioning and SIDS: positioning and SIDS. Pediatrics 1992;89:1120-6.
49. Turk AE, McCarthy JG, Thorne CH, et al. The "back to sleep campaign" and deformational plagiocephaly: is there cause for concern? J Craniofac Surg 1996;7:12-8.
50. Littlefield TR, Saba NM, Kelly KM. On the current incidence of deformational plagiocephaly: an estimation based on prospective registration at a single center. Semin Pediatr Neurol 2004;11:301-4.
51. Fearon JA. Evidence-based medicine: craniosynostosis. Plast Reconstr Surg 2014;133:1261-75.
52. Koshy JC, Chike-Obi CJ, Hatef DA, et al. The variable position of the ear in lambdoid synostosis. Ann Plast Surg 2011;66:65-8.
53. Menard RM, David DJ. Unilateral lambdoid synostosis: morphological characteristics. J Craniofac Surg 1998;9:240-6.
54. Pogliani L, Mameli C, Fabiano V, et al. Positional plagiocephaly: what the pediatrician needs to know. A review. Childs Nerv Syst 2011;27:1867-76.
55. Knight SJ, Anderson VA, Spencer-Smith MM, et al. Neurodevelopmental outcomes in infants and children with single-suture craniosynostosis: a systematic review. Dev Neuropsychol 2014;39:159-86.
56. Da Costa AC, Walters I, Savarirayan R, et al. Intellectual outcomes in children and adolescents with syndromic and nonsyndromic craniosynostosis. Plast Reconstr Surg 2006;118:175-81 [discussion: 182-3].
57. Noetzel MJ, Marsh JL, Palkes H, et al. Hydrocephalus and mental retardation in craniosynostosis. J Pediatr 1985;107:885-92.
58. Senarath-Yapa K, Chung MT, McArdle A, et al. Craniosynostosis: molecular pathways and future pharmacologic therapy. Organogenesis 2012;8: 103-13.
59. Cooper GM, Curry C, Barbano TE, et al. Noggin inhibits postoperative resynostosis in craniosynostotic rabbits. J Bone Miner Res 2007;22:1046-54.
60. Cooper GM, Usas A, Olshanski A, et al. Ex vivo Noggin gene therapy inhibits bone formation in a mouse model of postoperative resynostosis. Plast Reconstr Surg 2009;123:94S-103S.
61. Standards for cleft palate and craniofacial teams. Chapel Hill, NC: American Cleft Palate-Craniofacial Association; 2010. Available at: http://www.acpa-cpf.org/team_care/standards/. Accessed February 23, 2015.
62. Nelson P, Glenny AM, Kirk S, et al. Parents' experiences of caring for a child with a cleft lip and/or palate: a review of the literature. Child Care Health Dev 2012;38: 6-20.
63. Nelson PA, Kirk SA, Caress AL, et al. Parents' emotional and social experiences of caring for a child through cleft treatment. Qual Health Res 2012; 22:346-59.
64. Cloonan YK, Collett B, Speltz ML, et al. Psychosocial outcomes in children with and without non-syndromic craniosynostosis: findings from two studies. Cleft Palate Craniofac J 2013;50:406-13.
65. Bannink N, Maliepaard M, Raat H, et al. Health-related quality of life in children and adolescents with syndromic craniosynostosis. J Plast Reconstr Aesthet Surg 2010;63:1972-81.

66. Murray L, Arteche A, Bingley C, et al. The effect of cleft lip on socio-emotional functioning in school-aged children. J Child Psychol Psychiatry 2010;51: 94–103.
67. Berger ZE, Dalton LJ. Coping with a cleft: psychosocial adjustment of adolescents with a cleft lip and palate and their parents. Cleft Palate Craniofac J 2009;46:435–43.
68. Berger ZE, Dalton LJ. Coping with a cleft II: factors associated with psychosocial adjustment of adolescents with a cleft lip and palate and their parents. Cleft Palate Craniofac J 2011;48:82–90.

Structural Brain Defects

Matthew T. Whitehead, MD[a],*, Stanley T. Fricke, PhD[a],
Andrea L. Gropman, MD[b]

KEYWORDS

- Structural • Brain • Malformations • Genetic • Metabolic • MRI • Spectroscopy

KEY POINTS

- Structural brain abnormalities are not uncommon in the context of inborn errors of metabolism (IEM).
- IEM-associated brain injury tends to result in selective injury characterized by involvement of specific processes; this may be reflected by certain patterns seen on neuroimaging.
- Discovery of brain malformations should prompt a detailed search for signs of an underlying cause.
- Patients with suspected metabolic disease should be scrutinized for coexistent brain malformations.

INTRODUCTION

Many inborn errors of metabolism (IEM) are associated with structural brain defects that may add diagnostic specificity to an otherwise nonspecific clinical presentation. In the newborn period, the repertoire of clinical features of infants with IEM is limited and overlaps with one another and with non-genetic causes of encephalopathy. Clinically, these infants may present with seizures, hypothermia, acidosis, alkalosis, coma, hypotonia or hypertonia, or encephalopathy. The type of imaging abnormality depends on the timing of the insult in development, as well as its duration and severity. Although the pathophysiology of neurologic injury may not be known, shared mechanisms may be explanatory such as oxidative injury owing to overactivation of N-methyl-D-aspartate receptors with subsequent glutamatergic damage in some, or energy depletion or inflammation in others.

Neuroimaging has emerged as a useful clinical and research tool for studying the brain in a noninvasive manner. Several types of imaging exist to study neural networks underlying cognitive processes, white matter/myelin microstructure, and cerebral

Disclosures: None.
[a] Department of Radiology, Children's National Medical Center, 111 Michigan Avenue Northwest, Washington, DC 20010, USA; [b] Department of Neurology, Children's National Medical Center, 111 Michigan Avenue Northwest, Washington, DC 20010, USA
* Corresponding author.
E-mail address: MWhitehe@childrensnational.org

Clin Perinatol 42 (2015) 337–361
http://dx.doi.org/10.1016/j.clp.2015.02.007   **perinatology.theclinics.com**
0095-5108/15/$ – see front matter © 2015 Elsevier Inc. All rights reserved.

metabolism in vivo, and they may be used together to glean better understanding of the processes leading to the anatomic findings.

IEM-associated brain injury patterns may be characterized by whether the process primarily involves gray matter, white matter, or both. In addition, the affected gray matter may be subcortical or cortical. Although generally expected to be global insults, many IEMs tend to result in selective injury to a particular deep gray matter nucleus or to the white matter, such as the putamen (and to a lesser degree, the globus pallidi) in glutaric aciduria type 1,[1,2] putamen in certain mitochondrial cytopathies,[1,2] or the globus pallidus in methylmalonic acidemia.[3] There may be even more selectivity for particular cell types based on morphology or neurotransmitter systems (e.g., astrocytes/neuron: glutamatergic, GABA-ergic); however, this is currently poorly understood.

Patients with cortical gray matter involvement may present with seizures, encephalopathy, or dementia, whereas deep gray matter injury typically manifests with extrapyramidal findings of dystonia, chorea, athetosis, or other involuntary movement disorders when the basal ganglia are involved. White matter disorders feature pyramidal signs (spasticity, hyperreflexia) and visual findings. Involvement of the cerebellum or its connecting tracts may lead to ataxia.

Neurologic injury may be attributable to either a substrate intoxication or substrate depletion model of injury. Metabolic disorders caused by substrate intoxication include those in which there is a buildup of a compound such as in phenylketonuria, maple syrup urine disease, organic acidurias, and urea cycle disorders. Substrate depletion disorders include the creatine deficiencies (owing to guanidinoacetate methyltransferase and L-arginine:glycine amidinotransferase deficiency [GAMT and AGAT] or owing to mutations in the creatine transporter [SLC6A8]).

NEUROIMAGING THE BRAIN IN GENETIC DISORDERS

Neuroimaging in recent years has come to encompass a wide array of modalities that can be combined to gain complementary information regarding the brain's structural, functional and metabolic dimensions in both healthy and pathologic states. For example, routine structural MRI now includes not only T1- and T2-weighted sequences, but also fluid attenuation inversion recovery and voxel-based morphometry, all of which reveal macroscopic structure. Diffusion-weighted imaging and diffusion tensor imaging are used to study microstructural variance in white matter fiber tracts,[4] and MR spectroscopy (MRS) is used to measure brain metabolism in static and dynamic models.[5,6] Combining imaging platforms in multimodal assessment batteries gives investigators a complex and varied perspective into the structural, functional and biochemical parameters of the central nervous system in IEMs.

Magnetic Resonance Spectroscopy

^{1}H MRS is a robust,[7,8] versatile, noninvasive technique capable of producing information on a large number of brain chemicals.[9] Chemicals studied via the identification and integration of the spectral peaks found in the "proton" (^{1}H) spectra include *N*-acetylaspartate (NAA) for its role in mitochondrial oxidative metabolism, lipid synthesis (source of acetyl groups), and as a putative marker for neuronal viability; creatine and phosphocreatine as creatine to phosphocreatine energy conversion is mediated by creatine kinase; choline (Cho), a precursor for neurotransmitter acetylcholine, and membrane phospholipidsmyoinositol for neuronal signaling in the phophoinositide pathway, osmoregulation, cell nutrition, and detoxification; lactate, which is a byproduct of anaerobic metabolism, elevated concentrations resulting from glycolytic metabolism as happens in brain ischemia; glutamate and glutamine, which are major excitatory and inhibitory neurotransmitters in the central nervous system.

Single voxel spectroscopy is a technique used to acquire metabolic information from a localized region of brain tissue. To this end, a T1-weighted 3-dimensional image is obtained and segmented into gray matter, white matter and cerebrospinal fluid.[10,11] The single voxel spectroscopy voxel volume is mapped to the T1-weighted 3-dimensional image and weights of the partial volumes of each are understood in the context of the spectral data obtained in that volume. Furthermore, other imaging sequences can be equally mapped onto that voxel and onto the T1-weighted 3-dimensional image so that the effects of apparent diffusion coefficients, perfusion rates, and chemical concentrations will be estimated in that voxel from the data acquired. This step is essential because chemical concentration can affect the understood local diffusion and so forth. These data will then be used to interpret the condition of the brain.

Many, if not all, MRI equipment vendors offer the option to perform in vivo localized single voxel ^{1}H spectroscopy. There are a variety of pulse sequences from which to choose; however, industry has centered on the Short time to echo (TE) *ST*imulated-echo *A*cquisition *M*ode (STEAM) and the *P*oint *RES*olved *S*pectroscopy (PRESS) sequences. In this article, we primarily discuss the PRESS sequence. However, it should be noted that the STEAM sequence can often be more helpful than PRESS in the evaluation of metabolic disease owing to phase sensitivity issues of the PRESS sequence. This may seem counter intuitive, because the PRESS sequence typically renders more signal than the STEAM sequence; however, because of phase problems averaging of the PRESS sequence transients under large excursions of head movement, even 15 to 144 ms tau in the presence of the voxel selective gradients can significantly degrade signal to noise via canceling of signal through averaging.

Structural Brain Defects

Structural brain malformations occur when the normal cell proliferation, migration, and/or organization is perturbed. Various genetic, ischemic, infectious, and toxic insults may cause brain malformation. The extent of the resultant brain malformation is related directly to the severity, duration, and timing of the insult. The collective imaging pattern of brain abnormalities can provide additional clues to the underlying etiology, which is critical to understanding expected outcomes for these patients. This article focuses on common IEM-associated with structural brain defects. Selected metabolic diseases are reviewed; characteristic clinical and imaging manifestations that help to narrow the differential diagnosis are highlighted.

The association between structural brain malformations and specific inborn metabolic errors has been well-documented in the literature.[12–20] Structural brain abnormalities may be present in up to 14% of patients with congenital metabolic disease.[17] Because the placenta rids the fetus of toxic metabolites, most IEM have a postnatal onset. Structural brain abnormalities that occur in the context of genetic disease processes reflect a prenatal onset. The cause of this association remains debatable. Energy impairment, substrate insufficiency, cell membrane receptor and cell signaling abnormalities, and toxic byproduct accumulation are all possible.[14,16,19,20] In addition, concurrent defects in genes that encode for neuronal development and movement could cause structural brain anomalies. All in all, brain malformations seem to be more commonly associated with disorders of energy metabolism.[13,14,16]

The clinical expression of brain malformation depends on the type, location, and severity of the anomaly. For example, patients with perisylvian polymicrogyria may present with arthrogryposis and variable developmental delay given the involvement

Table 1
Disease specific locations of brain malformations associated with inborn metabolic errors

	Cer	CC	Cbl	BS	Vasc	Eye	CN	Cysts CSFS PVS	NAA	Cho	MI	Glx[a]	Ic	O
Zellweger	+++	+	+++	+++				GS	↓	↑	↓	↑	↑	Lipid
Neonatal ALD	+	+	+						↓	↑				Lipid
Infantile Refsum	+	+	+						↓	↑	↑			Lipid
RCDP	+									↓	↑			Lipid acetate
PDH	+	+++							↓					Acetate
NKH	+	+++	+											Glycine
S-L-O	+	+++	+++	+++				AC		↑				Lipid
Salla		+++	+++											
CDG	+	+++	+++	+++					↓	↓	↑			
Menkes	+	+++	+		+++							↑		
Walker–Warburg	+++	+	+++	+++		+++			↑					
Fukuyama	+++	+	+	+						↑				
M-E-B	+++	+	+++	+++		+++								
LAMA2	+++	+	+	+										
GA type 1	+							UO, AC, GC, MC	↓	↑	↑		↑	
GA type 2	+	+	+					UO, AC		↑				
Mucolipidoses		+++							↓					

										Other						
Krabbe										+++			↑	↑	↑	
MPS	+++	+++								PVS, SAS, VM	↓	↑	↑	↑	↑	
RC	+++	+	+++								↓	↑			↑	
FA	+	+++								UO, VM						
CPT2	+															
3HIBA	+	+														
BFED	+++	+++	+++													
D2HGA	+	+	+							GC, VM						
DHPDD	+++	+++														
3PGDD	+++	+++														
MMA	+										↓	↑	↑	↑	↑	
3MGA	+++	+++	+											↑	↑	

Commonly involved (+++), occasionally involved (+), ↑ (increased), ↓ (decreased).

Abbreviations: 3HIBA, 3-hydroxyisobutyric aciduria; 3MGA, 3-methylglutaconic aciduria; 3PGDD, 3-phosphoglycerate dehydrogenase deficiency; AC, arachnoid cysts; BFED, bifunctional enzyme deficiency; BS, brainstem; Cbl, cerebellum; CC, corpus callosum; CDG, congenital disorders of glycosylation; Cer, cerebrum; Cho, choline; CN, cranial nerves; CPT2, carnitine palmitoyltransferase II; CSFS, cerebrospinal fluid spaces; D2HGA, D-2-hydroxyglutaric aciduria; DHPDD, dihydropyrimidine dehydrogenase deficiency; FA, fumaric aciduria; GA, glutaric aciduria; Glx, glutamine/glutamate; GS, germinolytic cysts; LAMA2, merosin deficient muscular dystrophy; lc, lactate; MC, mesencephalic cistern enlargement; M-E-B, muscle–eye–brain disease; MI, myoinositol; MLIV, mucolipidosis type IV; MMA, methylmalonic aciduria; MPS, mucopolysacharidoses; NKH, nonketotic hyperglycinemia; O, other; PDH, pyruvate dehydrogenase deficiency; PVS, perivascular spaces; RC, respiratory chain disorders; RCDP, rhizomelic chondrodysplasia punctata; SAS, enlarged subarachnoid spaces; S-L-O, Smith–Lemli–Opitz; UO, underopercularization; Vasc, vasculature; VM, ventriculomegaly.

a Requires short time to echo.

of perirolandic cortex, language centers, and associative cortex among other regions. The MR appearance of brain malformations can be striking, potentially to the point of distracting the reader from a detailed evaluation of remainder of the brain, and depriving the reader from the detection of additional clues to the etiology. This situation has been called "satisfaction of search," and represents an unfortunate ever-present plague to the radiologist, a phenomenon that paradoxically worsens with loss of its awareness.[21] Moreover, if the observed brain malformation(s) are sufficient to explain the clinical symptoms, a detailed brain evaluation may be terminated prematurely. It is important for the reader to be mindful that many brain malformations are not sporadic, but rather represent interrupted areas of brain development from genetic, ischemic, infectious, and/or toxic processes. Brain malformation diagnoses should thus prompt the reader to initiate a search expedition through the remainder of the brain to find additional clues that could indicate a unifying diagnosis.[14]

Prenatal ultrasonography is a useful nonirradiating imaging modality that can be used in the initial workup of suspected brain abnormalities.[14] Neonatal head ultrasonography compares favorably with brain MRI in detection of structural brain anomalies and white matter disease.[22] However, the exquisite structural detail provided by a quality MR examination is unparalleled. A variety of MR pulse sequences can be prescribed to enhance signal detail and increase the contrast between normal and pathologic tissues. MRS can be employed in conjunction, potentially uncovering otherwise unknown metabolic brain deficits. In recent years, fetal MR has pushed the boundary of early diagnosis. Prenatal imaging manifestations of diseases such as Zellweger syndrome, nonketotic hyperglycinemia (NKH), pyruvate dehydrogenase deficiency, and glutaric aciduria type I have all been discovered by fetal MR.[12,23–25]

HETEROTOPIAS, DYSPLASIAS, AND OTHER MALFORMATIONS OF CORTICAL DEVELOPMENT

Gray matter heterotopias represent ectopic neuronal elements, arrested in suspended animation before or during migration. Cerebral neuronal migration commences in the first trimester and proceeds throughout the second trimester (approximately 6–24 gestational weeks).[26,27] It is during this time that specific genetic deficits affecting neuronal migration are realized. Peroxisomal disorders including Zellweger syndrome and its phenotypically milder relative, neonatal adrenoleukodystrophy, represent the most common inborn metabolic errors with concurrent gray matter heterotopia. Cerebellar malformations can be found histopathologically in infantile Refsum disease, a phenotypically mild peroxisomal disorder; however, no imaging correlates have been described.[28,29] Multiple additional genetic diseases have also been associated with heterotopias, cortical gyral abnormalities, polymicrogyria, pachygyria, lissencephaly, and cortical dysplasia (**Table 1**).[12–14,16,17] Incomplete opercularization (visibility of the insula from the brain surface) is found characteristically in glutaric aciduria types I/II and fumaric aciduria (see **Table 1**).[12]

PEROXISOMAL DISORDERS
Zellweger Syndrome

An archetypal peroxisomal assembly disorder, Zellweger syndrome is the most severe disease in the spectrum of peroxisomal defects. Peroxisomes are organelles necessary for normal anabolic and catabolic cellular processes. Because peroxisomes are integral components of nearly all bodily tissues, clinical manifestations are protean. The liver and brain tend to be affected profoundly in Zellweger syndrome; facial dysmorphia and skeletal manifestations are constant features. Typical neuroimaging manifestations include the triad of cerebral *polymicrogyria* (perirolandic and perisylvian predominant), germinolytic cysts, and diffuse cerebral white matter disease (**Fig. 1**).[12,13,30,31] Cerebellar dysplasia, inferior olivary nucleus dysplasia, and corpus callosum dysgenesis can also be found. MRS findings reflect hepatocellular dysfunction (elevated glutamine and glutamate, decreased myoinositol), decreased neurons and/or neuronal axonal integrity (decreased NAA:Cr) and findings of increased cell membrane turnover (elevated Cho:Cr; **Fig. 2**).[12,32,33] Elevated lactate and lipids can also be detected; the latter may reflect accumulation of lipids or myelin destruction. Fumaric aciduria is the main differential diagnosis on MR. However, ventriculomegaly and brainstem volume loss are more prominent in fumaric aciduria.[12,34]

Neonatal Adrenoleukodystrophy

Clinical and imaging signs are similar but less severe and extensive with respect to Zellweger syndrome. Facial dysmorphia is less obvious and skeletal manifestations are absent. A retinopathic "leopard spot" is specific.[35] On imaging, neuronal migrational anomalies often coexist with cerebral and cerebellar white matter disease; cerebellar malformations and corpus callosum thinning have also been described.[12] MRS demonstrates elevation of lipids, Cho, and to a lesser extent myoinositol with concurrently decreased NAA.[33]

Rhizomelic Chondrodysplasia Punctata

Malformations of cortical development, including polymicrogyria and pachygyria, have been described in this disorder of plasmalogen synthesis.[36] Shortened proximal limbs, epiphyseal calcifications, and cataracts are clinical hallmarks.[12,13] A case report of rhizomelic chondrodysplasia punctata described a unique spectroscopic profile: increased myoinositol/glycine, decreased Cho, increased lipid, and increased acetate.[37] Diminished Cho was speculated to be a consequence of decreased

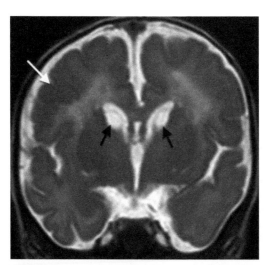

Fig. 1. Zellweger syndrome. Coronal T2 weighted image (repetition time ms/echo time ms, 5564/105) from a 4-day-old male with Zellweger syndrome demonstrating bilateral germinolytic cysts (*black arrows*) and polymicrogyria (*white arrow*). Excessive cerebral white matter hyperintensity reflects hypomyelination.

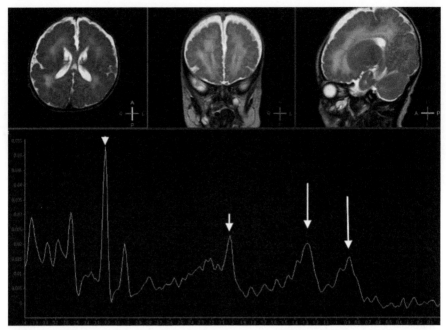

Fig. 2. Zellweger syndrome. Single voxel MR spectroscopy (MRS; 35-ms echo time) demonstrating typical alignment of the voxel placement in the brain, in this case, centered over the abnormal right frontal white matter (square box) in a 4-day-old male with Zellweger syndrome. Abnormal macromolecular peaks presumably reflecting elevated lipids are pronounced at 1.3 ppm and 0.9 ppm (long *arrows*). Decreased N-acetylaspartate (short *arrow*) and increased choline (*arrowhead*) are also present. Because glutamine/glutamate elevation and myoinositol disturbances are common in Zellweger syndrome, a short time to echo is essential in MRS examination. Note that the 3 localizer views allow for anatomic identification of brain region of interest. Other sections are also used, because "off-axis" voxels are required. Although isolated white matter analysis is the goal in this case, these images show that the voxel contains approximately 90% white matter and 10% gray matter, a fact that one should bear in mind during interpretation.

plasmalogen availability for myelin synthesis. Elevated myoinositol/glycine levels were felt to be a marker of activated glial cells.

Congenital Muscular Dystrophies

Although not technically IEM, neuromuscular disorders (dystroglycanopathies) such as Walker–Warburg syndrome, muscle–eye–brain disease, Fukuyama muscular dystrophy, and merosin-deficient muscular dystrophy (LAMA2) deserve special mention because they almost always manifest structural brain abnormalities.[12,13,38–43] Deficient muscular, retinal, meningeal, and brain specific proteins necessary for both normal muscular structure and neuronal guidance and organization result in concurrent skeletal muscle dysgenesis and central nervous system anomalies.[38] From a brain imaging perspective, these diseases share characteristics with peroxisomal disorders, namely, malformations of cortical development, cerebellar hypoplasia/dysplasia, white matter disease, and corpus callosum abnormalities. However, germinolytic cysts have not been described in dystroglycanopathies and cerebellar cysts are not present in peroxisomal diseases.[12]

Walker–Warburg Syndrome

Severe brain anomalies characterize this disorder, many of which are fairly specific to the disease. Extensive malformations of cortical development demonstrate a unique *"cobblestone" lissencephaly* pattern (type II lissencephaly) attributable to neuronal overmigration. True to form, abnormal cortex resembles cobblestone or piano keys on MRI (**Fig. 3**A, B). The typical "Z-shaped" brainstem morphology with a dorsal pontomesencephalic junction kink, marked pontine hypoplasia, and tectal plate thickening are major clues for the diagnosis, especially on fetal MR (see **Fig. 3**C). Cerebellar dysplasia and multifocal cysts are commonly present. Ocular changes are also seen, mainly persistent hyperplastic primary vitreous (see **Fig. 3**D).[38,39]

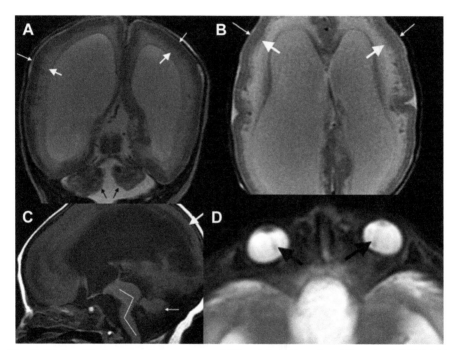

Fig. 3. Walker–Warburg syndrome. Coronal T2 weighted imaging (*A*) and axial T2WI (*B*; repetition time ms/echo time ms, 4050/90) from a 2-day-old female with Walker–Warburg syndrome showing "cobble-stone" lissencephaly. The brain surface is smooth (*thin white arrows*), whereas the corticomedullary interface is irregular (*thick white arrows*). Cerebellar dysplasia is also present (*black arrows*). Also note ventriculomegaly representing hydroceph-alus. (*C*) Sagittal T1WI (repetition time ms/echo time ms, 500/15) from a 2-day-old female with Walker–Warburg syndrome demonstrating a characteristic "Z-shape" brainstem configuration, marked pontine hypoplasia, and thickening of the midbrain associated with aqueductal stenosis or atresia. Cerebellar hypoplasia/dysplasia (*small arrow*), cobble-stone lissencephaly (*large arrow*), and ventriculomegaly representing hydrocephalus are also visible. (*D*) Axial T2WI (repetition time ms/echo time ms, 4040/80) through the orbits from a 7-day-old female with Walker–Warburg syndrome showing findings of bilateral persistent hyperplastic primary vitreous: microphthalmia, shallow anterior segments, and linear hypointense intravitreous structures coursing from the posterior globe margins to the lenses representing persistent hyaloid canals (*arrows*).

Fukuyama Muscular Dystrophy

A mixed cortical malformation pattern typifies Fukuyama muscular dystrophy. Polymicrogyria is present in the frontal lobes with or without temporoparietal lobe involvement.[38,40–43] Cobblestone lissencephaly is often found in the temporo-occipital lobes.[44] Cerebellar dysplasia with or without cysts is also characteristic.[40–43] The pons and vermis are generally hypoplastic. Diffuse central cerebral hypomyelination is present. Although ocular abnormalities may be present, the globes are usually normal on MRI.[41] Increased Cho demonstrable on MRS early in the disease process may resolve over time as white matter signal changes become less conspicuous.[43]

Muscle–Eye–Brain Disease

Brain malformations tend to be less severe than in Walker–Warburg syndrome. Variable ocular malformations are a necessary component of the disease, most commonly persistent hyperplastic primary vitreous. The cerebellum is dysplastic and may or may not have associated cysts. Diffuse cerebral cortical dysplasia, pontine and vermian hypoplasia, and corpus callosum dysgenesis are also common; hydrocephalus occurs on occasion.[38]

LAMA2-Related Muscular Dystrophy (Merosin-Deficient Muscular Dystrophy)

Occipitotemporal malformations of cortical development are common (**Fig. 4**). A fairly diffuse, frontal predominant cerebral white matter disease is also generally present. Mild hypoplasia of the pons and vermis may also be seen.[38]

CORPUS CALLOSUM

The corpus callosum is a midline cerebral structure composed of a collection of homotopic interhemispheric connecting white matter tracts. Thus, its appearance is influenced by the morphology, direction, and amount of its constituent fibers. Callosal thinning reflecting adjacent white matter volume loss or hypoplasia is present

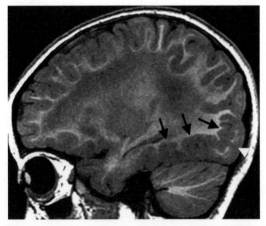

Fig. 4. Merosin-deficient muscular dystrophy (LAMA2). Sagittal spoiled gradient recalled acquisition in the steady state T1WI (repetition time ms/echo time ms/inversion time ms, 11/5/500) from a 5-year-old female with LAMA2-related muscular dystrophy showing occipitotemporal polymicrogyria (*arrows*). The occipital cortical surface is smooth (*arrowhead*). The imaged cerebral white matter is abnormally hypointense throughout, with relative sparing of the subcortical U fibers.

commonly in patients with IEMs, especially in later stages of disease. However, callosal dysgenesis implies incomplete formation or malformation, typically from an earlier event during its formation (11–12 weeks gestation) or growth in length (11–20 weeks).[45] This time range coincides with the neuronal migratory period, a concept that helps to explain the curious coincidence of gray matter heterotopia and corpus callosum dysgenesis. There are numerous genetic diseases associated with corpus callosum dysgenesis (see **Table 1**).

Pyruvate Dehydrogenase Deficiency

Pyruvate dehydrogenase is necessary for the conversion of pyruvate to acetyl-coenzyme A, integral for citric acid cycle energy production. Excessive pyruvate is converted to lactate, a considerably less useful fuel. Normal neuronal genesis, growth, migration, and organization require adequate energy production. Being a mitochondrial complex, pyruvate dehydrogenase defects can manifest with Leigh syndrome, which is defined by neurodegeneration caused by mitochondrial dysfunction and bilateral lesions in the central nervous system.[46]

On imaging, deep gray nuclear signal changes and white matter disease are typical. Cerebral white matter signal may be diffusely hyperintense on T2WI, occasionally without concurrent deep gray nuclei and brainstem involvement.[47] The corpus callosum can be dysgenetic (**Fig. 5**). Neuronal migration abnormalities and brainstem dysplasia may also be present.[16]

MRS most often shows abnormal lactate; however, its absence does not exclude the diagnosis (**Fig. 6**). Creatine can be increased, but NAA and Cho are often preserved.[48] Myoinositol may be increased. A novel MRS peak at 2.37 ppm has been described, attributable to pyruvate itself.[49] Acetate may also be detectable at 1.9 ppm.[48]

Nonketotic Hyperglycinemia

NKH is caused by a glycine cleavage defect. An interesting clinical pearl that can support the diagnosis of NKH is that of concomitant seizures and hypotonia. This is explained by

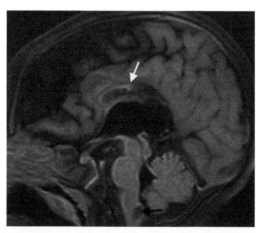

Fig. 5. Pyruvate dehydrogenase deficiency. Deficiency sagittal fat-saturated T2 fluid attenuation inversion recovery (repetition time ms/echo time/inversion time ms, 9000/94/2000) MRI from a 2-month-old female with pyruvate dehydrogenase deficiency showing a shortened, thinned corpus callosum compatible with dysgenesis (*white arrow*). Syringobulbia is partially visible (*black arrow*).

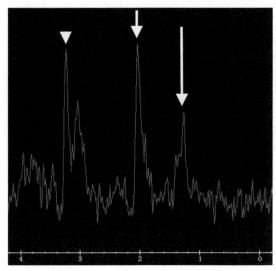

Fig. 6. MR spectroscopy (MRS). Single voxel MRS (288-ms echo time) with voxel of interest placed over the left basal ganglia demonstrates a lactate peak at 1.33 ppm (*long arrow*) consistent with ongoing anaerobic metabolism, common to mitochondrial disorders. *N*-acetylaspartate (*short arrow*) to creatine and choline (*arrowhead*) to creatine ratios are relatively normal for age.

the fact that glycine is excitatory in the brain and inhibitory in the spinal cord.[12] Glycine neurotoxicity could be responsible for structural brain abnormalities in NKH.

MRI discloses symmetric, hyperintense signal and reduced diffusion in myelinated or myelinating areas: internal capsules, ventrolateral thalami, posterior putamen, dorsal brainstem, cerebellar peduncles, and deep cerebellum (**Fig. 7**A). Although this pattern resembles findings seen in maple syrup urine disease, it is typically less severe and extensive. Deep cerebral white matter signal alteration is often encountered; its etiology is debatable and could represent myelination delay[12] or gliosis.[50] From a structural standpoint, the corpus callosum is always abnormal, either hypoplastic or frankly dysgenetic (see **Fig. 7**B).[12,20] Cortical gyral abnormalities and cerebellar hypoplasia have been reported.[20] In patients with typical MRI findings, MRS clinches the diagnosis: elevated glycine is found at 3.6 ppm (**Fig. 8**). Intermediate or long TE MRS is necessary as the normal myoinositol peak overlaps with this area on a short TE spectrum.

Smith–Lemli–Optiz Syndrome

In Smith–Lemli–Optiz syndrome, a cholesterol deficit is caused by deficiency in 7-dehydrocholesterol reductase. Cholesterol is necessary for normal prechordal mesoderm sonic hedgehog signaling.[51] Consequently, midline and especially ventral patterning may be interrupted. MRI confirms multiple midline anomalies, including *corpus callosum dysgenesis* (variable but often thickened), hypoplasia of cavum septum pellucidi, dysplastic fornices, inferior vermian hypoplasia, and extra-axial cysts (**Fig. 9**).[52] Holoprosencephaly has also been described.[51] In our experience, hypoplasia of the anterior commissure and medulla oblongata dysgenesis with anterior flattening and preolivary sulcus hypoplasia are also common. Reports of MRS abnormalities in Smith–Lemli–Optiz syndrome are sparse; increased lipid levels and Cho

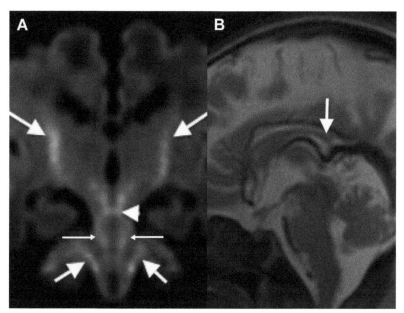

Fig. 7. Nonketotic hyperglycinemia. (*A*) Coronal diffusion weighted image (repetition time ms/echo time ms, 8000/85) from a 2-day-old female with nonketotic hyperglycinemia showing reduced diffusion manifested by hyperintensity in myelinating white matter tracts, including the corticospinal and thalamocortical (*long thick arrows*), dentatorubrothalamic (superior cerebellar peduncles = *short thin arrows*; superior cerebellar peduncle decussations = *arrowhead*), and inferior cerebellar peduncles (*short thick arrows*). (*B*) Sagittal T2 weighted image (repetition time ms/echo time ms, 2500/64) from a 2-day-old female with nonketotic hyperglycinemia reveals a thin, truncated corpus callosum consistent with dysgenesis (*arrow*).

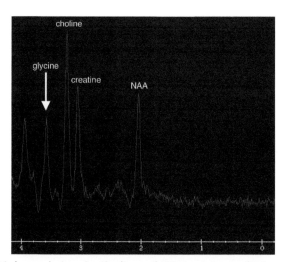

Fig. 8. Nonketotic hyperglycinemia. Single voxel MR spectroscopy (144 ms echo time) with voxel of interest placed over the left basal ganglia from a 2-day-old female with nonketotic hyperglycinemia demonstrates an abnormal peak at 3.6 ppm, representing glycine (*arrow*). Although myoinositol protons co-resonate in this portion of the spectrum, it is not expected to be present on intermediate echo time spectroscopy owing to its relatively short T2 relaxation time.

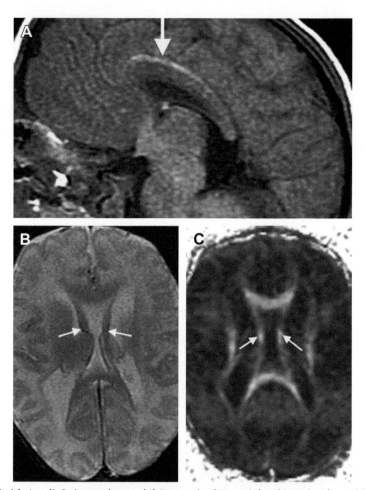

Fig. 9. Smith–Lemli–Opitz syndrome. (*A*) Parasagittal T1 weighted imaging (repetition time ms/echo time ms, 400/13) from a 16-day-old female with Smith–Lemli–Opitz syndrome demonstrating corpus callosum dysgenesis associated with a hyperintense filliform pericallosal lipoma (*arrow*). (*B*) Axial T2WI (repetition time ms/echo time ms, 3000/100) from a 16-day-old female with Smith–Lemli–Opitz syndrome demonstrating thickened forniceal bodies (*arrows*), unapposed at midline consistent with a cavum septum pellucidum and vergae. (*C*) Axial diffusion tensor image (repetition time ms/echo time ms, 10,000/86; 25 directions of encoding) from a 16-day-old female with Smith–Lemli–Opitz syndrome demonstrating thickened forniceal bodies with marked aniosotropy (*arrows*), unopposed at midline consistent with a cavum septum pellucidum and vergae.

have been reported in the cerebral white matter on short TE spectra, with improvement after cholesterol supplementation.[53]

Salla Disease

A mucolipidosis lysosomal storage disorder, Salla disease results from a genetic defect causing impaired sialic acid transport across lysosomal membranes.[12,44] The clinical phenotype is variable; hypotonia, ataxia, and nystagmus may be present.[44] Most reported cases were in Finnish patients. Brain MRI characteristically reveal marked thinning of the corpus callosum, cerebral white matter hypomyelination, and variable atrophy.[12,44] The etiology of the thin corpus callosum has been attributable to hypoplasia; however, the morphology and length are generally preserved, potentially indicating an acquired volume loss. Sonninen and colleagues[44] reported a patient with development of corpus callosum thinning on follow-up after a previously normal MR examination in an asymptomatic 1-month-old patient with Salla disease, reflecting volume loss or arrested development. MRS performed in the cerebral white matter is unique, demonstrating elevated NAA and creatine and decreased Cho.[54] NAA elevation may represent accumulated sialic acid (N-acetylneuraminic acid).[12,55]

CEREBELLAR AND BRAINSTEM DYSGENESIS

The cerebellum has rich connectivity with the cerebrum, brainstem, and spinal cord. Any process that disrupts the normal structure or function of these parenchymal elements may cause secondary cerebellar hypoplasia or volume loss, depending on the timing of the event. Moreover, the cerebellum can be affected primarily by various inborn metabolic errors, causing structural defects ranging from hypoplasia to dysplasia.[12,13,56,57] Hypertrophic olivary degeneration and olivary dysplasia has been described in a few IEMs (see **Table 1**).[12,13,58]

Congenital Disorders of Glycosylation

As glucose is the primary energy substrate for the brain, disorders of glucose metabolism like congenital disorders of glycosylation type I can result in structural defects chiefly affecting the cerebellum. Although other subtypes may not have radiologic correlates, this is a recently identified disease entity with sparsely described imaging findings. Pontine hypoplasia, combined cerebellar hypoplasia and atrophy, and cerebellar cortical/subcortical hyperintensity is typical of congenital disorders of glycosylation type Ia (**Fig. 10**).[59] Dandy–Walker malformation and corpus callosum hypoplasia have also been shown in congenital disorders of glycosylation.[60] Reported MRS findings include decreased NAA and Cho with increased myoinositol and glutamine/glutamate.[59,60]

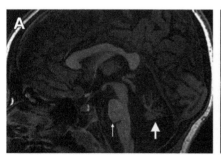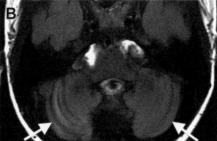

Fig. 10. Congenital disorder of glycosylation (CDG). (*A*) Sagittal fast spoiled gradient recalled acquisition in the steady state T1 weighted image (repetition time ms/echo time ms/inversion time ms, 8/3/450) from a 6-year-old male with CDG-1a demonstrating marked cerebellar atrophy (*long arrow*) and moderate pontine atrophy (*short arrow*). (*B*) Axial T2 fluid attenuation inversion recovery image (repetition time ms/echo time ms/inversion time ms, 10,000/144/2150) from a 6-year-old male with CDG-1a demonstrating marked cerebellar atrophy and hyperintensity (*arrows*), the so-called "shrunken, bright cerebellar sign."

VASCULAR DYSGENESIS

Neural crest cells and mesoderm contribute to the formation blood vessel walls in the ventral cephalic tree, and the dorsal cephalic tree is derived from mesoderm in extrapolation from chick chimera data.[61] Genetic defects modulating the development and migration of these elements can cause vascular dysgenesis. Perhaps the most widely recognized genetic disorder that presents with dysgenesis of the intracranial vasculature is Menkes disease. In this disorder, arteries of the anterior and posterior circulation are almost always ectatic and tortuous. D-2-hydroxyglutaric aciduria can also manifest vascular abnormalities, such as aneurysms and occlusive cerebrovascular disease.[62,63]

Menkes Disease

Menkes disease is an X-linked disorder of copper metabolism. In the brain, impaired copper transport results in copper accumulation in vessel walls and astrocytes and neuronal copper deficiency. The clinical disease hallmark, "kinky hair," may not be readily apparent in the first few months of life. Therefore, imaging plays an important role in the workup.

Imaging findings generally include arterial ectasia and tortuosity reflecting vascular dysplasia, vermian hypogenesis or agenesis, cerebral white matter changes, marked progressive atrophy, and development of subdural fluid collections (**Fig. 11**A, B).[16,56,64,65] Basal ganglia hyperintensity on T1WI can be present, reflecting concurrent hepatocellular disease.[64] Fleeting temporal lobe edema (see **Fig. 11**C) with temporary MRS alterations (decreased NAA, increased lactate) may be found on occasion.[66] Cerebellar hypoplasia has also been described.[56,67]

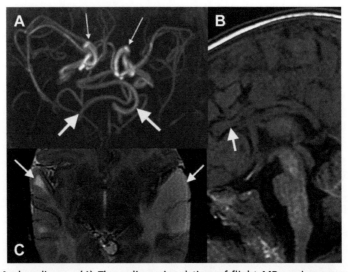

Fig. 11. Menkes disease. (*A*) Three-dimensional time-of-flight MR angiogram axial plane maximal intensity projection (repetition time ms/echo time ms/inversion time ms, 25/3/500) from a 5-month-old male with Menkes disease showing diffuse, marked intracranial arterial tortuosity and ectasia (*thick arrows* = vertebral arteries; *thin arrows* = internal carotid arteries). (*B*) Sagittal spoiled gradient recalled acquisition in the steady state T1 weighted image (repetition time ms/echo time ms/inversion time ms, 11/5/500) from a 5-month-old male with Menkes disease showing corpus callosum dysgenesis with deformity of the genu and rostrum (*arrow*). (*C*) Axial T2WI (repetition time ms/echo time ms, 3200/90) from a 5-month-old male with Menkes disease depicting bitemporal hyperintensity and swelling consistent with edema (*arrows*).

MISCELLANEOUS DISORDERS
Glutaric Aciduria

Glutaric aciduria types I and II present with brain signal changes and structural anomalies. Common to both disorders is temporal pole hypoplasia, enlarged temporal extra-axial spaces and/or temporal arachnoid cysts, open opercula, and cerebral white matter signal changes (**Fig. 12**A).[1,12] However, glutaric aciduria type I generally has basal ganglia (especially putamen; see **Fig. 12**A, B) and occasionally brainstem and dentate nucleus T2 prolongation and may have cerebellar heterotopia, whereas glutaric aciduria type II may have corpus callosum hypoplasia, vermian agenesis, and "warty dysplasia" of the cerebral cortex.[12,68–78] The mesencephalic cistern may also be expanded in more than 80% of patients with glutaric aciduria type I.[74] Caudothalamic groove germinolytic cysts and subdural hematomas may also be seen in glutaric aciduria type I. MRS may demonstrate decreased NAA and increased lactate in the basal ganglia representing anaerobic metabolism in glutaric aciduria type I (**Fig. 13**).[12,75] Cho and myoinositol are also elevated.[54] In glutaric aciduria type II, an increased Cho to creatine ratio can be found in abnormal cerebral white matter, suggesting demyelination.[76]

In glutaric aciduria type I, there is dose-related brain involvement and clinical symptomatology commensurate with diminished glutaryl-coenzyme A dehydrogenase enzymatic activity, a mitochondrial enzyme. Therefore, brain manifestations vary. Furthermore, biochemical assessment may be nondiagnostic or misleading, and clinical symptoms may not be present early in the disease, underscoring the importance of appropriate imaging in the diagnostic workup.[12,72] The diagnosis is, however, important because glutaric aciduria type I is treatable and permanent brain injury is preventable.[12]

LYSOSOMAL DISORDERS
Mucolipidoses

Intralysosomal accrual of mucopolysacharides and lipids defines the mucolipidoses. Type IV mucolipidosis may manifest structural brain abnormalities, including corpus callosum dysgenesis, white matter disease, and cerebral deep gray nuclei mineralization.[79] MRS tends to demonstrate decreased NAA compatible with neuronal loss or neuronal–axonal disintegrity.[80]

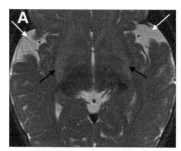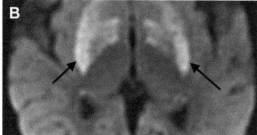

Fig. 12. Glutaric aciduria type I. (A) Axial T2 weighted image (repetition time ms/echo time ms, 3552/98) from an 11-month-old female with glutaric aciduria type I depicting open opercula (*white arrows*) and hyperintensity in the lentiform nuclei (*black arrows*). (B) Axial diffusion weighted image (repetition time ms/echo time ms, 10,000/90) from an 11-month-old female with glutaric aciduria type I showing reduced diffusion in the basal ganglia consistent with metabolic decompensation (*arrows*).

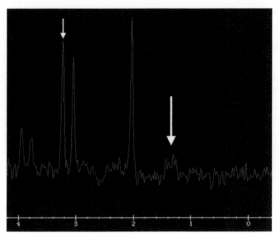

Fig. 13. Glutaric aciduria type I. Single voxel MR spectroscopy (288 ms echo time) with voxel of interest placed over the left basal ganglia in an 11-month-old patient with glutaric aciduria type I demonstrates abnormal metabolic peaks at 1.3 ppm, representing lactate (*long arrow*). The choline (*short arrow*) to creatine ratio is mildly increased for age.

Krabbe Disease (Globoid Cell Leukodystrophy)

In this lysosomal storage disease, a galactocerebroside β-galactosidase enzyme defect causes accumulation of the intermediate metabolite psychosine. Psychosine is toxic to oligodendrocytes, resulting in leukodystrophy that reflects combined hypomyelination and dysmyelination.[12] At the same time, multinuclear giant cells (globoid cells) gather on site and cause regional white matter enlargement, likely the cause of frequent optic pathway and other cranial nerve enlargement (**Fig. 14**A).[81–83] Characteristic MRI findings include optic pathway enlargement, deep cerebral white matter hyperintensity with a posteroanterior gradient on T2WI, brainstem and spinal cord signal alteration, and cerebellar white matter signal abnormality (see **Fig. 14**B, C).[12] The cerebellar white matter signal abnormality helps to distinguish Krabbe disease from the similar appearing leukodystrophies, metachromatic leukodystrophy (a lysosomal storage disorder) and X-linked adrenoleukodystrophy (a peroxisomal disorder). Dentate nuclei are characteristically spared (see **Fig. 14**C). Importantly, this is one of the few metabolic diseases in which CT is especially useful in narrowing the differential diagnosis. Thalamic mineralization causes hyperdensity, sometimes before more characteristic white matter changes (see **Fig. 14**D).[12] Gangliosidoses can also cause thalamic hyperdensity; however, these usually have additional basal ganglia T2 prolongation and white matter disease, if present, is less extensive. MR spectroscopic changes in the white matter include decreased NAA, increased Cho, increased myoinositol, and a lactate peak.[33,84]

Mucopolysacharidoses

Mucopolysacharidoses are types of lysosomal storage disorders characterized by an enzyme defect causing systemic glycosaminoglycan accumulation. Hepatosplenomegaly, skeletal anomalies, and brain enlargement are the result. Brain involvement causes MRI features such as hydrocephalus, enlarged perivascular spaces, and white matter disease of varying severity (**Fig. 15**).[85,86] When this imaging constellation is

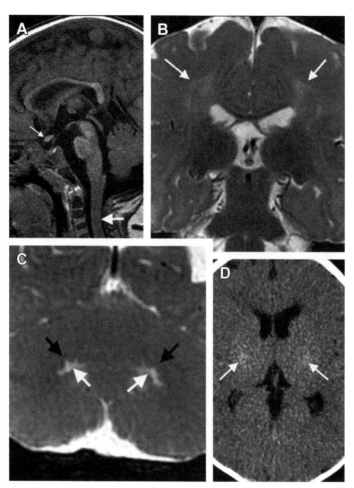

Fig. 14. Krabbe disease. (*A*) Sagittal spoiled gradient recalled acquisition in the steady state T1 weighted image (repetition time ms/echo time ms/inversion time ms, 11/5/500) from a 5-month-old female with Krabbe disease showing enlargement of the optic chiasm (*thin arrow*) and abnormal hypointense signal in the cervical spinal cord consistent with dysmyelination and/or demyelination (*thick arrow*). (*B*) Coronal fat-saturated T2WI (repetition time ms/echo time ms, 4000/90) from a 5-month-old female with Krabbe disease showing excessive hyperintensity in the deep parietal white matter for patient age (*arrows*). (*C*) Coronal fat-saturated T2WI (repetition time ms/echo time ms, 4000/90) from a 5-month-old female with Krabbe disease demonstrating abnormal hyperintensity in the hila of the dentate nuclei (*white arrows*). The dentate nuclei proper are spared (*black arrows*). (*D*) Axial CT image through the basal ganglia in a 5-month-old female with Krabbe disease showing ill-defined hyperattenuation consistent with mineralization in the lentiform nuclei, posterior internal capsules, and lateral thalami (*arrows*).

discovered, attention should be turned to the bones. Typical involvement of the axial and appendicular skeleton presents as concurrent dysostosis multiplex. These patients require dedicated cervical spine imaging because craniocervical junction instability and foramen magnum stenosis may coexist. Meningoencephalocele has also been described in mucopolysacharidosis.[87]

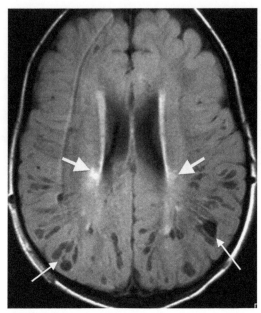

Fig. 15. Hurler syndrome. Axial T2 fluid attenuation inversion recovery image (repetition time ms/echo time ms, 11,000/125) from a 35-month-old male with Hurler syndrome (mucopolysacharidosis type I) demonstrating numerous enlarged perivascular spaces (*thin arrows*) and paraventricular white matter hyperintensity (*thick arrows*).

SUMMARY

Structural brain abnormalities are not uncommon in the context of IEM, especially those affecting energetics. Discovery of brain malformations should prompt a detailed search for signs of an underlying cause; symmetric brain signal abnormality may suggest an IEM in this setting. Likewise, patients with suspected metabolic disease should be scrutinized for coexistent brain malformations.

Best Practices

What is the current practice?

The imaging classification scheme of inborn errors of metabolism (IEM) is based mainly on the location of brain signal and/or attenuation abnormalities with little regard to concurrent structural brain anomalies. However, coexistent brain anomalies may represent a key element for the generation of a tailored differential diagnosis, adding diagnostic specificity to an otherwise nonspecific clinical presentation.

What changes in current practice are likely to improve outcomes?

Recognition of specific MRI and MR spectroscopy (MRS) disease patterns help to define and classify IEM-associated brain dysgenesis; the differential diagnosis can be narrowed and clues toward the underlying diagnosis can be revealed.

Major Recommendations

Discovery of either symmetric brain signal alteration or structural defects on brain MRI should prompt a detailed search the other.

Clinical Algorithm(s)

Brain MRI and MRS should be obtained in all patients with signs and symptoms referable to brain defects and/or inborn metabolic errors.

Bibliographic Source(s)

Patay Z. Metabolic disorders. In: Tortori-Donati P, Rossi A. Pediatric neuroradiology: brain, head, neck and spine. 1st edition. Berlin: Springer; 2009. p. 158–60.

Barkovich JA, Patay Z. Metabolic, toxic, and inflammatory brain disorders. In: Barkovich AJ, Raybaud C, editors Pediatric neuroimaging, 5th edition. Philadelphia: Lippincott Williams & Wilkins; 2012. p. 81–3.

Prasad AN, Malinger G, Lerman-Sagie T. Primary disorders of metabolism and disturbed fetal brain development. Clin Perinatol 2009;36(3):621–38.

Brassier A, Ottolenghi C, Boddaert N, et al. Prenatal symptoms and diagnosis of inherited metabolic diseases. Arch Pediatr 2012;19(9):959–69.

Nissenkorn A, Michelson M, Ben-Zeev B, et al. Inborn errors of metabolism: a cause of abnormal brain development. Neurology 2001;56:1265–72.

Bamforth FJ, Bamforth JS, Applegarth DA. Structural anomalies in patients with inherited metabolic diseases. J Inherit Metab Dis 1994;17(3):330–2.

Bamforth F, Bamforth S, Poskitt K, et al. Abnormalities of corpus callosum in patients with inherited metabolic diseases [letter]. Lancet 1988;2(8608):451.

Kolodny EH, Agenesis of the corpus callosum: a marker for inherited metabolic disease? Neurology 1989;39:847–8.

Dobyns WB. Agenesis of the corpus callosum and gyral malformations are frequent manifestations of nonketotic hyperglycinemia. Neurology 1989;39:817–20.

Summary Statement

IEM-associated brain dysgenesis manifests symmetric brain signal abnormality and concurrent brain dysgenesis. Specific patterns of brain signal alteration, structural defects, and spectroscopic abnormalities help narrow the differential diagnosis.

REFERENCES

1. Pérez-Dueñas B, De La Osa A, Capdevila A, et al. Brain injury in glutaric aciduria type I: the value of functional techniques in magnetic resonance imaging. Eur J Paediatr Neurol 2009;13(6):534–40.
2. Gropman AL. Neuroimaging in mitochondrial disorders. Neurotherapeutics 2013; 10(2):273–85.
3. Radmanesh A, Zaman T, Ghanaati H, et al. Methylmalonic acidemia: brain imaging findings in 52 children and a review of the literature. Pediatr Radiol 2008; 38(10):1054–61.
4. Basser PJ. Inferring microstructural features and the physiological state of tissues from diffusion-weighted images. NMR Biomed 1995;8(7–8):333–44.
5. Cakmakci H, Pekcevik Y, Yis U, et al. Diagnostic value of proton MR spectroscopy and diffusion-weighted MR imaging in childhood inherited neurometabolic brain diseases and review of the literature. Eur J Radiol 2010;74(3): e161–71.
6. Panigrahy A, Nelson MD Jr, Blüml S. Magnetic resonance spectroscopy in pediatric neuroradiology: clinical and research applications. Pediatr Radiol 2010; 40(1):3–30.

7. Brooks WM, Friedman SD, Stidley CA. Reproducibility of 1H-MRS in vivo. Magn Reson Med 1999;41(1):193–7.
8. Chard DT, McLean MA, Parker GJ, et al. Reproducibility of in vivo metabolite quantification with proton magnetic resonance spectroscopic imaging. J Magn Reson Imaging 2002;15(2):219–25.
9. Pfeuffer J, Tkac I, Provencher SW, et al. Toward an in vivo neurochemical profile: quantification of 18 metabolites in short-echo-time (1)H NMR spectra of the rat brain. J Magn Reson 1999;141(1):104–20.
10. Bowman C. A multiscale model for Bayesian image segmentation. IEEE Trans Med Imaging 1994;3:162–77.
11. Whitwell JL, Crum WR, Watt HC, et al. Normalization of cerebral volumes by use of intracranial volume: implications for longitudinal quantitative MR imaging. AJNR Am J Neuroradiol 2001;22(8):1483–9.
12. Patay Z. Metabolic disorders. In: Tortori-Donati P, Rossi A, editors. Pediatric neuroradiology: brain, head, neck and spine. Berlin: Springer; 2009. p. 158–60.
13. Barkovich JA, Patay Z. Metabolic, toxic, and inflammatory brain disorders. In: Barkovich AJ, Raybaud C, editors. Pediatric neuroimaging. 5th edition. Philadelphia: Lippincott Williams & Wilkins; 2012. p. 81–3.
14. Prasad AN, Malinger G, Lerman-Sagie T. Primary disorders of metabolism and disturbed fetal brain development. Clin Perinatol 2009;36(3):621–38.
15. Brassier A, Ottolenghi C, Boddaert N, et al. Prenatal symptoms and diagnosis of inherited metabolic diseases. Arch Pediatr 2012;19(9):959–69.
16. Nissenkorn A, Michelson M, Ben-Zeev B, et al. Inborn errors of metabolism: a cause of abnormal brain development. Neurology 2001;56:1265–72.
17. Bamforth FJ, Bamforth JS, Applegarth DA. Structural anomalies in patients with inherited metabolic diseases. J Inherit Metab Dis 1994;17(3):330–2.
18. Bamforth F, Bamforth S, Poskitt K, et al. Abnormalities of corpus callosum in patients with inherited metabolic diseases [letter]. Lancet 1988;2(8608):451.
19. Kolodny EH. Agenesis of the corpus callosum: a marker for inherited metabolic disease? Neurology 1989;39:847–8.
20. Dobyns WB. Agenesis of the corpus callosum and gyral malformations are frequent manifestations of nonketotic hyperglycinemia. Neurology 1989;39:817–20.
21. Fleck MS, Samei E, Mitroff SR. Generalized "satisfaction of search": adverse influences on dual-target search accuracy. J Exp Psychol Appl 2010;16(1):60–71.
22. Leijser LM, de Vries LS, Rutherford MA, et al. Cranial ultrasound in metabolic disorders presenting in the neonatal period: characteristic features and comparison with MR imaging. AJNR Am J Neuroradiol 2007;28(7):1223–31.
23. Mochel F, Grebille AG, Benachi A, et al. Contribution of fetal MR imaging in the prenatal diagnosis of Zellweger syndrome. AJNR Am J Neuroradiol 2006;27(2):333–6.
24. Robinson JN, Norwitz ER, Mulkern R, et al. Prenatal diagnosis of pyruvate dehydrogenase deficiency using magnetic resonance imaging. Prenat Diagn 2001;21(12):1053–6.
25. Righini A, Fiori L, Parazzini C, et al. Early prenatal magnetic resonance imaging of glutaric aciduria type 1: case report. J Comput Assist Tomogr 2010;34(3):446–8.
26. Volpe J. Neuronal proliferation, migration, organization and myelination. In: Volpe J, editor. Neurology of the newborn. 3rd edition. Philadelphia: WB Saunders; 1995. p. 43–94.
27. Montenegro MA, Gerreiro MM, Lopes-Cendes I, et al. Interrelationship of genetics and prenatal injury in the genesis of malformations of cortical development. Arch Neurol 2002;59:1147–53.

28. Choksi V, Hoeffner E, Karaarslan E, et al. Infantile refsum disease: case report. AJNR Am J Neuroradiol 2003;24:2082–4.
29. Cakirer S, Savas MR. Infantile refsum disease: serial evaluation with MRI. Pediatr Radiol 2005;35(2):212–5.
30. Barkovich AJ, Peck WW. MR of Zellweger syndrome. AJNR Am J Neuroradiol 1997;18(6):1163–70.
31. van der Knaap MS, Valk J. The MR spectrum of peroxisomal disorders. Neuroradiology 1991;33(1):30–7.
32. Bruhn H, Kruse B, Korenke GC, et al. Proton NMR spectroscopy of cerebral metabolic alterations in infantile peroxisomal disorders. J Compt Assist Tomogr 1992; 16(3):335–44.
33. Cecil KM, Lindquist DM. Leukodystrophies. In: Bluml S, Panigrahy A, editors. MR Spectroscopy of pediatric brain disorders. New York: Springer; 2013. p. 105–22.
34. Kerrigan JF, Aleck KA, Tarby TJ, et al. Fumaric aciduria: clinical and imaging features. Ann Neurol 2000;47(5):583–8.
35. Farrell DF. Neonatal adrenoleukodystrophy: a clinical, pathologic, and biochemical study. Pediatr Neurol 2012;47(5):330–6.
36. Goh S. Neuroimaging features in a neonate with rhizomelic chondrodysplasia punctata. Pediatr Neurol 2007;37(5):382–4.
37. Viola A, Confort-Gouny S, Ranjeva JP, et al. MR imaging and MR spectroscopy in rhizomelic chondrodysplasia punctata. AJNR Am J Neuroradiol 2002;23: 480–3.
38. Barkovich AJ. Neuroimaging manifestations and classification of congenital muscular dystrophies. AJNR Am J Neuroradiol 1998;19(8):1389–96.
39. Rhodes RE, Hatten HP Jr, Ellington KS. Walker-Warburg syndrome. AJNR Am J Neuroradiol 1992;13(1):123–6.
40. Aida N, Yagishita A, Takada K, et al. Cerebellar MR in Fukuyama congenital muscular dystrophy: polymicrogyria with cystic lesions. AJNR Am J Neuroradiol 1994;15(9):1755–9.
41. Aida N, Tamagawa K, Takada K, et al. Brain MR in Fukuyama congenital muscular dystrophy. AJNR Am J Neuroradiol 1996;17(4):605–13.
42. Yoshioka M, Saiwai S, Kuroki S, et al. MR imaging of the brain in Fukuyama-type congenital muscular dystrophy. AJNR Am J Neuroradiol 1991;12(1):63–5.
43. Kato Z, Morimoto M, Orii KE, et al. Developmental changes of radiological findings in Fukuyama-type congenital muscular dystrophy. Pediatr Radiol 2010; 40(Suppl 1):S127–9.
44. Sonninen P, Autti T, Varho T, et al. Brain involvement in Salla disease. AJNR Am J Neuroradiol 1999;20(3):433–43.
45. Raybaud C. The corpus callosum, the other great forebrain commissures, and the septum pellucidum: anatomy, development, and malformation. Neuroradiology 2010;52:447–77.
46. Baertling F, Rodenburg JR, Schaper J, et al. A guide to diagnosis and treatment of Leigh syndrome. J Neurol Neurosurg Psychiatry 2014;85:257–65.
47. Moroni I, Bugiani M, Bizzi A, et al. Cerebral white matter involvement in children with mitochondrial encephalopathies. Neuropediatrics 2002;33(2):79–85.
48. Rubio-Gozalbo ME, Heerschap A, Trijbels JM, et al. Proton MR spectroscopy in a child with pyruvate dehydrogenase complex deficiency. Magn Reson Imaging 1999;17(6):939–44.
49. Zand DJ, Simon EM, Pulitzer SB, et al. In vivo pyruvate detected by MR spectroscopy in neonatal pyruvate dehydrogenase deficiency. AJNR Am J Neuroradiol 2003;24(7):1471–4.

50. Mourmans J, Majoie CB, Barth PG, et al. Sequential MR imaging changes in non-ketotic hyperglycinemia. AJNR Am J Neuroradiol 2006;27(1):208–11.

51. Kelley RL, Roessler E, Hennekam RC, et al. Holoprosencephaly in RSH/Smith-Lemli-Opitz syndrome: does abnormal cholesterol metabolism affect the function of Sonic Hedgehog? Am J Med Genet 1996;66(4):478–84.

52. Lee RW, Conley SK, Gropman A, et al. Brain magnetic resonance imaging findings in Smith-Lemili-Opitz syndrome. Am J Med Genet A 2013;161(10):2407–19.

53. Caruso PA, Poussaint TY, Tzika AA, et al. MRI and 1H MRS findings in Smith-Lemli-Opitz syndrome. Neuroradiology 2004;46(1):3–14.

54. Cecil KM, Lindquist DM. Metabolic disorders. In: Bluml S, Panigrahy A, editors. MR spectroscopy of pediatric brain disorders. New York: Springer; 2013. p. 123–48.

55. Varho T, Komu M, Sonninen P, et al. A new metabolite contributing to N-acetyl signal in 1H MRS of the brain in Salla disease. Neurology 1999;52(8):1668–72 [Erratum appears in Neurology 1999;53(5):1162].

56. Aynaci FM, Mocan H, Bahadir S, et al. A case of Menkes' syndrome associated with deafness and inferior cerebellar vermian hypoplasia. Acta Paediatr 1997; 86(1):121–3.

57. Poretti A, Wolf NI, Boltshauser E. Differential diagnosis of cerebellar atrophy in childhood. Eur J Paediatr Neurol 2008;12(3):155–67.

58. Bindu PS, Taly AB, Sonam K, et al. Bilateral hypertrophic olivary nucleus degeneration on magnetic resonance imaging in children with Leigh and Leigh-like syndrome. Br J Radiol 2014;87(1034):20130478.

59. Feraco P, Mirabelli-Badenier M, Severino M, et al. The shrunken, bright cerebellum: a characteristic MRI finding in congenital disorders of glycosylation type 1a. AJNR Am J Neuroradiol 2012;33(11):2062–7.

60. Holzbach U, Hanefeld F, Helms G, et al. Localized proton magnetic spectroscopy of cerebral abnormalities in children with carbohydrate-deficient glycoprotein syndrome. Acta Paediatr 1995;84:781–6.

61. Etchevers HC, Vincent C, Le Douarin NM, et al. The cephalic neural crest provides pericytes and smooth muscle cells to all blood vessels of the face and forebrain. Development 2001;128(7):1059–68.

62. Eeg-Olofsson O, Zhang WW, Olsson Y, et al. D-2-hydroxyglutaric aciduria with cerebral, vascular, and muscular abnormalities in a 14-year-old boy. J Child Neurol 2000;15:488–92.

63. van der Knaap MS, Jakobs C, Hoffmann GF, et al. D-2-hydroxyglutaric aciduria: further clinical delineation. J Inherit Metab Dis 1999;22:404–13.

64. Takahashi S, Ishii K, Matsumoto K, et al. Cranial MRI and MR angiography in Menkes' syndrome. Neuroradiology 1993;35(7):556–8.

65. Jacobs DS, Smith AS, Finelli DA, et al. Menkes kinky hair disease: characteristic MR angiographic findings. AJNR Am J Neuroradiol 1993;14(5):1160–3.

66. Ito H, Mori K, Sakata M, et al. Transient left temporal lobe lesion in Menkes disease may influence the generation of tonic spasms. Brain Dev 2011;33(4):345–8.

67. Bekiesinska-Figatowska M, Rokicki D, Walecki J, et al. Menkes' disease with a Dandy-Walker variant: case report. Neuroradiology 2001;43(11):948–50.

68. Jamjoom ZA, Okamoto E, Jamjoom AH, et al. Bilateral arachnoid cysts of the sylvian region in female siblings with glutaric aciduria type I. Report of two cases. J Neurosurg 1995;82(6):1078–81.

69. Martinez-Lage JF, Casas C, FernÌÁndez MA, et al. Macrocephaly, dystonia, and bilateral temporal arachnoid cysts: glutaric aciduria type 1. Childs Nerv Syst 1994;10(3):198–203.

70. Lutcherath V, Waaler PE, Jellum E, et al. Children with bilateral temporal arachnoid cysts may have glutaric aciduria Type 1 (GAT1); operation without knowing that may be harmful. Acta Neurochir (Wien) 2000;142(9):1025–30.

71. Forstner R, Hoffmann GF, Gassner I, et al. Glutaric aciduria type I: ultrasonographic demonstration of early signs. Pediatr Radiol 1999;29(2):138–43.

72. Nunes J, Loureiro S, Carvalho S, et al. Brain MRI findings as an important diagnostic clue in glutaric aciduria type 1. Neuroradiol J 2013;26(2):155–61.

73. Santos CC, Roach ES. Glutaric aciduria type I: a neuroimaging diagnosis? J Child Neurol 2005;20(7):588–90.

74. Twomey EL, Naughten ER, Donoghue VB, et al. Neuroimaging findings in glutaric aciduria type 1. Pediatr Radiol 2003;33(12):823–30.

75. Oguz KK, Ozturk A, Cila A. Diffusion-weighted MR imaging and MR spectroscopy in glutaric aciduria type 1. Neuroradiology 2005;47(3):229–34.

76. Takanashi J, Fujii K, Sugita K, et al. Neuroradiologic findings in glutaric aciduria type II. Pediatr Neurol 1999;20(2):142–5.

77. Bohm N, Uy J, Kiessling M, et al. Multiple acyl-CoA dehydrogenation deficiency (glutaric aciduria type II), congenital polycystic kidneys, and symmetric warty dysplasia of the cerebral cortex in two newborn brothers. Morphology and pathogenesis. Eur J Pediatr 1982;139(1):60–5.

78. Neumaier-Probst E, Harting I, Seitz A, et al. Neuroradiological findings in glutaric aciduria type I (glutaryl-CoA dehydrogenase deficiency). Review. J Inherit Metab Dis 2004;27(6):869–76.

79. Frei KP, Patronas NJ, Crutchfield KE, et al. Mucolipidosis type IV: characteristic MRI findings. Neurology 1998;51(2):565–9.

80. Bonavita S, Virta A, Jeffries N, et al. Diffuse neuroaxonal involvement in mucolipidosis IV as assessed by proton magnetic resonance spectroscopic imaging. J Child Neurol 2003;18(7):443–9.

81. Patel B, Gimi B, Vachha B, et al. Optic nerve and chiasm enlargement in a case of infantile Krabbe disease: quantitative comparison with 26 age-matched controls. Pediatr Radiol 2008;38(6):697–9.

82. Beslow LA, Schwartz ES, Bonnemann CG. Thickening and enhancement of multiple cranial nerves in conjunction with cystic white matter lesions in early infantile Krabbe disease. Pediatr Radiol 2008;38(6):694–6.

83. Hittmair K, Wimberger D, Wiesbauer P, et al. Early infantile form of Krabbe disease with optic hypertrophy: serial MR examinations and autopsy correlation. AJNR Am J Neuroradiol 1994;15(8):1454–8.

84. Zarifi MK, Tzika AA, Astrakas LG, et al. Magnetic resonance spectroscopy and magnetic resonance imaging findings in Krabbe's disease. J Child Neurol 2001;16:522–6.

85. Alqahtani E, Huisman TA, Boltshauser E, et al. Mucopolysacharidoses type I and II: new neuroimaging findings in the cerebellum. Eur J Paediatr Neurol 2014; 18(2):211–7.

86. Zafeiriou DI, Batzios SP. Brain and spinal MR imaging findings in mucopolysaccharidoses: a review. AJNR Am J Neuroradiol 2013;34(1):5–13.

87. Manara R, Priante E, Grimaldi M, et al. Closed Meningo(encephalo)cele: a new feature in Hunter syndrome. AJNR Am J Neuroradiol 2012;33(5):873–7.

Neonatal Hypotonia

Susan E. Sparks, MD, PhD

KEYWORDS

- Hypotonia • Congenital • Weakness • Muscular dystrophy • Myotonia • Syndrome

KEY POINTS

- Determining the cause of hypotonia requires a detailed history and physical examination aided by diagnostic and laboratory evaluations.
- Medical genetic and neurologic consultations will help establish the diagnostic etiology of neonatal hypotonia.
- Advances in multidisciplinary medical care, home health care, and respiratory and nutritional support have led to longer lives at home for patients with severe hypotonia.

INTRODUCTION

Hypotonia, or low muscle tone, is defined by decreased resistance to passive movement, and may or may not be associated with decreased muscle strength or weakness. Recognition of hypotonia in the newborn may be straightforward, but determining the cause may be a challenge. The physical examination, including a detailed neurologic examination, is important in localizing the site of a defect within the nervous system (ie, central vs peripheral). History along with basic laboratory testing and imaging aids in the differential diagnosis. Identification of the cause is essential for determining the prognosis for the infant, associated morbidities, and the recurrence risk. Some disorders may have a specific treatment; however, the prevailing therapeutic modality comprises physical, occupational, speech/feeding, and respiratory therapy.[1–5]

CLINICAL PRESENTATION

A newborn term infant presents with poor respiratory effort and abnormal suck and swallow after a pregnancy complicated by decreased fetal movement. The baby

Disclosures: Dr S.E. Sparks receives grant funding from NIH (grant number P50 AR060836) and MDA. She is involved in clinical research studies with Genzyme, BioMarin, Sarepta, and Eli Lilly. She is on Advisory Boards for BioMarin and Sarepta.
Department of Pediatrics, Carolinas Healthcare System, 1000 Blythe Boulevard, Charlotte, NC 28203, USA
E-mail address: Susan.sparks@carolinashealthcare.org

was born by cesarean section because of breech presentation. Physical examination shows no dysmorphic features but significant hypotonia, with tongue fasciculations and absent deep tendon reflexes. The family history is negative for any muscle or neurologic disease, early infant deaths, or consanguinity. Examination of the mother is normal (specifically evaluating for signs of myotonia). What are the approaches to aid in the diagnosis and management of this infant? **Table 1** outlines the differential diagnosis and various evaluations that can be used in the diagnostic process.

DIAGNOSTIC ALGORITHM

Several approaches to a diagnostic algorithm for neonatal hypotonia have been proposed, consisting mainly of either a tree-structured approach based on the distinction between central and peripheral hypotonia[1,4–6] or a sequential method considering successively available tests according to their diagnostic yield.[7] Laugel and colleagues[8] proposed a combined approach involving the following:

1. History and physical examination
2. Neuroimaging/evaluation for congenital malformations
3. Medical genetic and neurogenetic evaluations (Oxford Medical Databases)
4. Karyotype, fluorescence in situ hybridization (FISH), microarray analysis
5. Biochemical evaluation (ammonia, lactate, amino acids, organic acids, very long chain fatty acids, carnitine/acylcarnitine profile, 7-dehydrocholesterol, transferrin isoelectric focusing, N- and O-glycan analysis, galactose-1-phosphate)
6. Muscle and nerve investigations (electromyography [EMG], nerve conduction velocity [NCV], muscle biopsy)
7. Other specific genetic testing

DIAGNOSTIC EVALUATION

Clinical evaluation of tone may be difficult in infants. Quantifiable measures, such as the Ashworth scales, may be useful in older children with serial measures, but reliability is questionable, especially in infants.[9] There are 4 standard maneuvers that can be used in assessing tone, particularly low tone, in infants. (1) "Pull to sit," whereby the infant is pulled by the arms from a supine to sitting position and a significant head lag is observed in the hypotonic infant. This reaction is also known as the traction response of the infant, whereby typically the infant attempts to counter this maneuver by flexion of the arms. (2) The "scarf sign," whereby an infant's arm is pulled across the chest to the opposite shoulder and there is minimal resistance, and the arm appears like a scarf across the hypotonic baby. (3) The hypotonic infant held under the arms requires significant support or the baby would slip through the evaluator's arms when held in "shoulder/axillary suspension." (4) "Vertical suspension," whereby the baby is suspended prone by the evaluator's hand under the abdomen/chest and the response of the baby's trunk, neck, and extremities are evaluated. Typically the baby will straighten the back, flex the limbs, and intermittently attempt to hold the head straight, whereas the hypotonic baby droops over the evaluator's palm loosely in the shape of a "U" with arms and legs dangling.[10]

Localization of hypotonia to central (ie, the brain and brainstem, either diffusely or focally) or peripheral (any component of the motor unit: anterior horn cell, peripheral nerve, neuromuscular junction, muscle itself) causes helps to further determine the cause of the hypotonia (**Table 2**).[11]

In the structured assessment of an infant with hypotonia, the history in conjunction with the physical examination may give clues to the cause. The history includes prenatal, perinatal/birth, and family history. Clues from the history can yield potential causes of the hypotonia (**Table 3**).

Physical examination will also determine whether there the hypotonia has a syndromic or nonsyndromic cause. If an infant with hypotonia has dysmorphic facial features, congenital malformations, or both, the standard of care is to obtain a chromosomal microarray (by either single nucleotide polymorphism or comparative genomic hybridization) to evaluate for chromosomal deletions and duplications. If the features are classic for a particular syndrome, such as Down syndrome or 22q11.2 deletion syndrome (velo-cardio-facial/Di George syndrome), a karyotype or specific FISH test, respectively, is more specific and cost effective (**Table 4**).

Once an infant is determined to be hypotonic and nondysmorphic, weakness or strength should be evaluated. This evaluation may be difficult if there are systemic symptoms (ie, infection, altered mental status) or if the baby is on systemic medications such as neuromuscular blocking agents (often needed because of respiratory failure), and sedatives. Strength is the voluntary resistance to a movement that for evaluation requires that the patient actively resist with maximum effort, which of course may be challenging in infants. There is no direct measurement of muscle strength in infants, but it may be assessed by observing the awake/alert infant. Typically an infant has many vigorous movements of the arms and legs, whereas a weak infant will have diminished or no spontaneous movements.[10]

LABORATORY AND OTHER TESTING

Laboratory testing of creatine kinase (CK) and aldolase may be helpful if there is a muscular dystrophy, but often is normal in infants with hypotonia. In addition, it can be falsely elevated after difficult deliveries. Elevated alanine aminotransferase (ALT) or aspartate aminotransferase (AST) may be an indication of muscle disease rather than liver disease. The diagnostic evaluation should also include assessment for infection (complete blood count, cultures, and so forth) and inborn errors of metabolism. Basic metabolic evaluations include blood gas and chemistries for metabolic acidosis and hypoglycemia, ammonia, orotic acid and plasma amino acids for urea cycle defects, urine organic acids and acyl carnitine profile for organic acidemias, plasma acyl carnitine and total carnitine for fatty acid oxidation defects, and plasma lactate and pyruvate for disorders of carbohydrate metabolism, defects of energy metabolism, and mitochondrial disorders. More specific biochemical testing can include very long chain fatty acids and plasmalogens for peroxisomal defects, 7-dehydrocholesterol for Smith-Lemli-Opitz syndrome, transferring isoelectric focusing/N-glycan and O-glycan analysis for congenital disorders of glycosylation, and specific lysosomal enzyme testing for Pompe disease, which presents with hypotonia and cardiomyopathy. Consultation with a clinical geneticist or metabolic physician is warranted to prioritize these evaluations.[5]

Chromosomal analysis (routine karyotype for Down syndrome [trisomy 21] and analysis for microdeletions/duplications either by chromosomal microarray or specific testing by FISH) may aid in the diagnosis when there are specific physical facial features or congenital malformations present. Methylation analysis of the chromosome region of 15q11-q13 for Prader-Willi syndrome (PWS) can detect 99% of the cases of PWS in comparison with FISH for deletion of chromosome 15q11-q13, which

Table 1
Differential diagnosis of hypotonia

Localization	Disorders	History and Physical Examination Features	Evaluations That Aid in Diagnosis
Central hypotonia may have altered mental status, increased deep tendon reflexes, Babinski sign, persistent infantile reflexes	HIE	Premature birth, difficult delivery	Brain MRI
	Intracranial hemorrhage		Brain MRI
	Cerebral malformations	May be noted on prenatal ultrasonography	Brain MRI
	Chromosomal abnormalities	Dysmorphic features, congenital malformations	Karyotype/array CGH
	Congenital infections	Prenatal history	Infectious cultures/evaluation
	Acquired infections		Infectious cultures
	Peroxisomal disorders	Dysmorphic features	Very long chain fatty acids
	Inborn errors of metabolism		Metabolic acidosis, hyperammonemia, hypoglycemia, lactic acidosis
	Maternal and infant drug effects	Prenatal and perinatal history of drug exposure	Toxicology screen
Spinal cord	Birth trauma	History of trauma	Brain MRI
	HIE		Spine MRI
	Syringomyelia		
Anterior horn cell	Spinal muscular atrophy	Diminished/absent deep tendon reflexes, muscle fasciculations	SMN1 copy number analysis

Neuromuscular junction	Myasthenia gravis: Transient acquired neonatal myasthenia Congenital myasthenia gravis	Easy fatigability, recurrent aspiration, feeding difficulty	EMG Responds to anticholinesterase Inhibitors
	Infantile botulism	Facial weakness and pupillary abnormality	ECG may show heart block Presence of toxin in food
	Drug toxicity (magnesium, aminoglycosides)	History of drug exposure	Plasma and urine drug levels
Peripheral nerves	Hereditary motor and sensory neuropathies	Diminished/absent DTRs, absent Babinski and infantile reflexes	EMG/NCV may be helpful; DNA sequencing
	Congenital hypomyelinating neuropathy	Family history	DNA sequencing
	Giant axonal neuropathy	Family history	DNA sequencing
Muscle	Muscular dystrophies	Family history	May have elevated serum CK and aldolase, ALT and AST may be elevated from muscle rather than liver; muscle biopsy
	Congenital myopathies	Family history	Muscle biopsy
	Metabolic myopathies	Family history	May have elevated serum CK, aldolase, ALT, and AST; muscle biopsy
	Congenital myotonic dystrophy	Family history; maternal myotonia	CTG-repeat analysis of DMPK

Abbreviations: ALT, alanine aminotransferase; AST, aspartate aminotransferase; CGH, comparative genomic hybridization; CK, creatine kinase; DTRs, deep tendon reflexes; ECG, electrocardiogram; EMG, electromyogram; HIE, hypoxic ischemic encephalopathy; MRI, magnetic resonance imaging; NCV, nerve conduction velocity.

Table 2
Central versus peripheral hypotonia

Characteristic	Central Hypotonia	Peripheral Hypotonia
Weakness	Mild to moderate	Significant
Deep tendon reflexes	Decreased or increased	Absent
Babinski sign	Present	Absent
Infantile reflexes	Persistent	Absent
Pull to sit	Some head lag	Marked head lag
Muscle mass	Normal or disuse atrophy	Prominent atrophy

only detects a deletion in 70% of the cases of PWS. In addition to hypotonia, individuals with PWS may have genital abnormalities and feeding difficulties alongside failure to thrive. Later complications include hyperphagia with obesity, short stature, and cognitive impairment.[12]

Imaging of the brain (computed tomography, magnetic resonance imaging [MRI], magnetic resonance spectroscopy) and spine (MRI) can be helpful in identifying structural changes that may contribute to the infant's hypotonia. Migration defects and

Table 3
Medical history and hypotonia

History	Feature	Comments
Prenatal	Maternal infection	
	Decreased movement	
	Teratogen exposure	
	Maternal diseases (diabetes/seizures)	Maternal systemic lupus erythematosus
	Breech presentation	Suggests decreased fetal movement
	Polyhydramnios	
	Shortened umbilical cord	Suggests decreased fetal movement
Birth	Trauma/delivery complications	
	Maternal Infection	Neonatal infection: Group B *Streptococcus*, *Escherichia coli*, etc
	Maternal delivery medications	
	Anoxia/hypoxia	
	Need for ventilator support	
Family	Neuromuscular disorders	
	Maternal myotonia (shake mom's hand to assess for myotonia; slow release)	Congenital myotonic dystrophy
	Parental age	Advanced maternal age is associated with increased risk of chromosomal aneuploidy
		Advanced paternal age is associated with increased risk of de novo mutations and new dominant diseases
	Consanguinity	Increased risk for autosomal recessive conditions
	Early infant deaths	

Table 4
Syndromes associated with hypotonia

Syndrome	Examination Feature	Diagnostic Test
Down syndrome (trisomy 21)	Characteristic facial features (microbrachycephaly, epicanthal folds, upslanting palpebral fissures, flat nasal bridge), short neck with redundant skin, single palmar creases, space between first and second toes; congenital heart defect	Peripheral blood karyotype
Prader-Willi syndrome	Feeding difficulties, failure to thrive, hypogonadism	Fluorescence in situ hybridization (FISH)/methylation analysis of SNRPN in chromosome region 15q11–13
Achondroplasia	Frontal bossing, rhizomelic shortening of bones	Molecular testing of FGFR3
Smith-Lemli-Opitz syndrome	Microcephaly, characteristic facial features (ptosis of eyelids, anteverted nostrils, low-set ears, micrognathia), 2–3 toe syndactyly	7-Dehydrocholesterol reductase deficiency with abnormal plasma elevations of 7-dehydrocholesterol
Trisomy 18	Intrauterine growth restriction, prominent occiput and bitemporal narrowing, low-set, malformed ears, narrow palate, micrognathia, clenched hands with index finger over third and fifth finger over fourth finger, hypoplastic nails, crossed legs and rocker bottom feet	Peripheral blood karyotype
Trisomy 13	Small size, holoprosencephaly, cleft lip/palate, scalp defects, multiple congenital anomalies	Peripheral blood karyotype
Other chromosomal deletions/duplications	Dysmorphic facial features, major/minor congenital anomalies	Comparative genomic hybridization/FISH for specific syndromes
Zellweger/other peroxisomal disorders	High forehead with flat facies, hepatomegaly	Very long chain fatty acids and plasmalogens
Congenital disorders of glycosylation	Inverted nipples, abnormal fat distribution, cerebellar hypoplasia on brain MRI	Transferrin isoelectric focusing/N-glycan analysis/O-glycan analysis

signal abnormalities in the white matter and basal ganglia, or certain structural abnormalities, may be pathognomonic for specific diagnoses.

NCV and EMG studies can be helpful in localizing the defect, but can be technically difficult and sometimes demanding to interpret in the newborn and young infant. EMG is very accurate in the diagnosis of spinal muscular atrophy,[13] and NCV is helpful in investigating hereditary motor sensory neuropathies by distinguishing between axonal and demyelinating conditions.[14] These studies can also be helpful in distinguishing between a neuronal and a myopathic process[15] and in the diagnosis of a neuromuscular transmission defect (congenital myasthenia gravis).[5] Though useful for muscular dystrophies and congenital myopathies, EMG has missed metabolic myopathies.[16]

Muscle biopsy is helpful if muscular dystrophy or myopathy is suspected.[17] Basic histology can identify myopathic, neuropathic, and dystrophic changes. Immunohistochemical techniques using antibodies against muscle-specific proteins are helpful in the diagnosis of muscular dystrophies and myopathies.[18] Electron microscopy can identify abnormalities of organelles (such as mitochondria), and identify inclusions and storage material.[19]

When screening tests and evaluations suggest a particular diagnosis, specific molecular and genetic testing can be done to confirm the diagnosis. However, without examination or evaluation clues to aid the clinician, deciding which tests to order may be difficult. Newer genetic testing with panels and whole exome analysis may be useful in the future. However, results may be difficult to interpret, as variants of unknown clinical significance are common until more research has been done. In addition, disorders such as chromosomal abnormalities (Down syndrome, microdeletion syndromes), congenital myotonic dystrophy (trinucleotide repeat disorder), spinal muscular atrophy (intragenic deletion), and PWS (methylation defect) are not identified by clinical exome analysis, which is sequence based.

Several studies have evaluated the diagnostic yield and etiology of neonatal hypotonia. In one such study,[8] a retrospective chart review of 144 neonates determined a cause in 83% of the cases, and a diagnostic algorithm was proposed. Other studies have had yields of 67% to 85%,[20–22] with a majority (80%) of the causes being identified by history and physical examination.

SUMMARY

Neonatal hypotonia can be daunting for a clinician, as there are many diagnostic possibilities. However, with a careful history and physical examination, accompanied by directed supplementary evaluations, a correct diagnosis can often be achieved. Adopting this approach is important for counseling parents with regard to anticipated outcomes and recurrence risk, and ensuring comprehensive management for the patient. Advances in multidisciplinary medical care, home health care, and respiratory and nutritional support have led to longer lives at home for patients with severe hypotonia.

REFERENCES

1. Crawford TO. Clinical evaluation of the floppy infant. Pediatr Ann 1992;21(6): 348–54.
2. Bodensteiner JB. The evaluation of the hypotonic infant. Semin Pediatr Neurol 2008;15(1):10–20.
3. Johnston HM. The floppy weak infant revisited. Brain Dev 2003;25(3):155–8.
4. Miller VS, Delgado M, Iannaccone ST. Neonatal hypotonia. Semin Neurol 1993; 13(1):73–83.

5. Prasad AN, Prasad C. The floppy infant: contribution of genetic and metabolic disorders. Brain Dev 2003;25(7):457–76.
6. Vasta I, Kinali M, Messina S, et al. Can clinical signs identify newborns with neuromuscular disorders? J Pediatr 2005;146(1):73–9.
7. Paro-Panjan D, Neubauer D. Congenital hypotonia: is there an algorithm? J Child Neurol 2004;19(6):439–42.
8. Laugel V, Cossee M, Matis J, et al. Diagnostic approach to neonatal hypotonia: retrospective study on 144 neonates. Eur J Pediatr 2008;167(5):517–23.
9. Kaufman HH, Bodensteiner J, Burkart B, et al. Treatment of spastic gait in cerebral palsy. W V Med J 1994;90(5):190–2.
10. Cohen W. Hypotonia and weakness. In: Kliegman RM, editor. Practical strategies in pediatric diagnosis and therapy. 1st edition. Philadelphia: W.B. Saunders Company; 1996. p. 590–610.
11. Harris SR. Congenital hypotonia: clinical and developmental assessment. Dev Med Child Neurol 2008;50(12):889–92.
12. Cassidy SB, Dykens E, Williams CA. Prader-Willi and Angelman syndromes: sister imprinted disorders. Am J Med Genet A 2000;97(2):136–46.
13. David WS, Jones HR Jr. Electromyography and biopsy correlation with suggested protocol for evaluation of the floppy infant. Muscle Nerve 1994;17(4): 424–30.
14. Lewis RA, Sumner AJ, Shy ME. Electrophysiological features of inherited demyelinating neuropathies: a reappraisal in the era of molecular diagnosis. Muscle Nerve 2000;23(10):1472–87.
15. Darras BT, Jones HR. Diagnosis of pediatric neuromuscular disorders in the era of DNA analysis. Pediatr Neurol 2000;23(4):289–300.
16. Ghosh PS, Sorenson EJ. Diagnostic yield of electromyography in children with myopathic disorders. Pediatr Neurol 2014;51(2):215–9.
17. Richer LP, Shevell MI, Miller SP. Diagnostic profile of neonatal hypotonia: an 11-year study. Pediatr Neurol 2001;25(1):32–7.
18. Bonnemann CG, Wang CH, Quijano-Roy S, et al. Diagnostic approach to the congenital muscular dystrophies. Neuromuscul Disord 2014;24(4):289–311.
19. North KN, Wang CH, Clarke N, et al. Approach to the diagnosis of congenital myopathies. Neuromuscul Disord 2014;24(2):97–116.
20. Birdi K, Prasad AN, Prasad C, et al. The floppy infant: retrospective analysis of clinical experience (1990–2000) in a tertiary care facility. J Child Neurol 2005; 20(10):803–8.
21. Dua T, Das M, Kabra M, et al. Spectrum of floppy children in Indian scenario. Indian Pediatr 2001;38(11):1236–43.
22. Trifiro G, Livieri C, Bosio L, et al. Neonatal hypotonia: don't forget the Prader-Willi syndrome. Acta Paediatr 2003;92(9):1085–9.

Genetics and Genetic Testing in Congenital Heart Disease

Jason R. Cowan, MS[a,b], Stephanie M. Ware, MD, PhD[b,*]

KEYWORDS

- Congenital anomaly • Cardiovascular malformation • Development • Genetics
- Genetic counseling • Genetic testing

KEY POINTS

- Congenital heart defects (CHDs) are the largest contributor to worldwide infant morbidity and mortality.
- Known genetic causes encompass single-gene mutations, complex chromosomal abnormalities, submicroscopic rearrangements, and whole-chromosome aneuploidies.
- Significant proportions of CHDs are associated with extracardiac malformations and/or occur as components of a genetic syndrome.
- Advancements in genetic testing technologies have facilitated improved diagnostics and identification of novel genetic causes of CHD.
- Genetic consultation and counseling are integral components of risk assessment and clinical care. Evaluation by a geneticist is essential when a possible syndrome is suspected.

INTRODUCTION

The impact of congenital heart defects (CHDs) is profound. With a traditionally cited incidence of 8 per 1000 live births ($\sim$1%), and a need for expert cardiologic intervention in 3 of every 1000 newborns,[1] CHDs are both the single largest cause of infant morbidity and mortality worldwide and a significant source of global economic burden.[2,3] Taking into account very high rates of CHDs in spontaneous abortuses[4] and subtle or subclinical abnormalities in another 1% to 2% of patients[5] the true overall incidence of CHDs is undoubtedly much greater. Although these figures effectively convey the large global clinical impact of CHDs, they fail to communicate both the

Disclosure: The authors have nothing to disclose.
[a] Division of Developmental Biology, Cincinnati Children's Hospital Medical Center, 3333 Burnet Avenue, Cincinnati, OH 45229, USA; [b] Department of Pediatrics and Medical and Molecular Genetics, Herman B Wells Center for Pediatric Research, Indiana University School of Medicine, 1044 West Walnut Street, Indianapolis, IN 46202, USA
* Corresponding author.
E-mail address: stware@iu.edu

enormous diversity of phenotypes among affected individuals and the emerging understanding of the complexity of genetic and developmental causes.

Research into the mechanisms that regulate heart development has advanced significantly in the last 20 years. Studies using a diverse array of model organisms, including mice, frogs, and zebrafish, have facilitated major insights into normal and abnormal cardiogenesis. Furthermore, systems biology approaches designed to assess functional convergence of causative CHD genes and associated transcriptional responders (genes with altered cardiac expression) have suggested that multiple CHD risk factors are more likely to act on different components of a common functional network than to directly converge on a common genetic or molecular target.[6,7] These findings, coupled with an ever-expanding list of CHD-associated gene mutations,[8] chromosomal abnormalities,[9] environmental causes,[10,11] and epigenetic insults,[12,13] hint at a significant complexity to both normal heart development and CHD pathogenesis. This article describes current understanding of the major embryologic events that shape the developing heart. It then provides a brief overview of key signaling and molecular concepts relevant to these developmental processes. Readers desiring additional details are directed to recent comprehensive reviews.[14–21]

Overview of Heart Development

Cell lineage is an important concept for heart development because distinct lineages support the development of specific cardiac compartments such that structural anomalies may result from dysregulation of a single cell lineage, multiple lineages, or specific inductive interactions between lineages. During the second and third weeks of human development, 2 mesodermal subpopulations, the first heart field (FHF) and second heart field (SHF) contribute cells to the developing heart. Although the FHF will ultimately contribute to the left ventricle and portions of the atria and right ventricle, the SHF supports development of the future outflow tract (OFT), ventricular septum, and the remainder of the atria and right ventricle.[22] Cells of the FHF originate in splanchnic mesoderm of the anterior lateral plate and in response to inductive signals from adjacent endoderm become the first cardiac precursors to differentiate.[23] Gastrulation movements help to position the cardiogenic mesoderm as bilateral folds alongside the prechordal plate. By 17 to 19 days, the cardiogenic folds coalesce anteriorly to form the cardiac crescent, a transient structure that fuses and detaches from the dorsal pericardial wall as a linear, bilaminar heart tube. Subsequent establishment of axial left-right asymmetries directs asymmetric growth and rightward looping of the heart tube, properly positioning the heart for future chamber and valve development. While these movements are occurring cells from the SHF have already begun migrating from positions dorsal and posterior to the heart tube to support elongation of the arterial and venous poles. During weeks 6 and 7 an epithelial to mesenchymal transition populates the common atrioventricular canal and OFT with loose mesenchymal cell populations called endocardial cushions. Mature valves arise through extensive cushion remodeling and become highly stratified into distinct layers. Meanwhile, neural crest cells delaminate from the dorsal neural tube and migrate into the developing OFT to support septation of the great vessels, as well as maturation of the aortic and pulmonary valves.[24] Significant cardiac contributions are also made by cells of the proepicardium, which originate from venous coelomic mesothelium and support development of the future epicardium and coronary vasculature.[25] As development nears completion the heart is refined into a muscular, 4-chambered organ capable of regulating incoming and outgoing blood

Table 1
Signaling pathways involved in heart development

Pathway	Developmental Roles
BMP	Cardiac mesoderm induction Cardiac progenitor specification/differentiation OFT septation Myocardial trabeculation AV canal development EC/valve development
EGF	Myocardial trabeculation EC/valve development
FGF	Cardiac mesoderm induction Cardiac progenitor specification/differentiation SHF development EC/valve development
Hedgehog	Cardiac progenitor specification Heart looping/L-R patterning SHF development/OFT septation AV septation EC/valve development NCC development
MAPK	Cardiac mesoderm induction OFT development EC/valve development NCC development
Notch	Cardiac progenitor specification/differentiation Heart looping/L-R patterning OFT development Myocardial trabeculation AV canal/EC/valve development NCC development
RA	Cardiac progenitor proliferation Heart tube formation/looping A-P cardiac patterning SHF development Myocardial trabeculation
TGF-β/Nodal	Cardiac mesoderm induction Cardiac progenitor specification Heart looping/L-R patterning
VEGF	OFT septation EC/valve development
Wnt (canonical)	Cardiac progenitor proliferation OFT septation EC/valve development
Wnt (noncanonical)	Cardiac mesoderm induction Cardiac progenitor specification SHF/OFT development

Abbreviations: A-P, anterior-posterior; AV, atrioventricular; BMP, bone morphogenetic protein; EC, endocardial cushion; EGF, epidermal growth factor; ERK, extracellular signal-regulated kinase; FGF, fibroblast growth factor; L-R, left-right; MAPK, mitogen-activated protein kinase; NCC, neural crest cell; RA, retinoic acid; TGF-β, transforming growth factor-beta; VEGF, vascular endothelial growth factor; Wnt, wingless type.

flow by way of divided inflow tracts and OFTs and mature valve and conduction systems.

Complex Signaling and Transcriptional Networks Regulate Heart Development

These embryonic events are tightly regulated by an extensive array of signaling pathways and transcription factors. Several recent publications have reviewed the roles of these networks throughout all major stages of cardiac development.[15–18,26] Therefore, the intent here is not to reproduce these comprehensive works, but rather to highlight general mechanisms.

Every major developmental pathway contributes in some capacity to heart development (**Table 1**), often through extensive cross-talk with other signals or molecular factors. The impact of a particular signal can vary dramatically as development proceeds, operating positively at one stage and negatively at another. For example, Bmp signaling is required to induce differentiation of early cardiac progenitors, but is inhibited at later stages by Smad6a to permit chamber development mediated by Tbx2 and Tbx20.[27] Similarly, mouse studies have shown that Wnt signals are critical for early cardiac precursor induction and proliferation, but later become inhibitory.[28,29] As previously mentioned, a diverse array of cardiac transcription factors acts in concert with these signals to specify, differentiate, and pattern the developing heart. Clinical genetic testing is available for many of these factors and is summarized in **Table 2**. The resulting web of interactions supports a highly complex milieu in which individual or multiple risk factors can act to disrupt normal heart morphogenesis. An ideal example is provided by the cardiac transcription factor, Nkx2.5, which has key functions in regulating proliferation of SHF cells through repression of Bmp2 signaling[30] and in conduction system development.[31] Nkx2.5 also physically and functionally interacts with the major cardiac transcription factors Gata4,[32] Tbx5,[33] and Mef2c,[34] each of which forms additional unique and shared connections with other molecular, genetic, and signaling components (**Fig. 1**). Such networks also hint at common disease–common variant hypotheses and the implication that some CHD phenotypes may result from additive effects of multiple low-effect susceptibility alleles. Following identification of two disease-associated haplotypes in large cohorts of white and African American people,[35] the SHF marker/Lim-homeodomain transcription factor, ISL1, has emerged as a possible susceptibility candidate. Although the pathogenicity of at least 1 of the reported variants remains uncertain,[36,37] these studies highlight a growing recognition of the potential for common alleles to contribute to CHD pathogenesis.

GENETICS AND RECURRENCE

Contemporary advancements in medical care, surgical interventions, and diagnostics have contributed to a well-characterized decrease in patient mortality and a concomitant increase in CHD prevalence among patients of reproductive age.[38–40] Recent analyses indicate that adults now constitute roughly two-thirds of the CHD population, representing a nearly 60% increase in CHD prevalence among adult patients since the year 2000.[38] The greatest increase in CHD prevalence has occurred among the 18-year-old to 40-year-old demographic,[38] which has clear implications for heritability.

Large-scale epidemiologic studies suggest that a genetic or environmental cause for CHD is identifiable in approximately 20% to 30% of cases.[41–43] Known genetic causes are extremely heterogeneous, encompassing not only mutations in cardiac-relevant genes but also more complex chromosomal abnormalities, submicroscopic

Table 2
Clinical testing availability for transcription factors associated with CHD

Gene	Protein	Associated Syndromes	Clinical Testing Available[a]
ALX3	Aristaless-like homeobox 3	Frontonasal dysplasia	Yes
ANKRD1	Ankyrin repeat domain 1	Dilated cardiomyopathy	Yes
ARX	Aristaless related homeobox	X-linked lissencephaly with ambiguous genitalia; epileptic encephalopathy, early infantile, 1; agenesis of corpus callosum with abnormal genitalia	Yes
CITED2	Cbp/P300-interacting transactivator, with Glu/Asp-rich carboxy-terminal domain, 2	Isolated CHD	No
ETS1	V-Ets avian erythroblastosis virus E26 oncogene homolog 1	Isolated CHD	No
EVC1	Ellis-van Creveld syndrome 1	Ellis-van Creveld syndrome; Weyers acrofacial dysostosis	Yes
EVC2	Ellis-van Creveld syndrome 2	Ellis-van Creveld syndrome	Yes
EYA1	Eyes absent homolog 1	Branchiootorenal syndrome; otofaciocervical syndrome	Yes
FOXC1	Forkhead box C1	Iridogoniodysgenesis, type 1; Axenfeld-Rieger syndrome, type 3	Yes
FOXC2	Forkhead box C2	Lymphedema-distichiasis syndrome	Yes
FOXH1	Forkhead box H1	Holoprosencephaly	Yes
FOXP1	Forkhead box P1	Mental retardation with language impairment and autistic features	Yes
GATA4	GATA binding protein 4	Isolated CHD	Yes
GATA5	GATA binding protein 5	Isolated CHD	Yes
GATA6	GATA binding protein 6	Isolated CHD	Yes
HAND1	Heart and neural crest derivatives expressed 1	Isolated CHD	No
HAND2	Heart and neural crest derivatives expressed 2	Isolated CHD	No
HOXA1	Homeobox A1	Athabaskan brain stem dysgenesis syndrome; Bosley-Salih-Alorainy syndrome	Yes
IRX4	Iroquois homeobox 4	Isolated CHD	No
MED12	Mediator complex subunit 12	FG syndrome type 1; Lujan-Fryns syndrome	Yes
MED13L	Mediator complex subunit 13-like	Isolated CHD	No
MEF2C	Myocyte enhancer factor 2C	Mental retardation, stereotypic movements, epilepsy, and/or cerebral malformations	Yes
MESP1	Mesoderm posterior 1 homolog	Isolated CHD	No
MYCN	V-Myc avian myelocytomatosis viral oncogene neuroblastoma-derived homolog	Feingold syndrome 1	Yes

(continued on next page)

Table 2
(continued)

Gene	Protein	Associated Syndromes	Clinical Testing Available[a]
MYOCD	Myocardin	Isolated CHD	No
NFATC1	Nuclear factor of activated T cells, cytoplasmic, calcineurin dependent 1	Isolated CHD	No
NKX2-5	NK2 homeobox 5	Isolated CHD	Yes
NKX2-6	NK2 homeobox 6	Isolated CHD	Yes
PAX3	Paired box 3	Waardenburg syndrome type I, type 3; craniofacial-deafness-hand syndrome	Yes
PITX2	Paired-like homeodomain 2	Axenfeld-Rieger syndrome	Yes
SALL1	Spalt-like transcription factor 1	Townes-Brocks syndrome	Yes
SALL4	Spalt-like transcription factor 4	Duane-radial ray syndrome; acrorenalocular syndrome	Yes
SETBP1	SET binding protein 1	Schinzel-Giedion midface retraction syndrome	Yes
SIX6	SIX homeobox 6	Microphthalmia with cataract 2	Yes
SOX2	Sex determining region Y-box 2	Anophthalmia/microphthalmia	Yes
SOX9	Sex determining region Y-box 9	Campomelic dysplasia	Yes
TBX1	T-box 1	22q11.2 deletion syndrome	Yes
TBX3	T-box 3	Ulnar-Mammary syndrome	Yes
TBX5	T-box 5	Holt-Oram syndrome	Yes
TBX20	T-box 20	Isolated CHD	Yes
TFAP2B	Transcription factor AP-2 beta	Char syndrome	Yes
TP63	Tumor protein P63	Acro-dermato-ungual-lacrimal-tooth (ADULT) syndrome, ectrodactyly, ectodermal dysplasia, and cleft lip/palate syndrome 3; Hay-Wells syndrome; limb-mammary syndrome; Rapp-Hodgkin syndrome	Yes
TWIST1	Twist family basic helix-loop-helix (BHLH) transcription factor 1	Saethre-Chotzen syndrome	Yes
ZEB2	Zinc finger E-box binding homeobox 2	Mowat-Wilson syndrome	Yes
ZFPM2	Zinc finger protein, FOG family member 2	Isolated CHD	Yes
ZIC3	Zic family member 3	Heterotaxy syndrome; VACTERL (anal atresia, cardiac defects, tracheo-esophageal fistula/atresia, renal/radial anomalies, limb defects)	Yes

[a] Accurate as of 7/24/2014.

Data from Genetests. Available at: http://www.genetests.org/. Accessed July 24, 2014.

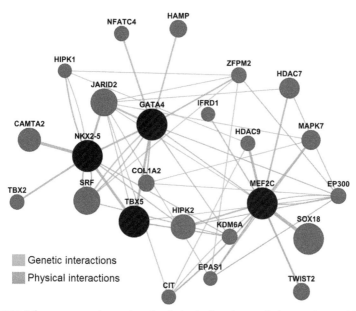

Fig. 1. NKX2-5 forms a complex network of physical and genetic interactions with GATA4, TBX5, and MEF2C. The network diagram was generated using GeneMANIA software (http://www.genemania.org/). "GATA4," "NKX-5," "TBX5," and "MEF2C" were used as query terms and results were weighted toward "biological process." To maximize readability, output was restricted to 20 related genes.

duplications/deletions, and whole-chromosome aneuploidies (**Table 3**). As genetic testing technologies have evolved to offer higher resolutions and greater diagnostic yields than those provided by conventional chromosomal analyses, copy number variants (CNVs) have emerged as important causes of both syndromic and nonsyndromic CHDs.[9] Moreover, an increasing recognition of contributing environmental[10,11] and epigenetic[12,13] factors has revealed a previously unanticipated breadth to the causes of CHD. Families with Mendelian inheritance have been useful for identifying monogenic causes, although mutations in identified genes have been infrequently detected in unrelated patient cohorts.[44] Autosomal dominant, autosomal recessive, and X-linked inheritance patterns have all been reported, often in the context of additional noncardiac malformations or syndromic disease, and each poses unique recurrence risks for affected families (**Table 4**). Improvements in diagnostic fidelity offered by chromosomal microarray analysis (CMA) and fluorescence in situ hybridization

Table 3 Causes of CHD		
Genetic Cause	**CHD Attributed (%)**	**References**
Single gene	3–5	96
Chromosomal/aneuploidy	8–10	96,97
Copy number Variation	3–25 (syndromic), 3–10 (isolated)	9
Environmental	2	11
Multifactorial	Unknown, estimated 80–85	97,98

Table 4
Examples of common syndromes associated with CHD

Syndrome	Live Birth Prevalence	Genetic Cause	Inheritance	Cardiac Phenotype (% Patients with CHD)
Aneuploidies				
Down syndrome	1 in 1000	Trisomy 21	Typically sporadic (RR ≤ 1%)	ASD, AVC, PDA, VSD (40–50)
Turner syndrome	1 in 2000–1 in 5000	45, X	Typically sporadic (RR ≤ 1%)	Left-sided defects: aortic dilatation, AS, BAV, CoA, HLHS, PAPVD (15–50)
Edward syndrome	1 in 6000	Trisomy 13	Typically sporadic (RR ≤ 1%)	ASD, PDA, polyvalvular disease, VSD (80–100)
Patau syndrome	1 in 10,000–1 in 20,000	Trisomy18	Typically sporadic (RR ≤ 1%)	ASD, PDA, polyvalvular disease, VSD (80–100)
Microdeletion/Duplication Syndromes				
22q11.2 Microdeletion syndrome	1 in 4000	22q11.2 deletion	Majority de novo, AD when inherited (RR = 50%)	Conotruncal defects: IAA type B, TrA, TOF, VSD (75–80)
Williams-Beuren syndrome	1 in 7500 to 1 in 20,000	7q11.23 del, incl. ELN gene	Majority de novo, AD when inherited (RR = 50%)	AS (especially SVAS), PPS, valve defects (80–100)
Singe Gene Disorders				
Noonan or Noonan-like syndrome	1 in 1000–1 in 2500	PTPN11, SOS1, RAF1, KRAS, HRAS, NRAS, BRAF, MAP2K1, MAP2K2, SHOC2	25%–70% de novo, AD when inherited (RR = 50%), rarely AR (RR = 25%)	ASD, HCM, PDA, PS, VSD (80–90)

CHARGE	1 in 8500–1 in 10,000	CHD7, SEMA3E	Majority de novo, AD when inherited (RR = 50%)	ASD, TOF, VSD (50–85)
Holt-Oram syndrome	1 in 100,000	TBX5	~85% de novo, AD (RR = 50%)	ASD, conduction defects VSD (75–85)
Alagille syndrome	1 in 100,000	JAG1, NOTCH2	50%–70% de novo, AD (RR = 50%)	AS, ASD, PPS, PS, TOF, VSD (85–95)
Costello syndrome	1 in 300,000–1 in 1,250,000	HRAS	Majority de novo, AD when inherited (RR = 50%)	Arrhythmias, HCM, PS (>60)
Char syndrome	Unknown, rare	TFAP2B	% De novo unknown, AD when inherited (RR = 50%)	PDA (100)
Cardiofaciocutaneous syndrome	Unknown, rare	BRAF, MAP2K1, MAP2K2, KRAS	Majority de novo, AD when inherited (RR = 50%)	ASD, HCM, PS, VSD (~70)

Abbreviations: AD, autosomal dominant; AR, autosomal recessive; AS, aortic stenosis; ASD, atrial septal defect; AVC, atrioventricular canal; BAV, bicuspid aortic valve disease; CHARGE, coloboma, heart defects, atresia of nasal choanae, retardation of growth/development, genital abnormalities, ear abnormalities/deafness; CoA, coarctation of the aorta; HCM, hypertrophic cardiomyopathy; HLHS, hypoplastic left heart syndrome; IAA, interrupted aortic arch; ; PAPVD, partial anomalous pulmonary venous drainage; PDA, patent ductus arteriosus; PPS, peripheral pulmonary stenosis; PS, pulmonary stenosis; RR, recurrence risk; SVAS, supravalvular aortic stenosis; TOF, tetralogy of Fallot; TrA, truncus arteriosus; VSD, ventricular septal defect.

Data from Refs.[8,19,99]

(FISH) have additionally facilitated rediagnosis of many patients with syndromic disease previously thought to have isolated CHD.[45] Establishment of an accurate genetic diagnosis is of critical importance, holding significant implications not only for medical management and long-term follow-up but also for communication of relevant reproductive risks and family planning.

In general, recurrence estimates are more precise for syndromic than for isolated CHDs because inheritance patterns for many CHD-associated genetic conditions are already well characterized (see **Table 4**). For dominantly inherited conditions, such as Noonan or Holt-Oram syndromes, individual recurrence risks for offspring with the syndrome is 50%. Genetic testing is also indicated for male offspring in families with X-linked heterotaxy caused by mutations in ZIC3 because they also have a 50% recurrence risk. Importantly, not all patients with a particular syndrome present with associated heart defects and the proportion that do can vary considerably depending on the specific diagnosis (see **Table 4**). The presence or severity of a CHD in a parent is also not predictive of the risk for offspring. The prevalence of CHDs in a population caused by a particular syndrome ultimately depends on the likelihood of affected individuals reaching reproductive age and the new mutation rate. Consequently, despite having high rates of associated CHDs, patients with lethal conditions such as Edwards syndrome (trisomy 18) or Patau syndrome (trisomy 13) contribute less to overall population CHD burden than patients with less severe but more prevalent conditions.

Recurrence risks for isolated CHDs can be difficult to assign, especially when the disease phenotype is complicated by reduced penetrance and variable expressivity, both of which are common. Dramatically different CHD phenotypes can be shown by patients with identical mutations, even among members of the same family. Nevertheless, consistent evidence of familial clustering and high heritability of isolated CHDs indicate that a strong genetic component exists, even for defects occurring without an obvious mode of inheritance.[46–49] Increased rates of CHDs among offspring of consanguineous unions have been noted in several populations and are commonly attributed to autosomal recessive mutations in associated disease genes (reviewed by Shieh and colleagues[50]). Long-standing CHD models consider a large subset of CHDs to be multifactorial in origin, resulting from combined interaction of several distinct environmental and genetic factors.[51] Several large-scale epidemiologic studies have examined rates of recurrence among first-degree relatives of patients with isolated CHDs and collectively suggest an overall risk of 5% to 10% for any CHD when either 1 parent or more than 2 siblings are affected.[52–54] This figure reduces to ~3% with a single affected child. Risk estimates for individual defects vary, but are generally estimated in the range of 2% to 6%, with higher risk afforded to children of affected mothers (**Table 5**). These figures are low relative to CHDs with demonstrable monogenic inheritance, but can still have potentially important implications, particularly with respect to future reproductive decision making and prospective screening of presumably unaffected family members.

DIAGNOSTIC EVALUATION
Genetic Testing Algorithm for Congenital Heart Defects

Genetic testing practices for CHDs have yet to be standardized in many centers and recommendations incorporating newer genetic testing technologies are, at present, poorly represented in the literature. In addition, there is evidence that genetic testing is frequently underused in infants with CHDs.[55,56] Nevertheless, the importance of genetic evaluation of patients with CHD has been emphasized in a position statement

Table 5
Recurrence risks for isolated (nonsyndromic) CHDs

Defect	Father Affected (%)	Mother Affected (%)	1 Sibling Affected (%)	2 Siblings Affected (%)
ASD	1.5–3.5	4–6	2.5–3	8
AVSD	1–4.5	11.5–14	3–4	10
VSD	2–3.5	6–10	3	10
AS	3–4	8–18	2	6
PS	2–3.5	4–6.5	2	6
TOF	1.5	2–2.5	2.5–3	8
CoA	2–3	4–6.5	2	6
PDA	2–2.5	3.5–4	3	10
HLHS	21[48]		2–9[a]	6
TGA	2[97]		1.5	5
L-TGA	3–5[97]		5–6	NR
EA	NR	6[97]	1	3
TrA	NR	NR	1	3
TA	NR	NR	1	3
PA	NR	NR	1	3

Merged cells indicate recurrence when 1 parent is affected, irrespective of gender, and are used in the absence of gender-stratified risks.

Abbreviations: AVSD, atrioventricular septal defect; EA, Ebstein anomaly; L-TGA, congenitally corrected transposition of the great arteries; NR, not reported/insufficient data; PA, pulmonary atresia; PDA, patent ductus arteriosus; PS, pulmonary stenosis; TA, tricuspid atresia; TGA, transposition of the great arteries.

[a] Eight percent recurrence risk HLHS, up to 22% recurrence risk for any CHD.[48]

Data from Refs.[52–54] except where otherwise noted.

from the American Heart Association,[57] which cites 4 specific reasons to pursue testing:

1. There may be other important organ system involvement
2. There may be prognostic information for clinical outcomes
3. There may be important genetic reproductive risks the family should know about
4. There may be other family members for whom genetic testing is appropriate

Fig. 2, suggests a genetic testing algorithm that could be instituted in infants with CHD to provide a more comprehensive and standardized approach. This algorithm is derived from extensive clinical experience and has been used at our institution since 2009. These recommendations were explicitly created to guide cardiac care practitioners in determining appropriate genetic testing and referral strategies for cardiac intensive care unit patients. Practitioners should evaluate guidelines that are most appropriate for their institution with a goal of practicing evidence-based medicine. In our center, geneticists consult on patients with syndromic or suspected syndromic CHD and genetic counselors facilitate genetic testing in patients with apparently isolated CHD for whom testing is indicated, and expedite appropriate cardiac screening in first-degree relatives. Ongoing multicenter registries designed to refine the interpretation of clinical CMA findings, such as the Clinical Genome Project and the Cytogenomics of Cardiovascular Malformations Consortium, will continue to improve the diagnostic yield and interpretation of abnormal CMA in patients with CHD.

Proposed genetic testing algorithm for infants with CHD

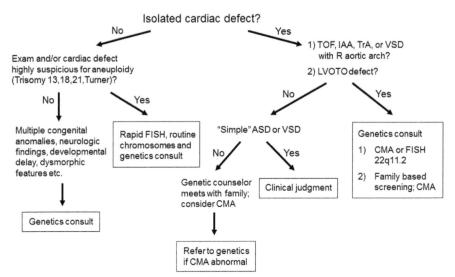

Fig. 2. Proposed genetic testing algorithm for infants with CHD. Genetic testing and referral decisions are determined based on the nature of the cardiac defect. If the defect is associated with features suggestive of a common chromosomal aneuploidy, karyotyping and FISH are undertaken and the patient is referred for evaluation by genetics. Likewise, patients with multiple congenital anomalies, neurologic findings, developmental delay, and/or dysmorphic features all receive a genetics referral. Patients with isolated CHDs are stratified based on the nature of their individual phenotypes. Those with conotruncal defects have testing for 22q11.2 deletion syndrome via CMA or targeted FISH testing depending on the level of suspicion. Apparently nonsyndromic patients with LVOTO, RVOTO, AVSD, heterotaxy, and other complex defects have a detailed pedigree and CMA testing, as indicated. First-degree relatives of patients with LVOTO defects are referred for cardiac screening. ASD, atrial septal defect; AVSD, atrioventricular septal defect; IAA, interrupted aortic arch; LVOTO/RVOTO, left/right ventricular outflow tract obstruction; TOF, tetralogy of Fallot; TrA, truncus arteriosus; VSD, ventricular septal defect.

Genetic Services and Counseling

Recent surveys of adult CHD populations have shown that most patients lack proper understanding of their personal recurrence risks, but that provision and recall of genetic information can be significantly improved by incorporating genetic services into routine cardiovascular care.[58,59] Genetic counselors skilled in cardiovascular genetics have, consequently, become an invaluable clinical asset, helping not only to provide accurate recurrence risks but also to obtain family and medical histories, facilitate appropriate genetic testing, interpret test results, make necessary subspecialty referrals, and provide attendant psychosocial support for patients and their families.[60] The importance of cardiologists in promoting genetic services cannot be understated: most patients first hear about the possibility of genetic consultation from their cardiologist and most of these patients retroactively view the resulting genetics appointments positively.[58,59] These findings are particularly relevant in light of results from a nonscientific poll recently conducted at the 21st Annual International Adult Congenital Heart Disease (ACHD) course, which suggest that only 18% of ACHD practitioners regularly refer their patients for genetic evaluation and that only 25% regularly work alongside genetic counselors and clinical geneticists.[60] Continued integration of genetic professionals into existing and new cardiovascular programs will undoubtedly help to improve use of increasingly comprehensive and affordable genetic services.

GENETIC TESTING AND EMERGING TECHNOLOGIES
Chromosomal Analyses and Copy Number Variation

Genetic testing technologies have progressed considerably in recent years with novel sequencing and chromosome-based methods improving both the speed and breadth of available testing options. Although karyotyping remains the gold standard for diagnosis of aneuploidies and other large chromosomal abnormalities, cytogenetic methods such as FISH and CMA have proved invaluable in identifying microdeletion and duplication syndromes resulting from abnormalities too small to be detected by conventional chromosomal analyses (**Table 6**). These developments are significant: an ever-growing body of studies indicate that pathogenic CNVs are a major cause of CHDs, occurring in 3% to 25% of patients with extracardiac abnormalities and in 3% to 10% of patients with isolated heart defects (reviewed by Lander and Ware[9]). In practice, the limited resolutions of karyotyping and FISH have rendered them insufficient to detect a genetic cause in most patients with CHDs of uncertain cause[55] and in nearly half of all patients with syndromic CHD.[61] Therefore, use of CMA as a higher fidelity option for first-line CHD genetic testing has been recommended, particularly when extracardiac features are present and a suspected diagnosis is lacking.[61]

This opinion has been strongly supported by additional clinical and research studies assessing diagnostic yields in selected cohorts.[55,56,62–65] In our retrospective analysis, CMA testing detected cytogenetic abnormalities of clinical or unknown significance in 35 of 121 (29%) infants with CHD,[56] representing rates on par with those observed in patients undergoing testing for intellectual disability,[66,67] for which CMA is already a first-line diagnostic test. Because most causal CNVs in patients with syndromic

Table 6				
Types of genetic tests for CHDs				
Test	**Type**	**Target**	**Resolution**	**Detects**
Karyotyping	Cytogenetic	Genome	>10 Mb	Aneuploidies, chromosomal abnormalities
FISH	Cytogenetic	Chromosomal region	>20 kb	Aneuploidies, chromosomal abnormalities
CMA (aCGH, SNP arrays)	Molecular	Genome	5 kbp	SNPs, CNVs, and other submicroscopic rearrangements
Sanger sequencing	Molecular	Gene specific	Single base	SNPs, indels
WGS/WES	Molecular	Genome/exome	Single base	SNPs, indels, CNVs[a]

Abbreviations: aCGH, array comparative genomic hybridization; SNPs, single nucleotide polymorphisms; WES, whole exome sequencing; WGS, whole genome sequencing.

[a] Detection of indels and CNVs can be difficult using current technology. Bioinformatics capabilities are emerging.

CHD are readily detectable by even low-resolution CMAs, and because significant increases in CMA resolution may not always translate to higher diagnostic yields,[68] physicians encountering patients with potentially syndromic phenotypes but normal CMA results should rule out the possibility of a previously missed monogenic cause. Supporting this recommendation, Breckpot and colleagues[55] identified 7% of patients in their cohort with normal CMA results who were later found to have a single-gene disorder on follow-up.

Next-Generation Sequencing and Whole Exome Analysis

Genetic technologies are advancing at such a rapid pace that keeping abreast of methodological advancements and emerging clinical applications has become both more essential and more challenging than ever before. Arguably the most significant development in recent years has been the advent of massively parallel next-generation sequencing (NGS) technologies, which encompass an assortment of commercially and methodologically distinct services that share similar foundations in repeated sequencing of DNA fragments (reviewed by Dorn and colleagues,[69] with a focus on CHD). Millions of individual sequences (called reads) are generated in simultaneous reactions and are subsequently aligned to form a completed sequence. These techniques facilitate considerably greater depths of coverage, faster turnaround times, and increased cost-effectiveness compared with traditional capillary-based sequencing methods.[70,71] Although Sanger sequencing remains the gold standard for targeted analyses of specific genes or familial mutations, it requires a priori knowledge of causative disease genes or sequences and does not contribute to novel gene discovery. In addition, most gene panels are disease specific, necessitating implementation of large numbers of distinct assays. In contrast, like CMA, NGS approaches provide greater diagnostic utility for suspected genetic disease of uncertain cause and for genetically heterogeneous conditions stemming from mutations in larger numbers of causative loci. One of the biggest benefits of this technology has been its scalability, both to large-scale whole genome/exome analyses and to smaller gene-specific targeted studies. This flexibility has initiated a paradigm shift toward adoption of NGS in both clinical and research settings and has, even in its infancy, greatly benefited novel disease gene discovery and patient diagnosis.[72–76]

Nowhere is this shift more apparent than in the increased clinical implementation of whole exome sequencing (WES).[73] In contrast to whole genome sequencing (WGS), which interrogates every base in the genome, WES specifically targets protein-encoding genomic regions and makes the implicit assumption that a significant proportion of uncharacterized genetic disease can be explained by sequence variation in coding DNA. This assumption is reasonable for many inherited conditions because most mutations resulting in Mendelian disease have traditionally been detected in protein-coding regions.[77–79] In addition, the current ability to interpret the functional significance of variants in noncoding regions is primitive.[57] Importantly, WES has been shown to be both robust and cost-effective,[80] necessitating only 5% of the total sequencing required by GWS.[81] Adoption of WES has consequently been swift: since its clinical debut in 2011, most major genetic centers have established WES as a testing option for patients with complex phenotypes for whom traditional single-gene and multigene panels were unrevealing, prohibitively expensive, or otherwise unavailable. Although these programs are still young, initial studies have reported deleterious mutation detection rates in the range of 20% to 50%,[72,82,83] indicating significant potential for high diagnostic yields. WES has already been used successfully to identify genetic defects associated with a diverse spectrum of CHDs.[84–87] However, interpretation of detected variants remains a major challenge because

WES identifies, on average, 12,000 unique coding variants per exome sequenced[88] and potentially pathogenic variants are observed even in apparently healthy individuals.[89–91] Reporting laboratories are expected to perform a thorough literature review for all variants of potential clinical relevance and properly classify each as having known or uncertain significance.

Although WES is clearly beneficial in multiple settings, its use as a first-tier test has generated debate, with concerns raised over not only interpretation and reporting of clinically relevant mutations but also return of incidental findings, availability of insurance coverage, and cost-effectiveness relative to existing multigene panels.[72,92] Thus, it is important that care providers familiar with both the strengths and limitations of WES and its applicability to the patient's phenotypes be involved in facilitating testing. It is anticipated that the already widespread application of WES will lead to improvements in existing technologies, decreasing overall costs and increasing insurance coverage.

Future Developments

To date, clinical application of NGS has largely been restricted to analysis of genomic variation. Nevertheless, the same technologies used for DNA-based analyses can be used to interrogate a variety of other disease-relevant processes, including RNA expression, alterations in splicing, epigenetic regulation, and protein-nucleotide interactions (eg, transcription factor binding).[93] These applications hold considerable future diagnostic and clinical potential and are already providing great utility for investigators applying comprehensive system-based approaches to the study of CHD.[94,95] The recognition that multiple independent insults are likely to contribute to at least a subset of CHD phenotypes indicates that systems-based approaches will be necessary to understand CHD risk factor networks and properly contextualize many genetic testing results, particularly in the absence of extracardiac features or clear syndromic diagnoses.

SUMMARY

CHD genetics is progressing at a rapid pace. The last decade in particular has witnessed unprecedented improvements in genetic testing technologies that have greatly assisted gene discovery and helped to reshape standards of patient care. These trends are likely to continue as testing costs continue to decline and genetic services become further integrated into new and existing cardiovascular programs. With the functional significance of much of the genome still undefined and the mechanisms driving both normal and abnormal heart development incompletely understood, interpretation and reporting of clinically relevant mutations will remain a major challenge for the foreseeable future. Accordingly, clinical geneticists and genetic counselors will need to play increasingly key roles in patient care, ensuring accurate diagnosis and effective communication of inheritance and recurrence risks. Despite, or perhaps because of, such challenges, this new era of unbiased, genome-based and exome-based testing is an exciting one. Recent efforts integrating results from animal modeling studies with systems biology approaches indicate great potential for future developmental research, whereas collaborative endeavors such as the National Heart, Lung, and Blood Institute's Bench to Bassinet program (http://www.benchtobassinet.com/) are designed to bridge the gap between basic research and clinical practice. The wealth of genetic data anticipated from these and other forward-thinking studies promises to power novel hypotheses for future experimentation and to generate new avenues for potential therapeutic intervention.

Best Practices

What is the current practice?

Genetic testing in congenital heart disease:

- Genetic testing practices for CHDs have yet to be standardized in many centers.
- Recommendations incorporating newer genetic testing methods are poorly represented in the literature.
- Genetic testing is frequently underused for infants with CHD.

Genetic testing options:

- Chromosome analysis is the gold standard for diagnosis of aneuploidies and other large chromosomal abnormalities.
- CMA and FISH permit identification of microdeletion and duplication syndromes resulting from abnormalities too small to be detected by conventional chromosome analyses.
- Sanger sequencing is the gold standard for targeted molecular analysis of specific genes or familial mutations. Gene panels are available for many CHD-associated syndromes, but are limited by knowledge of causative disease genes. NGS panels for CHD continue to emerge but diagnostic yield is not yet well established.

What changes in current practice are likely to improve outcomes?

- Continued integration of genetic testing services into cardiovascular practice will improve diagnostic and prognostic accuracy and will support risk assessment and family planning initiatives.
- Emerging NGS technologies promise to greatly benefit patient diagnosis and gene discovery efforts.

Is there a clinical algorithm?

- Our proposed genetic testing algorithm is presented in **Fig. 2**.
- In our center, geneticists consult patients with known or suspected syndromic CHDs and genetic counselors facilitate genetic testing in patients with apparently isolated CHDs and expedite appropriate screening in first-degree relatives.

Major recommendations:

Genetic testing and referral decisions should be determined based on the nature of the cardiac defect:

1. Patients with defects suggesting a common chromosomal aneuploidy should undergo karyotyping and FISH testing. These patients should be referred for further genetic evaluation.
2. Patients with multiple congenital anomalies, neurologic findings, developmental delay, and/or dysmorphic features should also be referred for further genetics evaluation.
3. Depending on the level of suspicion, patients with conotruncal defects should undergo CMA and/or targeted FISH testing for 22q11.2 deletion syndrome.
4. A detailed pedigree should be obtained and CMA testing should be pursued for patients with apparently nonsyndromic left ventricular OFT obstruction (LVOTO), right ventricular OFT obstruction (RVOTO), atrioventricular septal defect (AVSD), heterotaxy, or other complex defects. Abnormal test results warrant referral for further genetics evaluation.

Rating for the strength of the evidence:

C recommendation based on consensus, usual practice, expert opinion, disease-oriented evidence, and case series for studies of diagnosis, treatment, prevention, or screening

References

Pierpont ME, Basson CT, Benson DW Jr, et al. Genetic basis for congenital heart defects: current knowledge: a scientific statement from the American Heart Association Congenital Cardiac Defects Committee, Council on Cardiovascular Disease in the Young: endorsed by the American Academy of Pediatrics. Circulation 2007;115:3015–38.

Summary

1. Improvements in genetic testing technologies have assisted gene discovery and helped to reshape standards of patient care. These trends are expected to continue as testing costs decline and genetic services become further integrated into new and existing cardiovascular programs.

REFERENCES

1. Hoffman JI, Kaplan S. The incidence of congenital heart disease. J Am Coll Cardiol 2002;39:1890–900.
2. Centers for Disease Control and Prevention (CDC). Hospital stays, hospital charges, and in-hospital deaths among infants with selected birth defects–United States, 2003. MMWR Morb Mortal Wkly Rep 2007;56:25–9.
3. Boneva RS, Botto LD, Moore CA, et al. Mortality associated with congenital heart defects in the United States: trends and racial disparities, 1979-1997. Circulation 2001;103:2376–81.
4. Hoffman JI. Incidence of congenital heart disease: II. Prenatal incidence. Pediatr Cardiol 1995;16:155–65.
5. Srivastava D. Making or breaking the heart: from lineage determination to morphogenesis. Cell 2006;126:1037–48.
6. Lage K, Greenway SC, Rosenfeld JA, et al. Genetic and environmental risk factors in congenital heart disease functionally converge in protein networks driving heart development. Proc Natl Acad Sci U S A 2012;109:14035–40.
7. Lage K, Mollgard K, Greenway S, et al. Dissecting spatio-temporal protein networks driving human heart development and related disorders. Mol Syst Biol 2010;6:381.
8. Stenson PD, Ball EV, Mort M, et al. Human gene mutation database (HGMD): 2003 update. Hum Mutat 2003;21:577–81.
9. Lander J, Ware S. Copy number variation in congenital heart defects. Curr Genet Med Rep 2014. http://dx.doi.org/10.1007/s40142-014-0049-3.
10. Jenkins KJ, Correa A, Feinstein JA, et al. Noninherited risk factors and congenital cardiovascular defects: current knowledge: a scientific statement from the American heart Association Council on Cardiovascular Disease in the Young: endorsed by the American Academy of Pediatrics. Circulation 2007;115:2995–3014.
11. Kuciene R, Dulskiene V. Selected environmental risk factors and congenital heart defects. Medicina (Kaunas) 2008;44:827–32.
12. Vallaster M, Vallaster CD, Wu SM. Epigenetic mechanisms in cardiac development and disease. Acta Biochim Biophys Sin (Shanghai) 2012;44:92–102.
13. Chang CP, Bruneau BG. Epigenetics and cardiovascular development. Annu Rev Physiol 2012;74:41–68.
14. Lalani SR, Belmont JW. Genetic basis of congenital cardiovascular malformations. Eur J Med Genet 2014;57:402–13.
15. Bruneau BG. Signaling and transcriptional networks in heart development and regeneration. Cold Spring Harb Perspect Biol 2013;5:a008292.
16. Rochais F, Mesbah K, Kelly RG. Signaling pathways controlling second heart field development. Circ Res 2009;104:933–42.

17. Rana MS, Christoffels VM, Moorman AF. A molecular and genetic outline of cardiac morphogenesis. Acta Physiol (Oxf) 2013;207:588–615.
18. Kodo K, Yamagishi H. A decade of advances in the molecular embryology and genetics underlying congenital heart defects. Circ J 2011;75:2296–304.
19. Fahed AC, Gelb BD, Seidman JG, et al. Genetics of congenital heart disease: the glass half empty. Circ Res 2013;112:707–20.
20. Wagner M, Siddiqui MA. Signal transduction in early heart development (II): ventricular chamber specification, trabeculation, and heart valve formation. Exp Biol Med (Maywood) 2007;232:866–80.
21. Wagner M, Siddiqui MA. Signal transduction in early heart development (I): cardiogenic induction and heart tube formation. Exp Biol Med (Maywood) 2007;232:852–65.
22. Meilhac SM, Esner M, Kelly RG, et al. The clonal origin of myocardial cells in different regions of the embryonic mouse heart. Dev Cell 2004;6:685–98.
23. Schultheiss TM, Xydas S, Lassar AB. Induction of avian cardiac myogenesis by anterior endoderm. Development 1995;121:4203–14.
24. Jiang X, Rowitch DH, Soriano P, et al. Fate of the mammalian cardiac neural crest. Development 2000;127:1607–16.
25. Ratajska A, Czarnowska E, Ciszek B. Embryonic development of the proepicardium and coronary vessels. Int J Dev Biol 2008;52:229–36.
26. McCulley DJ, Black BL. Transcription factor pathways and congenital heart disease. Curr Top Dev Biol 2012;100:253–77.
27. de Pater E, Ciampricotti M, Priller F, et al. Bmp signaling exerts opposite effects on cardiac differentiation. Circ Res 2012;110:578–87.
28. Naito AT, Shiojima I, Akazawa H, et al. Developmental stage-specific biphasic roles of Wnt/beta-catenin signaling in cardiomyogenesis and hematopoiesis. Proc Natl Acad Sci U S A 2006;103:19812–7.
29. Kwon C, Arnold J, Hsiao EC, et al. Canonical Wnt signaling is a positive regulator of mammalian cardiac progenitors. Proc Natl Acad Sci U S A 2007;104:10894–9.
30. Prall OW, Menon MK, Solloway MJ, et al. An Nkx2-5/Bmp2/Smad1 negative feedback loop controls heart progenitor specification and proliferation. Cell 2007;128:947–59.
31. Jay PY, Harris BS, Maguire CT, et al. Nkx2-5 mutation causes anatomic hypoplasia of the cardiac conduction system. J Clin Invest 2004;113:1130–7.
32. Lee Y, Shioi T, Kasahara H, et al. The cardiac tissue-restricted homeobox protein Csx/Nkx2.5 physically associates with the zinc finger protein GATA4 and cooperatively activates atrial natriuretic factor gene expression. Mol Cell Biol 1998;18:3120–9.
33. Hiroi Y, Kudoh S, Monzen K, et al. Tbx5 associates with Nkx2-5 and synergistically promotes cardiomyocyte differentiation. Nat Genet 2001;28:276–80.
34. Vincentz JW, Barnes RM, Firulli BA, et al. Cooperative interaction of Nkx2.5 and Mef2c transcription factors during heart development. Dev Dyn 2008;237:3809–19.
35. Stevens KN, Hakonarson H, Kim CE, et al. Common variation in ISL1 confers genetic susceptibility for human congenital heart disease. PLoS One 2010;5:e10855.
36. Cresci M, Vecoli C, Foffa I, et al. Lack of association of the 3'-UTR polymorphism (rs1017) in the ISL1 gene and risk of congenital heart disease in the white population. Pediatr Cardiol 2013;34:938–41.
37. Xue L, Wang X, Xu J, et al. ISL1 common variant rs1017 is not associated with susceptibility to congenital heart disease in a Chinese population. Genet Test Mol Biomarkers 2012;16:679–83.

38. Marelli AJ, Ionescu-Ittu R, Mackie AS, et al. Lifetime prevalence of congenital heart disease in the general population from 2000 to 2010. Circulation 2014; 130:749–56.
39. Engelfriet P, Boersma E, Oechslin E, et al. The spectrum of adult congenital heart disease in Europe: morbidity and mortality in a 5 year follow-up period. The Euro Heart Survey on Adult Congenital Heart Disease. Eur Heart J 2005;26:2325–33.
40. Marelli AJ, Mackie AS, Ionescu-Ittu R, et al. Congenital heart disease in the general population: changing prevalence and age distribution. Circulation 2007;115: 163–72.
41. Ferencz C, Boughman JA, Neill CA, et al. Congenital cardiovascular malformations: questions on inheritance. Baltimore-Washington infant study group. J Am Coll Cardiol 1989;14:756–63.
42. Grech V, Gatt M. Syndromes and malformations associated with congenital heart disease in a population-based study. Int J Cardiol 1999;68:151–6.
43. Meberg A, Hals J, Thaulow E. Congenital heart defects–chromosomal anomalies, syndromes and extracardiac malformations. Acta Paediatr 2007;96:1142–5.
44. Posch MG, Perrot A, Schmitt K, et al. Mutations in GATA4, NKX2.5, CRELD1, and BMP4 are infrequently found in patients with congenital cardiac septal defects. Am J Med Genet A 2008;146A:251–3.
45. Erdogan F, Larsen LA, Zhang L, et al. High frequency of submicroscopic genomic aberrations detected by tiling path array comparative genome hybridisation in patients with isolated congenital heart disease. J Med Genet 2008;45:704–9.
46. Burn J, Brennan P, Little J, et al. Recurrence risks in offspring of adults with major heart defects: results from first cohort of British collaborative study. Lancet 1998; 351:311–6.
47. Cripe L, Andelfinger G, Martin LJ, et al. Bicuspid aortic valve is heritable. J Am Coll Cardiol 2004;44:138–43.
48. Hinton RB Jr, Martin LJ, Tabangin ME, et al. Hypoplastic left heart syndrome is heritable. J Am Coll Cardiol 2007;50:1590–5.
49. Insley J. The heritability of congenital heart disease. Br Med J (Clin Res Ed) 1987; 294:662–3.
50. Shieh JT, Bittles AH, Hudgins L. Consanguinity and the risk of congenital heart disease. Am J Med Genet A 2012;158A:1236–41.
51. Nora JJ. Multifactorial inheritance hypothesis for the etiology of congenital heart diseases. The genetic-environmental interaction. Circulation 1968;38:604–17.
52. Calcagni G, Digilio MC, Sarkozy A, et al. Familial recurrence of congenital heart disease: an overview and review of the literature. Eur J Pediatr 2007;166:111–6.
53. Nora JJ. From generational studies to a multilevel genetic-environmental interaction. J Am Coll Cardiol 1994;23:1468–71.
54. Nora JJ, Nora AH. Update on counseling the family with a first-degree relative with a congenital heart defect. Am J Med Genet 1988;29:137–42.
55. Breckpot J, Thienpont B, Peeters H, et al. Array comparative genomic hybridization as a diagnostic tool for syndromic heart defects. J Pediatr 2010;156:810–7, 817.e1–817.e4.
56. Connor JA, Hinton RB, Miller EM, et al. Genetic testing practices in infants with congenital heart disease. Congenit Heart Dis 2014;9:158–67.
57. Pierpont ME, Basson CT, Benson DW Jr, et al. Genetic basis for congenital heart defects: current knowledge: a scientific statement from the American Heart Association Congenital Cardiac Defects Committee, Council on Cardiovascular Disease in the Young: endorsed by the American Academy of Pediatrics. Circulation 2007;115:3015–38.

58. van Engelen K, Baars MJ, Felix JP, et al. The value of the clinical geneticist caring for adults with congenital heart disease: diagnostic yield and patients' perspective. Am J Med Genet A 2013;161A:1628–37.

59. van Engelen K, Baars MJ, van Rongen LT, et al. Adults with congenital heart disease: patients' knowledge and concerns about inheritance. Am J Med Genet A 2011;155A:1661–7.

60. Parrott A, Ware SM. The role of the geneticist and genetic counselor in an ACHD clinic. Prog Pediatr Cardiol 2012;34:15–20.

61. Breckpot J, Thienpont B, Arens Y, et al. Challenges of interpreting copy number variation in syndromic and non-syndromic congenital heart defects. Cytogenet Genome Res 2011;135:251–9.

62. Baker K, Sanchez-de-Toledo J, Munoz R, et al. Critical congenital heart disease–utility of routine screening for chromosomal and other extracardiac malformations. Congenit Heart Dis 2012;7:145–50.

63. Richards AA, Santos LJ, Nichols HA, et al. Cryptic chromosomal abnormalities identified in children with congenital heart disease. Pediatr Res 2008;64:358–63.

64. Thienpont B, Mertens L, de Ravel T, et al. Submicroscopic chromosomal imbalances detected by array-CGH are a frequent cause of congenital heart defects in selected patients. Eur Heart J 2007;28:2778–84.

65. Goldmuntz E, Paluru P, Glessner J, et al. Microdeletions and microduplications in patients with congenital heart disease and multiple congenital anomalies. Congenit Heart Dis 2011;6:592–602.

66. Schoumans J, Ruivenkamp C, Holmberg E, et al. Detection of chromosomal imbalances in children with idiopathic mental retardation by array based comparative genomic hybridisation (array-CGH). J Med Genet 2005;42:699–705.

67. Thuresson AC, Bondeson ML, Edeby C, et al. Whole-genome array-CGH for detection of submicroscopic chromosomal imbalances in children with mental retardation. Cytogenet Genome Res 2007;118:1–7.

68. Wincent J, Anderlid BM, Lagerberg M, et al. High-resolution molecular karyotyping in patients with developmental delay and/or multiple congenital anomalies in a clinical setting. Clin Genet 2011;79:147–57.

69. Dorn C, Grunert M, Sperling SR. Application of high-throughput sequencing for studying genomic variations in congenital heart disease. Brief Funct Genomics 2014;13:51–65.

70. Shendure J, Ji H. Next-generation DNA sequencing. Nat Biotechnol 2008;26:1135–45.

71. Mardis ER. A decade's perspective on DNA sequencing technology. Nature 2011;470:198–203.

72. Atwal PS, Brennan ML, Cox R, et al. Clinical whole-exome sequencing: are we there yet? Genet Med 2014;16:717–9.

73. Bamshad MJ, Ng SB, Bigham AW, et al. Exome sequencing as a tool for Mendelian disease gene discovery. Nat Rev Genet 2011;12:745–55.

74. Iglesias A, Anyane-Yeboa K, Wynn J, et al. The usefulness of whole-exome sequencing in routine clinical practice. Genet Med 2014;16:922–31.

75. Levenson D. Whole-exome sequencing emerges as clinical diagnostic tool: testing method proves useful for diagnosing wide range of genetic disorders. Am J Med Genet A 2014;164A:ix–x.

76. Schuler BA, Prisco SZ, Jacob HJ. Using whole exome sequencing to walk from clinical practice to research and back again. Circulation 2013;127:968–70.

77. Chen CT, Wang JC, Cohen BA. The strength of selection on ultraconserved elements in the human genome. Am J Hum Genet 2007;80:692–704.

78. Kryukov GV, Pennacchio LA, Sunyaev SR. Most rare missense alleles are deleterious in humans: implications for complex disease and association studies. Am J Hum Genet 2007;80:727–39.

79. Ahituv N, Zhu Y, Visel A, et al. Deletion of ultraconserved elements yields viable mice. PLoS Biol 2007;5:e234.

80. Lupski JR, Gonzaga-Jauregui C, Yang Y, et al. Exome sequencing resolves apparent incidental findings and reveals further complexity of SH3TC2 variant alleles causing Charcot-Marie-Tooth neuropathy. Genome Med 2013;5:57.

81. Ng SB, Turner EH, Robertson PD, et al. Targeted capture and massively parallel sequencing of 12 human exomes. Nature 2009;461:272–6.

82. Yang Y, Muzny DM, Reid JG, et al. Clinical whole-exome sequencing for the diagnosis of mendelian disorders. N Engl J Med 2013;369:1502–11.

83. Need AC, Shashi V, Hitomi Y, et al. Clinical application of exome sequencing in undiagnosed genetic conditions. J Med Genet 2012;49:353–61.

84. Al Turki S, Manickaraj AK, Mercer CL, et al. Rare variants in NR2F2 cause congenital heart defects in humans. Am J Hum Genet 2014;94:574–85.

85. Arrington CB, Bleyl SB, Matsunami N, et al. Exome analysis of a family with pleiotropic congenital heart disease. Circ Cardiovasc Genet 2012;5:175–82.

86. Francis C, Prapa S, Abdulkareem N, et al. 95 identification of likely pathogenic variants in patients with bicuspid aortic valve: correlation of complex genotype with a more severe aortic phenotype. Heart 2014;100(Suppl 3):A55–6.

87. Tariq M, Belmont JW, Lalani S, et al. SHROOM3 is a novel candidate for heterotaxy identified by whole exome sequencing. Genome Biol 2011;12:R91.

88. Ng PC, Levy S, Huang J, et al. Genetic variation in an individual human exome. PLoS Genet 2008;4:e1000160.

89. Marth GT, Yu F, Indap AR, et al. The functional spectrum of low-frequency coding variation. Genome Biol 2011;12:R84.

90. Tennessen JA, Bigham AW, O'Connor TD, et al. Evolution and functional impact of rare coding variation from deep sequencing of human exomes. Science 2012; 337:64–9.

91. Li Y, Vinckenbosch N, Tian G, et al. Resequencing of 200 human exomes identifies an excess of low-frequency non-synonymous coding variants. Nat Genet 2010;42:969–72.

92. Kaye J, Boddington P, de Vries J, et al. Ethical implications of the use of whole genome methods in medical research. Eur J Hum Genet 2010;18:398–403.

93. Morozova O, Marra MA. Applications of next-generation sequencing technologies in functional genomics. Genomics 2008;92:255–64.

94. MacLellan WR, Wang Y, Lusis AJ. Systems-based approaches to cardiovascular disease. Nat Rev Cardiol 2012;9:172–84.

95. Sperling SR. Systems biology approaches to heart development and congenital heart disease. Cardiovasc Res 2011;91:269–78.

96. van der Bom T, Zomer AC, Zwinderman AH, et al. The changing epidemiology of congenital heart disease. Nat Rev Cardiol 2011;8:50–60.

97. Roos-Hesselink JW, Kerstjens-Frederikse WS, Meijboom BR, et al. Inheritance of congenital heart disease. Neth Heart J 2005;13:4.

98. Blue GM, Kirk EP, Sholler GF, et al. Congenital heart disease: current knowledge about causes and inheritance. Med J Aust 2012;197:155–9.

99. Bernier FP, Spaetgens R. The geneticist's role in adult congenital heart disease. Cardiol Clin 2006;24:557–69, v–vi.

Disorders of Sexual Development

Bonnie McCann-Crosby, MD[a],*, V. Reid Sutton, MD[b]

KEYWORDS

- Disorders of sexual development (DSDs) • Ambiguous genitalia • Sex assignment
- Neonates

KEY POINTS

- Disorders of sexual development (DSDs) are classified into 3 categories: 46,XX DSD, 46,XY DSD, and sex chromosome DSD. There are many genes that are involved in normal sexual development, and mutations in most of these genes have been identified in individuals with DSD.
- Initial evaluation of a neonate with ambiguous genitalia must include a thorough history, physical examination, and laboratory evaluation including routine chromosomal analysis to identify the underlying cause. This process is of the utmost urgency to arrive at a diagnosis for treatment and gender assignment. It is critical to evaluate for life-threatening conditions such as congenital adrenal hyperplasia (CAH) in any infant presenting with ambiguous genitalia.
- A multidisciplinary team, including a neonatologist, pediatric urologist, endocrinologist, gynecologist, geneticist, medical ethicist, and psychologist, must be involved in the diagnosis and management of any neonate with a suspected DSD.

INTRODUCTION

Disorders of Sexual Development (DSDs) encompass a large group of congenital conditions in which there is abnormal development of chromosomal, gonadal, or anatomic sex.[1] In these disorders, anatomic sex and hormonal sex are discordant with sex chromosomes. DSDs commonly present in the newborn period because of the presence of ambiguous genitalia. The differential diagnosis is often broad, and management of DSDs can be challenging. These challenges are both medical/scientific and psychological and require the collaborative efforts of an experienced multidisciplinary team, including a neonatologist, pediatric urologist, endocrinologist, gynecologist, geneticist, medical ethicist, and psychologist. DSDs are classified broadly into 3 categories based on the

Disclosure statement: The authors of this article declare that they have nothing to disclose.
a Division of Pediatric Endocrinology, Baylor College of Medicine, Texas Children's Hospital, 6701 Fannin Street, Houston, TX 77030, USA; b Department of Molecular and Human Genetics, Baylor College of Medicine, Texas Children's Hospital, 6701 Fannin Street, Houston, TX 77030, USA
* Corresponding author.
E-mail address: mccann@bcm.edu

underlying cause: 46,XX DSD, 46,XY DSD, and sex chromosome DSD. Specific diagnoses can often be made within each of the major categories based on further investigation, although occasionally a specific diagnosis or cause remains elusive. Ambiguous genitalia in a neonate should be treated as an emergency, and a thorough evaluation should take place to establish the diagnosis and gender assignment of the infant. This article focuses on the clinical presentation, diagnostic evaluation, and differential diagnoses of DSDs.

NORMAL SEXUAL DEVELOPMENT

Normal sexual development is a complex process that relies on proper expression of specific genes as well as normal hormone production/function. In early development, the gonads and internal genital structures are bipotential, meaning that they can further differentiate into male or female depending on the gene expression that occurs.[2,3] In early embryology, the bipotential gonad develops from the urogenital ridge. Germ cells migrate from the yolk sac to the bipotential gonad around the fourth or fifth week of gestation and intermingle with pre-Sertoli and pregranulosa cells.

NORMAL MALE DEVELOPMENT

Expression of the sex determining region on the Y chromosome (SRY) around the sixth week of gestation leads to the organization of pre-Sertoli cells and germ cells into primitive sex cords. Further sex-determining genes and transcription factors such as *SOX9, SF1,* and *WT1* lead to further maturation and development of the testes.[4] The primitive testes begin to produce hormones beginning at approximately 8 weeks of gestation. The Sertoli cells produce anti-Müllerian hormone (AMH) and inhibin B, whereas the Leydig cells produce insulinlike factor 3 (INSL3) and testosterone. AMH leads to regression of the Müllerian (female) ducts. INSL3 is important in the transabdominal phase of testicular descent.[5] Production of testosterone leads to development of the wolffian (male) ducts into the epididymis, vas deferens, and seminiferous tubules. Further differentiation of the urogenital sinus into external male genitalia occurs from the activity of dihydrotestosterone (DHT), which is converted from testosterone locally in the sexual skin by the enzyme 5-α reductase. In the presence of DHT, the genital tubercle differentiates into the penis, the urogenital slit fuses to form the urethra, and the labioscrotal folds fuse to form the scrotum.

NORMAL FEMALE DEVELOPMENT

In the absence of proper SRY expression, the bipotential gonad develops into an ovary. If AMH is insufficient or absent, the Wolffian ducts regress and the Müllerian structures develop into the upper part of the vagina, uterus, and fallopian tubes. In the absence of circulating testosterone, DHT, or normal androgen receptors, the genital tubercle becomes a clitoris, the urogenital folds become the labia minora, and the labia majora form from the labioscrotal swelling, leading to a female external phenotype. Thus, the presence or absence of SRY leads to determination of gonadal sex (testes or ovary), followed by sex differentiation, which under normal circumstances, leads to either a male or female phenotype.

CLINICAL PRESENTATION OF DISORDERS OF SEXUAL DEVELOPMENT

Infants who have the following clinical features should be evaluated for a DSD:

- Micropenis with bilateral nonpalpable testes
  - Micropenis is defined as stretched penile length less than 2.5 cm in full-term infants

- Clitoromegaly
  - Clitoral length greater than 9 mm or clitoral width greater than 6 mm in full-term infant[6]
- Apparent female genitalia with an inguinal or labial mass
- Hypospadias with unilateral nonpalpable testes
- Penoscrotal or perineoscrotal hypospadias with undescended testes
- Posterior labial fusion
  - The anogenital ratio is measured as the distance between the anus and the posterior fourchette divided by the distance between the anus and the base of the phallus. If the ratio is greater than 0.5, it suggests a component of female differentiation and virilization with posterior labial fusion.[7]
- Discordant genitalia and prenatal chromosome complement

DIAGNOSTIC EVALUATION

Initial evaluation of an infant with suspected DSD should include a thorough history, physical examination, and laboratory/imaging studies.

History

- Maternal
  - Previous pregnancy history
  - Drug use during pregnancy that could suggest an exogenous source of androgen leading to virilization of a female fetus
  - Maternal virilization that could suggest excess androgen production (androgen secreting ovarian or adrenal tumors)
  - Results of prenatal tests, such as chromosome/genetic studies, maternal serum estriol levels, and prenatal ultrasound imaging
- Familial
  - Consanguinity of the parents (increasing risk of autosomal recessive disorders such as CAH)
  - History of urologic or genital anomalies such as ambiguous genitalia
  - Female infertility and amenorrhea
  - Neonatal deaths (of concern for undiagnosed salt-wasting CAH)

Physical Examination

- General examination
  - Assess for dysmorphic features or malformations that may suggest an underlying genetic syndrome (eg, Smith-Lemli-Opitz syndrome [SLOS]).
  - Assess for midline defects such as cleft lip/cleft palate that could indicate a hypothalamic-pituitary cause of hypogonadism.
  - Assess state of hydration and blood pressure to evaluate for CAH. Defects in adrenal steroid biosynthesis can be associated with salt wasting, ambiguous genitalia, or hypertension.
  - Assess for hyperbilirubinemia, which can be an indication of thyroid or cortisol deficiency.
- Examination of the external genitalia
  - Assess the development of the genital tubercle (which forms the penis in males and the clitoris in females) and the genital folds (which form the scrotum in the male and the labia in the female).

○ Evaluate for the size and location of the gonads. It is important to look for palpable gonads in the labioscrotal folds or inguinal region. Palpable external gonads are most commonly testes but can also be ovotestes.

○ Evaluate phallic length and width. A stretched penile length less than 2.5 cm is consistent with a micropenis.

○ Evaluate for hypospadias and chordee.

○ Evaluate for the presence of a urogenital sinus, location of urethral meatus, and presence of a vaginal opening.

○ Evaluate the degree of labioscrotal fusion and note the texture and pigmentation of the genital skin, including rugosity.

○ Evaluate for clitoromegaly.

Several scoring systems have been developed to help characterize the appearance of the external genitalia including Prader staging and the external masculinization score (EMS). The Prader scale ranges from 1 to 5, depending on the degree of virilization of the external genitalia. The EMS developed by Ahmed and colleagues[8] is an objective measure of the degree of virilization of the genitalia. The EMS takes into account individual features of the genitalia, including labioscrotal fusion, microphallus, location of urethreal meatus, and location of each gonad. The score ranges from 0 to 12, with 12 representing a normally virilized male (**Fig. 1**).

Initial Laboratory and Imaging Studies

- Genetic testing (see **Figs. 2** and **3** for diagnostic algorithms)
  ○ Routine chromosome analysis should be obtained immediately on all patients with ambiguous genitalia to guide further investigation.
  ○ Chromosome microarray analysis should be performed.

The laboratory should be notified of the urgency of the situation so that the studies can be expedited. Both analyses are required, as chromosome microrray analysis may have limited ability to detect sex chromosome mosaicism in certain conditions; in addition, small deletions or duplications, such as deletion of *SRY*, are not detected on routine chromosome analysis.

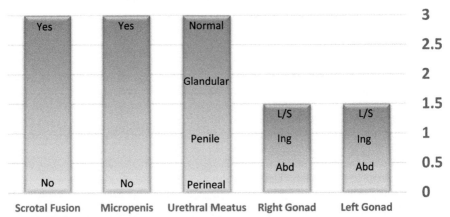

Fig. 1. External masculinization score. Abd, abdominal; Ing, inguinal; L/S, labial/scrotal. (*Data from* Ahmed SF, Khwaja O, Hughes IA. The role of a clinical score in the assessment of ambiguous genitalia. BJU Int 2000;85:120–4.)

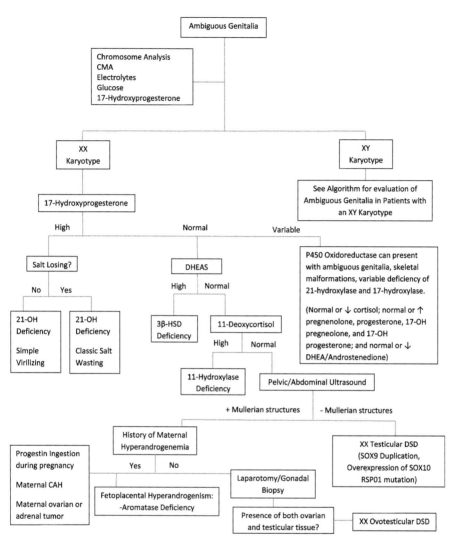

Fig. 2. Diagnostic algorithm for patients with ambiguous genitalia. 13β-HSD, hydroxysteroid dehydrogenase; DHEA, dehydroepiandrosterone; DHEAS, dehydroepiandrosterone sulfate.

- Hormonal testing
  - Evaluation for CAH
    - 17-Hydroxyprogesterone level is elevated in cases of CAH caused by 21-hydroxylase deficiency.
    - Serum electrolytes: evaluate for hyponatremia or hyperkalemia, which may be suggestive of salt-wasting CAH.
    - Adrenocorticotropic hormone (ACTH) stimulation testing should be performed if the 17-hydroxyprogesterone levels are not conclusive or there remains concern about a potential diagnosis of CAH.
  - Basal luteinizing hormone (LH) and follicle-stimulating hormone (FSH) levels should be determined.
  - Testosterone level should be determined.

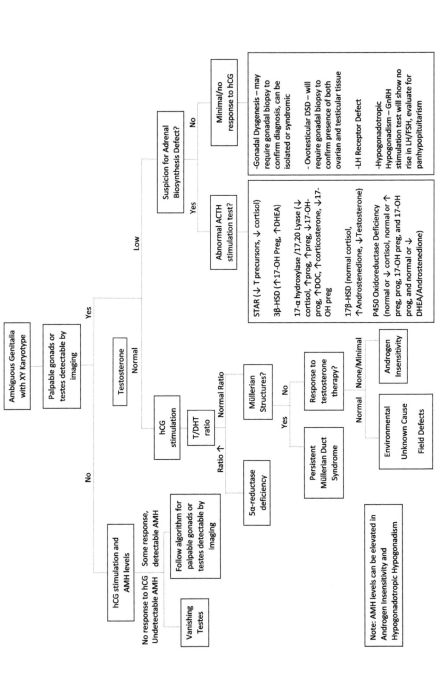

Fig. 3. Diagnostic algorithm for ambiguous genitalia with XY karyotype. DHEA, dehydroepiandrosterone; DOC, Deoxycorticosterone; FSH, follicle-stimulating hormone; GnRH, gonadotropin-releasing hormone; hCG, human chorionic gonadotropin; HSD, hydroxysteroid dehydrogenase; LH, leutinizing hormone; preg, pregnenolone; prog, progesterone; T, testosterone.

○ AMH concentration should be determined.
- The serum concentration of AMH is a reliable indicator of the presence and function of testes. Undetectable levels indicate the absence of testicular tissue, whereas normal or high levels are suggestive of a defect in androgen synthesis or an androgen receptor defect.[9,10]
○ Human chorionic gonadotropin (hCG) stimulation testing should be performed.
● Imaging
○ Pelvic/abdominal ultrasonography or MRI should be performed to evaluate internal anatomy and position of gonads.

CATEGORIES OF DISORDERS OF SEXUAL DEVELOPMENT

As mentioned previously, DSD is classified into 3 broad categories:
● 46,XX DSD
● 46,XY DSD
● Sex chromosome DSD

These 3 categories are further subdivided based on further investigation including laboratory and imaging studies.

46,XX DISORDERS OF SEXUAL DEVELOPMENT

46,XX DSDs are subdivided into disorders of gonadal (ovarian) development and androgen excess.[1] Genes involved in 46,XX DSD are listed in **Table 1**.

Table 1
Genes involved in 46,XX DSD

Phenotype	Gene (Locus)	Protein	Inheritance	Associated Disorders
Overvirlization of 46,XX individual Normal ovary	CYP11B1 (8q24)	11β-Hydroxylase	AR	Congenital adrenal hyperplasia
	CYP21 (6p21–23)	21-Hydroxylase	AR	Congenital adrenal hyperplasia
	CYP19 (15q21)	Aromatase	AR	—
	HSD3B2 (1p13.1)	3β-Hydroxysteroid dehydrogenase type 2	AR	Congenital adrenal hyperplasia
	POR (P450 oxidoreductase) (7q11.2)	CYP enzyme electron donor	AR	May have congenital adrenal hyperplasia
Testicular development in a 46,XX individual	SOX9 (17q24)	Transcription factor	Duplication	—
Testicular or ovotesticular development in a 46,XX individual	SRY (Yp11.3)	Transcription factor	Translocation	—

Abbreviation: AR, autosomal recessive.

Disorders of Gonadal (Ovarian) Development

Ovotesticular disorders of sexual development

Ovotesticular DSD is a rare condition in which an individual has the presence of both testicular and ovarian tissue. Most patients with ovotesticular DSD have a 46,XX karyotype; however, ovotesticular DSD has also been associated with other karyotypes, including 46,XY and sex chromosome mosaicism such as 46,XX/46,XY.[11] Patients can present with a wide range of genital ambiguity, as well as a mixture of both Müllerian and Wolffian structures. The mechanisms in the formation of ovotestes are unclear; however, the *SRY* gene does seem to play a role, including the instances of mosaicism with a Y cell line in the gonad.[12]

Testicular disorders of sexual development (SRY gene translocation, duplicate SOX9)

46,XX testicular DSD is a rare condition that is characterized by the development of both gonads as testes without the presence of ovarian tissue or Müllerian structures. Many patients are phenotypically normal males who present later in life because of infertility, but other cases may present with genital ambiguity. Patients may present with hypospadias, undescended testes, hypogonadism, short stature, and gynecomastia.[13] Most cases are caused by *SRY* gene translocation to the X chromosome during paternal meiosis; however, in approximately 10% of cases *SRY* is not present. The cause of *SRY*-negative testicular DSD remains unclear in most cases; however, there have been case reports describing duplication of *SOX9*, overexpression of *SOX10*, and mutations in the R-spondin 1 (*RSP01*) gene leading to this condition.[14–16]

Gonadal dysgenesis

Gonadal dysgenesis is a heterogeneous condition of abnormal gonadal (ovarian) development in patients who have a 46,XX karyotype. Patients have a normal female phenotype and typically present in adolescence because of lack of female secondary sexual characteristics and lack of menarche. Evaluation reveals streak gonads and elevated gonadotropins. Although most patients with XX gonadal dysgenesis have a defect that is restricted to the gonad, some forms can be associated with somatic abnormalities such as sensorineural hearing loss, as seen in Perrault syndrome.[17]

Androgen Excess

Adrenal steroid biosynthesis defects

CAH is a group of autosomal recessive disorders characterized by defects in the synthesis of cortisol. CAH is the most common cause of ambiguous genitalia in the 46,XX female. Three forms of CAH can present with virilization of a female fetus, including 21-hydroxylase deficiency (accounting for 95% of cases of CAH), 11-hydroxylase deficiency, and 3β-hydroxysteroid dehydrogenase (3β-HSD) deficiency. Mutations of these enzymes leads to deficient cortisol production, causing increased ACTH production, stimulation of the adrenal cortex, and accumulation of cortisol precursors, which are diverted to adrenal androgen production. The excess production of fetal adrenal androgens leads to virilization of the female external genitalia. Patients with 46,XX CAH have normal development of female internal genitalia. In cases of severe 21-hydroxylase deficiency, there is deficient aldosterone production and patients may present with salt-wasting crisis (hyponatremia, hyperkalemia, hypovolemia, and shock). Biochemically, patients with 21-hydroxylase deficiency have elevated levels of 17-hydroxyprogesterone, patients with 11-hydroxylase deficiency have accumulation of 11-deoxycortisol, and patients with 3β-HSD deficiency have elevated levels of 17-hydroxypregnenolone and dehydroepiandrosterone. Borderline or nondiagnostic results may require more definitive evaluation with ACTH stimulation. Genetic testing may also be helpful in establishing the diagnosis.[18] Newborns with classic CAH require treatment with maintenance hydrocortisone, sodium chloride supplementation, and fludrocortisone.[19]

Aromatase deficiency

Aromatase deficiency is a rare disorder in which patients cannot synthesize endogenous estrogen from androgen precursors. In the absence of aromatase, dehydroepiandrosterone sulfate produced by the fetal adrenal glands cannot be converted into estrogen by the placenta and is converted in the placenta to androstenedione and testosterone.[20,21] The excess androgen levels leads to virilization of both the fetus and the mother.

P450 oxidoreductase deficiency

This condition is a rare, autosomal recessive form of CAH in which there is a mutation in the electron donor enzyme P450 oxidoreductase (POR). POR deficiency causes partial deficiency of 21-hydroxylase and 17α-hydroxylase/17,20 lyase activities.[22] Affected females can present with virilization of the external genitalia, glucocorticoid deficiency, and skeletal malformations such as craniosynostosis, midface hypoplasia, radiohumeral synostosis, and phalangeal abnormalities.[23] There is no progression of virilization after delivery, and postnatal androgen concentrations are low or normal. Maternal virilization can also occur during pregnancy but is reversed after delivery. Undervirilization of an XY male can also be seen with POR deficiency.

Maternal causes

Maternal ingestion of progestins or androgens is a rare cause of virilization of the 46,XX female. Other causes of excessive maternal androgens are virilizing adrenocortical tumors, ovarian tumors, or luteomas.[24] A careful history including signs of maternal virilization during pregnancy should be obtained when evaluating an infant with ambiguous genitalia.

46,XY DISORDERS OF SEXUAL DEVELOPMENT

46,XY DSDs are subdivided into disorders of gonadal (testicular) development (**Table 2**) and disorders of androgen synthesis or action (**Fig. 4**).[1]

Disorders of Gonadal (Testicular) Development

Complete gonadal dysgenesis (Swyer syndrome)

In 46,XY complete gonadal dysgenesis (CGD), no testicular development occurs and therefore patients present as completely phenotypic females because of the lack of any gonadal steroid production. These individuals have normal Müllerian structures and bilateral streak gonads. They typically present in adolescence with delayed puberty or primary amenorrhea. Mutations and deletions in the SRY gene account for 10% to 20% of cases of 46,XY CGD.[25,26] Other mutations in genes involved in gonadal development have been described, but in many cases, the cause of XY CGD remains unknown. Evaluation typically reveals a 46,XY karyotype and hypergonadotropic hypogonadism with elevated levels of LH and FSH. Imaging studies demonstrate the presence of a uterus and may show bilateral streak gonads.

Partial gonadal dysgenesis

XY partial gonadal dysgenesis includes a heterogeneous group of individuals with varying degrees of clinical phenotypes depending on the degree of testicular development that has occurred. Patients can have a spectrum of presentations, including females with a Turner syndrome phenotype, ambiguous genitalia, undervirilized

Table 2
Genes involved in 46,XY DSD

Phenotype	Gene (Locus)	Protein	Inheritance	Associated Disorders
Dysgenetic testes	ATRX (Xq13.3)	Transcription factor	X	Mental retardation, α-thalassemia
	DAX1 (Xp21.3)	Transcription factor, nuclear receptor protein	Duplication	Adrenal hypoplasia congenita
	DHH (12q13.1)	Signaling molecule	AR	—
	DMRT1 (9p24.3)	Transcription factor	Deletion	—
	SF1 (9q33)	Transcription factor, nuclear receptor	AD/AR	Adrenal failure
	SRY (Yp11.3)	Transcription factor	Deletion, point/missense mutation	—
	WNT4 (1p35)	Signaling molecule	Duplication	—
	WT1 (11p13)	Transcription factor	AD	Denys-Drash syndrome, Frasier syndrome, Wilms tumor
Dysgenetic testes or ovotestes	SOX9 (17q24.3-25.1)	Transcription factor	AD	Campomelic dysplasia
Persistent Müllerian Duct Syndrome	AMH (19p13.3-13.2)	Signaling molecule	AR	—
	AMH receptor (12q12–13)	Serine-threonine kinase receptor	AR	—
Undervirilized XY individuals	AR (Xq11–12)	Androgen receptor, ligand transcription factor	X	—
	CYP17 (10q24–25)	17α-Hydroxylase and 17,20 lyase	AR	Congenital adrenal hyperplasia
	DHCR7 (11q12–13)	7-Dehydrocholesterol reductase	AR	Smith-Lemli-Opitz
	HSD3B2 (1p13.1)	3β-Hydroxysteroid dehydrogenase type 2	AR	Congenital adrenal hyperplasia
	HSD17B3 (9q22)	17β-Hydroxysteroid dehydrogenase	AR	—
	LHGCR (2p21)	G-protein receptor	AR	—
	POR (P450 oxidoreductase) (7q11.2)	CYP enzyme electron donor	AR	May be associated with congenital adrenal hyperplasia
	SRD5A2 (5p15)	5α-reductase	AR	SRD5A2 (5p15)
	StAR (8p11.2)	Steroidogenic acute regulatory protein	AR	Congenital lipoid adrenal hypoplasia

Abbreviations: AD, autosomal dominant; AR, autosomal recessive.

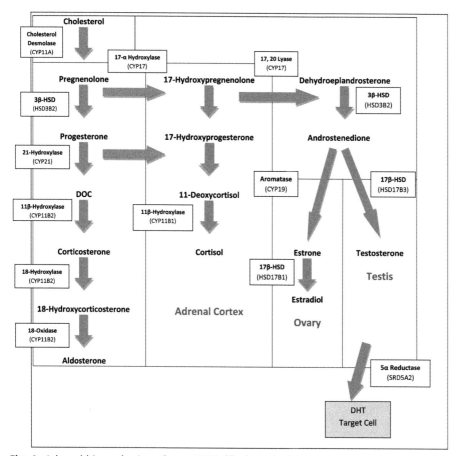

Fig. 4. Adrenal biosynthesis pathway. DHT, dihydrotestosterone.

males, or normal phenotypic females.[3] The most common karyotype is 45,X/46,XY as seen in mosaic Turner syndrome, but many other sex chromosome complements may be seen, such as 46,XY or 45,X/47,XYY. Imaging shows absent to fully developed Müllerian structures, depending on the degree of testicular dysgenesis. Gonadal histology may reveal either bilateral dysgenetic testes or one streak gonad and a contralateral dysgenetic or normal-appearing testis. Hormonal evaluation typically shows decreased levels of AMH and testosterone, as well as minimal to no elevation in testosterone level in response to hCG stimulation.

Several disorders, including camptomelic dysplasia, Denys-Drash syndrome, and Frasier syndrome, are associated with XY gonadal dysgenesis, so a thorough evaluation for any dysmorphic features or malformations must be done when a patient presents with ambiguous genitalia.

Gonadal regression or vanishing testes syndrome

Vanishing testes syndrome is characterized by the absence of gonads in an XY individual. The cause of this syndrome is unclear but thought to be related to perinatal vascular thrombosis, torsion, or endocrinopathy.[27] The degree of virilization of the patient depends on the timing of testicular regression in utero. Loss of testes before 8 weeks' gestation leads to completely female internal and external genitalia, with either no gonads or streak gonads. A loss of testes between 8 to 10 weeks leads to ambiguous genitalia with variable internal sexual ductal development. After 12 to 14 weeks' gestation, most of the male development is complete, so loss of testes after this time results in a normal external male phenotype with absence of testes internally.[28] Most cases of vanishing testes syndrome are sporadic, but there have been reports of familial cases in the literature.[29]

Ovotesticular disorders of sexual development

As discussed previously, ovotesticular DSD is a condition in which an individual has the presence of both ovarian and testicular tissue. Although the most common karyotype is 46,XX, about 10% of cases have a 46,XY karyotype. Patients can present with variable phenotypes, although the most common is ambiguous genitalia or severe hypospadias. The cause of XY ovotesticular DSD remains largely unclear; however, mutations in *SRY* have been identified in several patients.[30]

Disorders of Androgen Synthesis or Action

Defects in androgen action including complete or partial androgen insensitivity syndrome

Androgen insensitivity syndrome results from a mutation in the androgen receptor gene on the long arm of the X chromosome in XY individuals. This X-linked-recessive condition is inherited in 70% of cases, and so there is often a family history of maternal aunts with infertility and amenorrhea.[31] Patients with complete androgen insensitivity have female external genitalia with a blind vaginal pouch, internally located testes, and absence of Müllerian structures because of the action of AMH.[32] Patients typically present in adolescence with primary amenorrhea but can also be discovered in infancy with inguinal or labial swellings containing testes. Patients with partial androgen insensitivity may present with a wide range of phenotypes depending on the degree of responsiveness to androgen activity. Hormonal evaluation reveals normal to elevated testosterone levels and elevated LH levels. Patients with complete androgen insensitivity are raised as females, whereas patients with partial androgen insensitivity are typically raised as males.

Testosterone biosynthesis enzyme defects

Testosterone is derived from cholesterol; therefore, defects in the synthesis of cholesterol can lead to undervirilization of a 46,XY individual. In addition, there are 5 enzymatic steps that are required in the conversion of cholesterol to testosterone.

SLOS is caused by a deficiency of 7-dehydrocholesterol reductase, which is an enzyme that is necessary for the synthesis of cholesterol.[33] This condition is inherited as an autosomal recessive disorder and can present with variable phenotypes, including genital ambiguity in 46,XY males ranging from hypospadias to female external genitalia.[34] Biochemically, patients with SLOS have low blood cholesterol levels and elevated levels of 7-dehydrocholesterol.

The first step in the conversion of cholesterol to hormonal steroids is catalyzed by the steroidogenic acute regulatory (StAR) protein and P450scc, which converts cholesterol to pregnenolone.[35,36] Mutations in StAR result in severe salt-losing CAH, as well as lipid accumulation and enlargement of the adrenal glands. In general, patients are phenotypic females with underdeveloped male internal organs, although some patients can have mild virilization. Deficiencies of P450scc result in a phenotype similar to that of StAR mutations, although they do not always have CAH.

3β-HSD type II converts dehydroepiandrosterone into androstenedione, which is the next step in testosterone biosynthesis.[37] 46,XY individuals with a deficiency of 3β-HSD present with ambiguous genitalia, such as micropenis, perineal hypospadias, bifid scrotum, and a blind vaginal pouch.[38] 3β-HSD deficiency presents with cortisol deficiency and can have mineralocorticoid deficiency as well.

17α-Hydroxylase converts pregnenolone to 17α-hydroxypregnenolone in both adrenal and gonadal tissues. Male patients with a deficiency of 17α-hydroxylase present with female or slightly virilized external genitalia with a blind vaginal pouch and cryptorchidism.[39]

17,20 Lyase is an enzyme that occurs only in the gonadal tissue and is necessary for the production of testosterone. 17,20 Lyase and 17α-hydroxylase activities are shared by the *CYP17A1* gene product on chromosome 10. Patients with isolated 17,20 lyase deficiency present with ambiguous genitalia, including micropenis, perineal hypospadias, and cryptorchidism, but do not have adrenal hypofunction, as this enzyme is limited to the gonadal tissue only.[40]

The final biosynthetic step that converts androstenedione to testosterone is catalyzed by the type III 17β-hydroxysteroid dehydrogenase, located on chromosome 9q22.[41] The phenotype of 46,XY individuals can vary from female to ambiguous genitalia, with cryptorchid testes.[42] Virilization can occur at the age of puberty if the gonads remain in situ.

Persistent Müllerian duct syndrome

Persistent Müllerian duct syndrome is characterized by the presence of Müllerian derivatives (uterus, fallopian tubes) in otherwise normally virilized 46,XY males.[43] This condition can be caused either by mutations in the AMH gene leading to inadequate levels of AMH or by mutations in the AMH2 receptor.[44] There can be variable testicular descent, and the diagnosis is often made at the time of inguinal hernia repair or orchidopexy when Müllerian structures are identified.

Leydig cell aplasia or hypoplasia

As described previously, the testicular Leydig cells produce testosterone, which is critical for differentiation of the Wolffian ducts and external male genitalia. Leydig cells are stimulated by hCG and LH, which act by binding to a common receptor (luteinizing hormone/choriogonadotropin receptor [LHCGR]). Mutations in the LHCGR gene have been identified in patients with Leydig cell hypoplasia, and this is an autosomal recessive condition.[45] Patients can present with a wide variety of phenotypes depending on the degree of Leydig cell hypoplasia. The complete form of Leydig cell hypoplasia presents with female external genitalia, small undescended testes, absence of Müllerian structures, presence of seminiferous tubules, vas deferens, and epididymis. Partial forms of Leydig cell hypoplasia can present with undervirilization including micropenis or hypospadias. Many patients with the complete form of Leydig cell hypoplasia are not identified until they fail to develop secondary sex characteristics at the time of puberty.

5α-Reductase deficiency

Patients with 5α-reductase deficiency have a defect in converting testosterone to DHT, which is necessary for virilization of the external genitalia. This condition is inherited in an autosomal recessive manner and is due to a mutation on chromosome 2, which causes a defect in the type II 5α-reductase enzyme.[46] Patients present with ambiguous genitalia or undervirilization in the newborn period but have normal testes and normal internal Wolffian structures because of normal testosterone levels. During puberty, significant virilization occurs because of the increased testosterone levels. An elevated testosterone:DHT ratio following hCG stimulation is characteristic of 5α-reductase deficiency.[47]

SEX CHROMOSOME DISORDERS OF SEXUAL DEVELOPMENT

Sex chromosome DSD encompasses entities such as Turner syndrome (45,X), Klinefelter syndrome (47,XXY), and mosaic karyotypes such as 45,X/46,XY, and 46,XX/46,XY.[1] In most cases, Turner syndrome and Klinefelter syndrome present later in childhood or in adolescence and do not have genital ambiguity. Some individuals with mosaic cell lines 45,X/46,XY or 46,XX/46,XY can present with a wide range of genital ambiguity depending on the degree of testicular development and function.

Psychosocial Considerations

Genital ambiguity in a newborn can be quite distressing for parents, and although families are eager to announce the sex of their baby, it is critical that the sex assignment is not made prematurely. It is best to delay sex assignment until the newborn has had a thorough anatomic, endocrinologic, and genetic evaluation under the supervision of an experienced multidisciplinary team. During the initial evaluation, the use of gender-neutral terms such as "baby" is preferable when discussing the infant rather than "she" or "he." Similarly, generic terms such as genital tubercle, genital folds, and gonads should be used rather than gender-specific terms (penis/clitoris, labia/scrotum, and testes/ovaries). Open communication with the family at regular intervals is important, and families should always be included in the decision-making process with respect to sex assignment. We suggest to parents that when individuals inquire about the sex of the baby that they reply that the genital development is incomplete and that doctors are performing tests to determine the sex. A psychologist should be part of the multidisciplinary team to provide support and assist families who may be having difficulty coping with the diagnosis of genital ambiguity in their child.[48] Any surgical intervention should be delayed until a clear diagnosis is established and must take into account both the best interest of the patient and the families' values and preferences.[49,50] If medical or surgical interventions are not necessary for the health of the infant, they should be delayed until the child is old enough to make an informed decision. In general, the benefits must outweigh the risks for any surgical procedure to be deemed necessary. Factors that should be evaluated in making a gender assignment should be based on what is known about a specific diagnosis or findings from the diagnostic evaluation and include the following:

- Anticipated gender preference of the child
- Ability to achieve sexual intercourse and orgasm as male or female
- Potential for reproductive function
- Whether sex-partner preference is likely to be the same or opposite sex
- Gender role behavior

As an example, females with 21-hydroxylase deficiency should always be raised as female, even if external genitalia are completely virilized, because, although they may have more masculine gender role behaviors, it is well established that gender preference, reproductive function, and other measures listed earlier are female.

SUMMARY/DISCUSSION

Evaluation and diagnostic workup for patients with DSDs in the newborn period is challenging to health care providers and families. A thorough investigation with the expertise of a multidisciplinary team, including specialists in pediatric endocrinology, urology, gynecology, genetics, ethics, and psychology, must be initiated on all newborns who present with ambiguous genitalia. Initial evaluation must rule out life-threatening conditions such as CAH. Most patients can be classified into 1 of the 3 broad categories of DSD (46,XX DSD, 46,XY DSD, and sex chromosome DSD), and further testing can be tailored to each individual patient thereafter to establish a more specific diagnosis. It is of utmost importance to involve the family in all decisions regarding sex assignment and definitive surgical management.

Best Practices

What is the current practice?

DSDs are complex and require the expertise of a multidisciplinary team for evaluation and management.

What changes in current practice are likely to improve outcomes?

An approach to evaluation and management that involves a multidisciplinary team and open communication with the family is necessary when evaluating infants with ambiguous genitalia. Guidelines and algorithms can be used to help standardize the evaluation of patients who have a DSD.

Is there a clinical algorithm?

The evaluation of an infant with ambiguous genitalia involves a thorough history, physical examination, laboratory tests, and imaging. It is critical to rule out life-threatening conditions such as CAH in any infant who presents with ambiguous genitalia. Algorithms provided in this article can be used to guide the diagnostic evaluation of infants with ambiguous genitalia. Specific gene mutations have been identified in most cases of DSD.

Summary statement

The evaluation and management of DSDs is challenging to health care providers and families. Understanding the differential diagnosis of DSDs is important to guide the diagnostic workup and management.

REFERENCES

1. Lee PA, Houk CP, Ahmed SF, et al. Consensus statement on management of intersex disorders. International Consensus Conference on Intersex. Pediatrics 2006;118:e488–500.
2. Brennan J, Capel B. One tissue, two fates: molecular genetic events that underlie testis versus ovary development. Nat Rev Genet 2004;5:509–21.
3. Cools M, Looijenga LH, Wolffenbuttel KP, et al. Disorders of sex development: update on the genetic background, terminology and risk for the development of germ cell tumors. World J Pediatr 2009;5:93–102.
4. Fleming A, Vilain E. The endless quest for sex determination genes. Clin Genet 2005;67:15–25.
5. Ferlin A, Foresta C. Insulin-like factor 3: a novel circulating hormone of testicular origin in humans. Ann N Y Acad Sci 2005;1041:497–505.
6. Oberfield SE, Mondok A, Shahrivar F, et al. Clitoral size in full-term infants. Am J Perinatol 1989;6:453–4.
7. Callegari C, Everett S, Ross M, et al. Anogenital ratio: measure of fetal virilization in premature and full-term newborn infants. J Pediatr 1987;111:240–3.
8. Ahmed SF, Khwaja O, Hughes IA. The role of a clinical score in the assessment of ambiguous genitalia. BJU Int 2000;85:120–4.

9. Lee MM, Donahoe PK, Silverman BL, et al. Measurements of serum Mullerian inhibiting substance in the evaluation of children with nonpalpable gonads. N Engl J Med 1997;336:1480–6.

10. Josso N, Picard JY, Rey R, et al. Testicular anti-Mullerian hormone: history, genetics, regulation and clinical applications. Pediatr Endocrinol Rev 2006;3: 347–58.

11. Josso N, De Grouchy J, Auvert J, et al. True hermaphroditism with XX-XY mosaicism, probably due to double fertilization of the ovum. J Clin Endocrinol Metab 1965;25:114–26.

12. Ortenberg J, Oddoux C, Craver R, et al. SRY gene expression in the ovotestes of XX true hermaphrodites. J Urol 2002;167:1828–31.

13. Vorona E, Zitzmann M, Gromoll J, et al. Clinical, endocrinological, and epigenetic features of the 46,XX male syndrome, compared with 47,XXY Klinefelter patients. J Clin Endocrinol Metab 2007;92:3458–65.

14. Huang B, Wang S, Ning Y, et al. Autosomal XX sex reversal caused by duplication of SOX9. Am J Med Genet 1999;87:349–53.

15. Seeherunvong T, Perera EM, Bao Y, et al. 46,XX sex reversal with partial duplication of chromosome arm 22q. Am J Med Genet A 2004;127A:149–51.

16. Parma P, Radi O, Vidal V, et al. R-spondin1 is essential in sex determination, skin differentiation and malignancy. Nat Genet 2006;38:1304–9.

17. Meyers CM, Boughman JA, Rivas M, et al. Gonadal (ovarian) dysgenesis in 46,XX individuals: frequency of the autosomal recessive form. Am J Med Genet 1996;63:518–24.

18. Nordenstrom A, Thilen A, Hagenfeldt L, et al. Genotyping is a valuable diagnostic complement to neonatal screening for congenital adrenal hyperplasia due to steroid 21-hydroxylase deficiency. J Clin Endocrinol Metab 1999;84: 1505–9.

19. Speiser PW, Azziz R, Baskin LS, et al. Congenital adrenal hyperplasia due to steroid 21-hydroxylase deficiency: an Endocrine Society clinical practice guideline. J Clin Endocrinol Metab 2010;95:4133–60.

20. Bulun SE. Clinical review 78: aromatase deficiency in women and men: would you have predicted the phenotypes? J Clin Endocrinol Metab 1996;81:867–71.

21. Jones ME, Boon WC, Mcinnes K, et al. Recognizing rare disorders: aromatase deficiency. Nat Clin Pract Endocrinol Metab 2007;3:414–21.

22. Arlt W, Walker EA, Draper N, et al. Congenital adrenal hyperplasia caused by mutant P450 oxidoreductase and human androgen synthesis: analytical study. Lancet 2004;363:2128–35.

23. Krone N, Dhir V, Ivison HE, et al. Congenital adrenal hyperplasia and P450 oxidoreductase deficiency. Clin Endocrinol (Oxf) 2007;66:162–72.

24. Kousta E, Papathanasiou A, Skordis N. Sex determination and disorders of sex development according to the revised nomenclature and classification in 46,XX individuals. Hormones (Athens) 2010;9:218–31.

25. Rocha VB, Guerra-Junior G, Marques-De-Faria AP, et al. Complete gonadal dysgenesis in clinical practice: the 46,XY karyotype accounts for more than one third of cases. Fertil Steril 2011;96:1431–4.

26. Michala L, Creighton SM. The XY female. Best Pract Res Clin Obstet Gynaecol 2010;24:139–48.

27. Pirgon O, Dundar BN. Vanishing testes: a literature review. J Clin Res Pediatr Endocrinol 2012;4:116–20.

28. Lambert SM, Vilain EJ, Kolon TF. A practical approach to ambiguous genitalia in the newborn period. Urol Clin North Am 2010;37:195–205.

29. De Grouchy J, Gompel A, Salomon-Bernard Y, et al. Embryonic testicular regression syndrome and severe mental retardation in sibs. Ann Genet 1985;28:154–60.

30. Maier EM, Leitner C, Lohrs U, et al. True hermaphroditism in an XY individual due to a familial point mutation of the SRY gene. J Pediatr Endocrinol Metab 2003;16: 575–80.

31. Hughes IA, Deeb A. Androgen resistance. Best Pract Res Clin Endocrinol Metab 2006;20:577–98.

32. Hughes IA, Davies JD, Bunch TI, et al. Androgen insensitivity syndrome. Lancet 2012;380:1419–28.

33. Tint GS, Irons M, Elias ER, et al. Defective cholesterol biosynthesis associated with the Smith-Lemli-Opitz syndrome. N Engl J Med 1994;330:107–13.

34. Joseph DB, Uehling DT, Gilbert E, et al. Genitourinary abnormalities associated with the Smith-Lemli-Opitz syndrome. J Urol 1987;137:719–21.

35. Bose HS, Sugawara T, Strauss JF 3rd, et al. The pathophysiology and genetics of congenital lipoid adrenal hyperplasia. N Engl J Med 1996;335:1870–8.

36. Kim CJ, Lin L, Huang N, et al. Severe combined adrenal and gonadal deficiency caused by novel mutations in the cholesterol side chain cleavage enzyme, P450scc. J Clin Endocrinol Metab 2008;93:696–702.

37. Rheaume E, Simard J, Morel Y, et al. Congenital adrenal hyperplasia due to point mutations in the type II 3 beta-hydroxysteroid dehydrogenase gene. Nat Genet 1992;1:239–45.

38. Bongiovanni AM. The adrenogenital syndrome with deficiency of 3 beta-hydroxysteroid dehydrogenase. J Clin Invest 1962;41:2086–92.

39. Yanase T, Simpson ER, Waterman MR. 17 alpha-hydroxylase/17,20-lyase deficiency: from clinical investigation to molecular definition. Endocr Rev 1991;12: 91–108.

40. Geller DH, Auchus RJ, Mendonca BB, et al. The genetic and functional basis of isolated 17,20-lyase deficiency. Nat Genet 1997;17:201–5.

41. Geissler WM, Davis DL, Wu L, et al. Male pseudohermaphroditism caused by mutations of testicular 17 beta-hydroxysteroid dehydrogenase 3. Nat Genet 1994;7:34–9.

42. Boehmer AL, Brinkmann AO, Sandkuijl LA, et al. 17Beta-hydroxysteroid dehydrogenase-3 deficiency: diagnosis, phenotypic variability, population genetics, and worldwide distribution of ancient and de novo mutations. J Clin Endocrinol Metab 1999;84:4713–21.

43. Knebelmann B, Boussin L, Guerrier D, et al. Anti-Mullerian hormone Bruxelles: a nonsense mutation associated with the persistent Mullerian duct syndrome. Proc Natl Acad Sci U S A 1991;88:3767–71.

44. Imbeaud S, Belville C, Messika-Zeitoun L, et al. A 27 base-pair deletion of the anti-Mullerian type II receptor gene is the most common cause of the persistent Mullerian duct syndrome. Hum Mol Genet 1996;5:1269–77.

45. Mendonca BB, Costa EM, Belgorosky A, et al. 46,XY DSD due to impaired androgen production. Best Pract Res Clin Endocrinol Metab 2010;24:243–62.

46. Thigpen AE, Davis DL, Milatovich A, et al. Molecular genetics of steroid 5 alpha-reductase 2 deficiency. J Clin Invest 1992;90:799–809.

47. Ahmed SF, Rodie M. Investigation and initial management of ambiguous genitalia. Best Pract Res Clin Endocrinol Metab 2010;24:197–218.

48. Douglas G, Axelrad ME, Brandt ML, et al. Consensus in guidelines for evaluation of DSD by the Texas Children's Hospital multidisciplinary gender medicine team. Int J Pediatr Endocrinol 2010;2010:919707.

49. Maharaj NR, Dhai A, Wiersma R, et al. Intersex conditions in children and adolescents: surgical, ethical, and legal considerations. J Pediatr Adolesc Gynecol 2005;18:399–402.
50. Wiesemann C, Ude-Koeller S, Sinnecker GH, et al. Ethical principles and recommendations for the medical management of differences of sex development (DSD)/intersex in children and adolescents. Eur J Pediatr 2010;169:671–9.

Inborn Errors of Metabolism

Ayman W. El-Hattab, MD, FAAP, FACMG

KEYWORDS

- Metabolic • Acidosis • Hypoglycemia • Hyperammonemia • Fatty acid oxidation
- Urea cycle • Organic acidemia

KEY POINTS

- Inborn errors of metabolism (IEMs) are not uncommon; their overall incidence is more than 1:1000.
- Neonates with IEMs usually present with nonspecific signs; therefore, maintaining a high index of suspicion is extremely important for early diagnosis of IEMs.
- Metabolic acidosis with hyperammonemia is suggestive of organic acidemias.
- Hypoglycemia without ketosis is suggestive of fatty acid oxidation defects.
- Hyperammonemia with respiratory alkalosis is suggestive of urea cycle defects.
- Liver failure can be caused by galactosemia and tyrosinemia type I.
- Cardiomyopathy can be caused by glycogen storage disease type II and fatty acid oxidation defects.
- Adequate caloric intake and early introduction of the appropriate enteral feeding are important in managing acute metabolic decompensation in neonates with IEMs.

INTRODUCTION

Inborn errors of metabolism (IEMs) are a group of disorders each of which results from deficient activity of a single enzyme in a metabolic pathway. Although IEMs are individually rare, they are collectively common, with an overall incidence of more than 1:1000.[1] More than 500 IEMs have been recognized, with approximately 25% of them having manifestations in the neonatal period.[2,3] Neonates with IEMs are usually healthy at birth with signs typically developing in hours to days after birth. The signs are usually nonspecific, and may include decreased activity, poor feeding, respiratory distress, lethargy, or seizures. These signs are common to several other neonatal conditions, such as sepsis and cardiopulmonary dysfunction. Therefore, maintaining a high index of suspicion is

Disclosure: None.
Division of Clinical Genetics and Metabolic Disorders, Pediatric Department, Tawam Hospital, P.O. Box 15258, Al-Ain, United Arab Emirates
E-mail address: elhattabaw@yahoo.com

important for early diagnosis and the institution of appropriate therapy, which are mandatory to prevent death and ameliorate complications from many IEMs.[3]

The vast majority of IEMs are inherited in an autosomal recessive manner. Therefore, a history of parental consanguinity or a previously affected sibling should raise the suspicion of IEMs. Some IEMs, such as ornithine transcarbamylase (OTC) deficiency, are X-linked. In X-linked disorder, typically male patients have severe disease, whereas female patients are either asymptomatic or have milder disease.

Pathophysiologically, IEMs can be divided into three groups. The first includes IEMs causing intoxication because of defects in the intermediary metabolic pathway, resulting in the accumulation of toxic compounds proximal to the metabolic block; examples are urea cycle defects and maple syrup urine disease (MSUD). The second group includes IEMs resulting in energy deficiency and includes mitochondrial respiratory chain defects. The third group is IEMs resulting in defects in the synthesis or the catabolism of complex molecules in certain cellular organelles, such as lysosomal storage disorders.[3]

CLINICAL MANIFESTATIONS

After an initial symptom-free period, neonates with IEMs can start deteriorating for no apparent reasons and do not respond to symptomatic therapies. The interval between birth and clinical symptoms may range from hours to weeks, depending on the enzyme deficiency. Neonates with IEMs can present with 1 or more of the following clinical groups.[4,5]

Neurologic Manifestations

Deterioration of consciousness is one of the common neonatal manifestations of IEMs that can occur due to metabolic derangements, including acidosis, hypoglycemia, and hyperammonemia. Neonates with these metabolic derangements typically exhibit poor feeding and decreased activity that progress to lethargy and coma. Other common neurologic manifestations of IEMs in the neonatal period are seizures, hypotonia, and apnea (**Box 1**).

Hepatic Manifestations

Neonates with IEMs can present with hepatomegaly and hypoglycemia, cholestatic jaundice, or liver failure presenting with jaundice, coagulopathy, elevated transaminases, hypoglycemia, and ascites (**Box 2**).

Cardiac Manifestations

Some IEMs can present predominantly with cardiac diseases, including cardiomyopathy, heart failure, and arrhythmias (**Box 3**).

Abnormal Urine Odor

An abnormal urine odor is present in IEMs in which volatile metabolites accumulate (**Box 4**).

Distinctive Facial Features

Several IEMs can present with distinctive facial features (**Box 5**).

Hydrops Fetalis

Several lysosomal storage diseases can present with hydrops fetalis (**Box 6**).

Box 1
IEMs associated with neurologic manifestations in neonates

- Deterioration in consciousness
  - Metabolic acidosis
    - Organic acidemias
    - Maple syrup urine disease (MSUD)
    - Disorders of pyruvate metabolism
    - Fatty acid oxidation defects
    - Fructose-1,6-bisphosphatase deficiency
    - Glycogen storage disease type 1
    - Mitochondrial respiratory chain defects
    - Disorders of ketolysis
    - 3-hydroxy-3-methylglutaryl coenzyme A (HMG CoA) lyase deficiency
  - Hypoglycemia
    - Fatty acid oxidation defects
    - Fructose-1,6-bisphosphatase deficiency
    - Glycogen storage disease type 1
    - Organic acidemias
    - Mitochondrial respiratory chain defects
    - HMG CoA lyase deficiency
  - Hyperammonemia
    - Urea cycle disorders
    - Organic acidemias
    - Disorders of pyruvate metabolism
- Seizures
  - Biotinidase deficiency
  - Pyridoxine-dependent epilepsy
  - Pyridoxal phosphate-responsive epilepsy
  - Glycine encephalopathy
  - Mitochondrial respiratory chain defects
  - Zellweger syndrome
  - Sulfite oxidase/molybdenum cofactor deficiency
  - Disorders of creatine biosynthesis and transport
  - Neurotransmitter defects
  - Congenital disorders of glycosylation
  - Purine metabolism defects
- Hypotonia
  - Mitochondrial respiratory chain defects
  - Zellweger syndrome
  - Glycine encephalopathy

- ○ Sulfite oxidase/molybdenum cofactor deficiency
- Apnea
  - ○ Glycine encephalopathy
  - ○ MSUD
  - ○ Urea cycle disorders
  - ○ Disorders of pyruvate metabolism
  - ○ Fatty acid oxidation defects
  - ○ Mitochondrial respiratory chain defects

Box 2
IEMs associated with neonatal hepatic manifestations

- Liver failure
  - ○ Galactosemia
  - ○ Tyrosinemia type I
  - ○ Hereditary fructose intolerance
  - ○ Mitochondrial respiratory chain defects
- Cholestatic jaundice
  - ○ Citrin deficiency
  - ○ Zellweger syndrome
  - ○ Alpha-1-antitrypsin deficiency
  - ○ Niemann-Pick disease type C
  - ○ Inborn errors of bile acid metabolism
  - ○ Congenital disorders of glycosylation
- Hepatomegaly with hypoglycemia
  - ○ Fructose-1,6-bisphosphatase deficiency
  - ○ Glycogen storage disease type 1

Box 3
IEMs associated with neonatal cardiomyopathy

- Glycogen storage diseases type II (Pompe disease)
- Fatty acid oxidation defects
  - ○ Very long chain acyl-CoA dehydrogenase (VLCAD) deficiency
  - ○ Long-chain hydroxyacyl-CoA dehydrogenase (LCHAD) deficiency/Trifunctional protein deficiency
  - ○ Carnitine-acylcarnitine translocase (CAT) deficiency
  - ○ Carnitine palmitoyltransferase II (CPT II) deficiency
  - ○ Systemic primary carnitine deficiency
- Mitochondrial respiratory chain defects
- Congenital disorders of glycosylations
- Tricarboxylic acid cycle defects: α-Ketoglutarate dehydrogenase deficiency

Box 4
IEMs associated with abnormal urine odor

- Maple syrup
  - MSUD
- Sweaty feet
  - Isovaleric acidemia
  - Glutaric acidemia type II
- Sulfur
  - Cystinuria
  - Tyrosinemia type I
- Boiled cabbage
  - Tyrosinemia type I
- Old fish
  - Trimethylaminuria
  - Dimethylglycine dehydrogenase deficiency
- Cat's urine
  - Multiple carboxylase deficiency
- Mousy
  - Phenylketonuria

Box 5
IEMs associated with distinctive facial features

- Zellweger syndrome: large fontanelle, prominent forehead, flat nasal bridge, epicanthal folds, hypoplastic supraorbital ridges.
- Pyruvate dehydrogenase deficiency: epicanthal folds, flat nasal bridge, small nose with anteverted flared alae nasi, long philtrum.
- Glutaric aciduria type II: macrocephaly, high forehead, flat nasal bridge, short anteverted nose, ear anomalies, hypospadias, rocker-bottom feet.
- Cholesterol biosynthetic defects (Smith-Lemli-Opitz syndrome): epicanthal folds, flat nasal bridge, toe 2/3 syndactyly, genital abnormalities, cataracts.
- Congenital disorders of glycosylation: inverted nipples, lipodystrophy.

Box 6
IEMs associated with hydrops fetalis

- Lysosomal disorders
  - Mucopolysaccharidosis types I, IVA, and VII
  - Sphingolipidosis (Gaucher disease, Farber disease, Niemann-Pick disease A, GM1 gangliosidosis, multiple sulfatase deficiency)
  - Lipid storage diseases (Wolman and Niemann-Pick disease C)
  - Oligosaccharidosis (galactosialidosis), sialic acid storage disease, mucolipidoses I (sialidosis), mucolipidoses II (I cell disease).
- Zellweger syndrome
- Glycogen storage disease type IV
- Congenital disorders of glycosylation
- Mitochondrial respiratory chain defects

PRINCIPLES OF MANAGEMENT

Early diagnosis and the institution of appropriate therapy are mandatory in IEMs to prevent death and ameliorate complications. Management of suspected IEMs should be started even before birth.[3,5]

Before or During Pregnancy

When a previous sibling has an IEM, the following can be done:

- Prenatal counseling regarding the possibility of having an affected infant.
- Considering intrauterine diagnosis by measurement of abnormal metabolites in the amniotic fluid or by enzyme assay or molecular genetic analysis of amniocytes or chorionic villus cells.
- Planning for delivery in a facility equipped to handle potential metabolic or other complications.

Initial Evaluation

If an IEM is suspected in a neonate, initial laboratory studies should be obtained immediately (**Box 7**). The results of these tests can help to narrow the differential diagnosis and determine which specialized tests are required.

Box 7
Laboratory evaluation for newborns suspected of having IEMs

- Initial laboratory studies
  - Complete blood count
  - Blood gas
  - Blood glucose and electrolytes
  - Plasma ammonia
  - Plasma lactate
  - Liver function tests: transaminases, total and direct bilirubin, albumin, and coagulation profile
  - Urine reducing substances, pH, and ketones
  - Plasma amino acids
  - Urine organic acids
  - Plasma carnitine and acylcarnitine profile
- Additional laboratory studies considered in neonatal seizures
  - Cerebrospinal fluid (CSF) amino acids
  - CSF neurotransmitters
  - Sulfocysteine in urine
  - Very long chain fatty acids

Management of Acute Metabolic Decompensation

Several IEMs can present with acute metabolic decompensation during the neonatal period, such as urea cycle defects and organic acidemias. The principles of managing acute metabolic decompensation are as follows:

- Decrease production of the toxic intermediates by holding enteral intake for 24 to 48 hours and suppressing catabolism. Reversal of catabolism and promotion of anabolism can be achieved by:
  - Providing adequate caloric intake, which is at least 20% greater than the ordinary maintenance. Adequate calories can be achieved parenterally by intravenous (IV) glucose and intralipid and enterally by giving protein-free formula or special formula appropriate for the IEM.
  - Insulin is a potent anabolic hormone and can be administered as a continuous infusion (0.05–0.1 unit/kg/hour) with adjusting the IV glucose to maintain a normal blood glucose.
  - Providing adequate hydration and treating infections aggressively.
  - Introducing enteral feeding as early as possible. The period of enteral feed restriction should not exceed 24 to 48 hours; after that a special formula appropriate for the suspected IEM should be introduced if there are no contraindications for enteral feeding.
- Elimination of toxic metabolites. Toxic metabolites can be eliminated by:
  - IV hydration, which can promote renal excretion of toxins.
  - The use of specific medications that create alternative pathways. For example, carnitine can bind organic acid metabolites and enhance their excretion in urine in organic acidemias. Another example is sodium benzoate, which is used in glycine encephalopathy and urea cycle defects, because it binds to glycine forming hippurate, which is excreted in urine.
  - Hemodialysis is indicated in cases of unresponsive hyperammonemia (>500 mg/dL) in urea cycle defects and hyperleucinemia in MSUD.
- Additional treatments include metabolic acidosis correction with sodium bicarbonate, which can be given as a bolus followed by a continuous infusion, hypoglycemia correction of with IV glucose, and the administration of pharmacologic doses of appropriate cofactors in cases of vitamin-responsive enzyme deficiencies (eg, thiamine in MSUD).

Monitoring

Neonates with IEMs should be monitored closely for any mental status changes, fluid imbalance, evidence of bleeding (if thrombocytopenic), and symptoms of infection (if neutropenic). Biochemical parameters that need to be followed include electrolytes, glucose, ammonia, blood gases, complete blood cell count, and urine ketones.

Long-term Management

Several IEMs require dietary restrictions (eg, leucine-restricted diet in isovaleric acidemia). If hypoglycemia occurs, then frequent feeding and the use of uncooked cornstarch is advised. Cofactors are used in vitamin-responsive IEMs (eg, pyridoxine in pyridoxine-dependent epilepsy). Examples of other oral medications used in chronic management of IEMs are carnitine for organic acidemias, sodium benzoate for urea cycle defects, and nitisinone in tyrosinemia type I.

INBORN ERRORS OF METABOLISM WITH METABOLIC ACIDOSIS

Metabolic acidosis is an important feature of many IEMs (see **Box 1**). The presence or absence of ketosis in metabolic acidosis can help in guiding the diagnostic workup (**Fig. 1**).

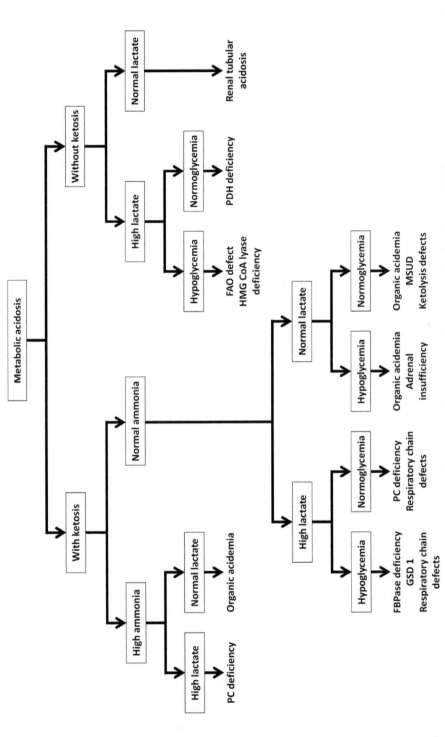

Fig. 1. Approach to neonatal metabolic acidosis. FAO, fatty acid oxidation; FBPase, fructose-1,6-bisphosphatase deficiency; GSD I, glycogen storage disease type 1; HMG CoA, 3-hydroxy-3-methylglutaryl coenzyme A; MSUD, maple syrup urine disease; PC, pyruvate carboxylase; PDH, pyruvate dehydrogenase. Note that although a significant elevation in lactate is more associated with mitochondrial respiratory chain defects and pyruvate metabolism disorders, milder lactate elevations can be seen in organic acidemia and MSUD.

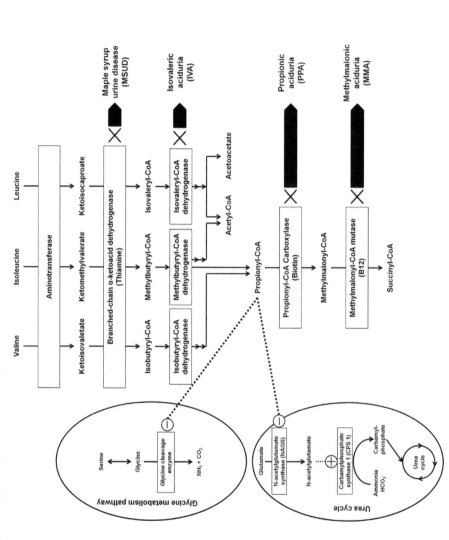

Fig. 2. Branched-chain amino acid metabolic pathways with related IEMs. Note that propionic acid inhibits glycine cleavage enzyme and NAGS resulting in elevated glycine and hyperammonemia, respectively in propionic and methylmalonic acidemias.

Organic Acidemias

Organic acidemias are characterized by the excretion of organic acids in urine. Isovaleric acidemia (IVA), propionic acidemia (PPA), and methylmalonic acidemia (MMA) result from enzymatic defects in the branched-chain amino acids metabolism (**Fig. 2**). The organic acid intermediate metabolites are toxic to brain, liver, kidney, pancreas, retina, and other organs.

Manifestations
Infants with organic acidemias usually present in the neonatal period with poor feeding, vomiting, decreased activity, truncal hypotonia with limb hypertonia, seizures, hypothermia, unusual odor (see **Box 4**), lethargy progressing to coma, and multiorgan failure.

Diagnosis
In addition to metabolic acidosis and ketosis, initial laboratory evaluation can reveal hypoglycemia and elevated transaminases. Hyperammonemia and hyperglycinemia can result from the inhibition of N-acetylglutamate synthase and glycine cleavage enzyme, respectively by propionic acid (see **Fig. 2**). Organic acids also can suppress bone marrow, resulting in neutropenia or pancytopenia. The specific diagnosis can be reached by performing urine organic acid analysis, serum acylcarnitine profile, enzyme assay, and molecular genetic testing (**Table 1**).

Table 1
Enzyme deficiency, genes, and biochemical abnormalities in organic acidemias

Organic acidemias	Enzymes	Genes	Urine Organic Acid Analysis	Plasma Acylcarnitine Profile
Propionic academia (PPA)	Propionyl-CoA carboxylase	*PCCA* and *PCCB*	Elevated hydroxypropionic acid, methylcitric acid, and propionyl glycine	Elevated propionylcarnitine (C3)
Methylmalonic acidemia (MMA)	Methylmalonyl-CoA mutase	*MUT*	Elevated methylmalonic, hydroxypropionic, and methylcitric acids	Elevated propionylcarnitine (C3)
Isovaleric academia (IVA)	Isovaleryl-CoA dehydrogenase	*IVD*	Elevated hydroxyisovaleric acid and isovalerylglycine	Elevated isovalerylcarnitine (C5)

Management
Management of acute decompensation includes holding protein intake, suppressing catabolism with glucose and insulin infusions, correcting acidosis with sodium bicarbonate infusion, and administering carnitine (100–300 mg/kg/d) to enhance the excretion of organic acids in urine. Hemodialysis may be considered if these measures fail. Chronic treatment includes oral carnitine and dietary restrictions. A diet low in amino acids producing propionic acid (isoleucine, valine, methionine, and threonine) is used for PPA and MMA, and a leucine-restricted diet is used for IVA. Biotin is a cofactor for propionyl-CoA carboxylase and can rarely be beneficial in PPA.

Vitamin B12 (adenosylcobalamin) is a cofactor for methylmalonyl-CoA mutase, and hydroxycobalamin injection (1 mg daily) can be given as a trial in MMA. Glycine (150–250 mg/kg/d) enhances the excretion of isovaleric acid in urine and should be used in IVA.[6,7]

Maple Syrup Urine Disease

MSUD is caused by decreased activity of the branched-chain α-ketoacid dehydrogenase (BCKAD), which catalyzes the second step in the metabolic pathway of the branched-chain amino acids (BCAAs) (leucine, isoleucine, and valine) (see **Fig. 2**). Decreased activity of BCKAD results in the accumulation of BCAAs and corresponding ketoacids in tissues and plasma. The pathophysiology in MSUD can be explained by the neurotoxicity of leucine, which interferes with the transport of other large neutral amino acids across the blood-brain barrier leading to cerebral amino acid deficiency that has adverse consequences for brain growth and neurotransmitter synthesis.

Manifestations
Neonates with classic MSUD typically present in the first week of life with poor feeding, irritability, ketosis, maple syrup odor of urine and cerumen (see **Box 4**), lethargy, opisthotonus, stereotyped movements (fencing and bicycling), coma, and apnea.

Diagnosis
MSUD can be diagnosed biochemically by the identification of elevated plasma alloisoleucine and the BCAAs with perturbation of the normal 1:2:3 ratio of isoleucine:leucine:valine. Ketoacids and hydroxyacids can be detected in urine organic acid analysis or the dinitrophenylhydrazine (DNPH) test. Enzyme activity and molecular testing for the genes coding BCKAD subunits (*BCKDHA*, *BCKDHB*, and *DBT*) are available.

Management
Management of acute presentation includes holding protein intake and suppressing catabolism with glucose and insulin infusions. Isoleucine and valine supplementations (20–120 mg/kg/d) and adequate caloric intake also are needed. Hemodialysis can be considered for rapid correction of hyperleucinemia. Thiamine, a cofactor for BCKAD, can be tried for 4 weeks at a dosage of 10 mg/kg/d. Long-term management requires a BCAA-restricted diet.[8]

Disorders of Pyruvate Metabolism

Defects in pyruvate metabolism cause the accumulation of pyruvate in plasma, which is subsequently converted into lactate causing an elevated plasma lactate and metabolic acidosis. Disorders of pyruvate metabolism include pyruvate dehydrogenase (PDH) and pyruvate carboxylase (PC) deficiencies (**Fig. 3**).

Pyruvate dehydrogenase deficiency
PDH catalyzes the conversion of pyruvate to acetyl-CoA and is composed of E1α, E1β, E2, E3, and E3BP subunits (see **Fig. 3**). PDH deficiency occurs mostly due to defects in E1α, which is encoded by the *PDHA1* gene located on chromosome X. Therefore, PDH deficiency is usually X-linked with the most severe illness occurs in male infants.

Manifestations Neonates with PDH deficiency typically present with severe lactic acidosis, hypotonia, seizures, apnea, distinctive facial features (see **Box 5**), lethargy,

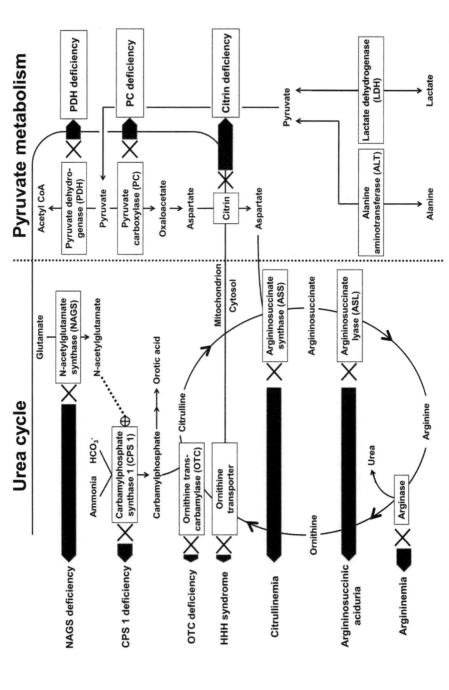

Fig. 3. Metabolic pathways for urea cycle and pyruvate with the related IEMs. HHH, hyperornithinemia-hyperammonemia-homocitrullinemia.

coma, and brain changes, including cerebral atrophy, hydrocephaly, corpus callosum agenesis, cystic lesions, gliosis, and hypomyelination.

Diagnosis Diagnosis is confirmed by enzyme studies and molecular genetic testing.

Management The prognosis is very poor, and treatment is not effective. Acidosis correction with bicarbonate and hydration with glucose infusion are needed during the acute presentation. However, excess administration of glucose may worsen the acidosis, and a ketogenic diet may reduce the lactic acidosis. Thiamin, a cofactor for PDH, can be used (10 mg/kg/d).[9]

Pyruvate carboxylase deficiency
PC catalyzes the conversion of pyruvate to oxaloacetate (see **Fig. 3**).

Manifestations Neonates with severe form of PC deficiency present with severe lactic acidosis, seizures, hypotonia, lethargy, and coma.

Diagnosis Biochemical profile of PC deficiency includes lactate acidosis, ketosis, hyperammonemia, hypercitrullinemia, and low aspartate. Oxaloacetate is the precursor of aspartate. Therefore, impaired oxaloacetate synthesis in PC deficiency results in low aspartate leading to urea cycle inhibition (see **Fig. 3**). Enzyme studies and molecular gene sequencing for *PC* gene are necessary for a definitive diagnosis.

Management The prognosis is poor, and treatment is not effective. Correction of acidosis with bicarbonate and hydration with glucose infusion are needed during the acute presentation. Biotin is a cofactor for PC and can be given (5-20 mg/d).[9,10]

INBORN ERRORS OF METABOLISM WITH HYPOGLYCEMIA

Hypoglycemia is a frequent finding in neonates. The suspicion of an IEM should be raised if the hypoglycemia is severe and persistent without any other obvious etiology (see **Box 1**). The presence or absence of ketosis can help in guiding the diagnostic workup (**Fig. 4**).

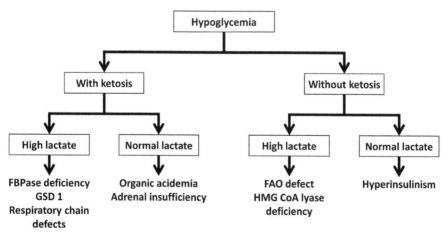

Fig. 4. Approach to neonatal hypoglycemia. FAO, fatty acid oxidation; FBPase: fructose-1,6-bisphosphatase; GSD I: glycogen storage disease type 1; HMG CoA, 3-hydroxy-3-methylglutaryl coenzyme A.

Fatty Acid Oxidation Defects

Fatty acids are transported into the mitochondria where they are catabolized through β-oxidation to yield acetyl-CoA units. Disorders of fatty acid oxidation result from defects in the mitochondrial transfer or β-oxidation. When fat cannot be used, glucose is consumed, resulting in a hypoketotic hypoglycemia. In addition, the released fat from adipose tissue accumulates in the liver, skeletal muscle, and heart, resulting in hepatopathy and skeletal and cardiac myopathy. Diagnosis is based on abnormalities in acylcarnitine profile, enzyme assay, and molecular testing (**Table 2**).

Very long chain acyl-CoA dehydrogenase deficiency

Very long chain acyl-CoA dehydrogenase (VLCAD) catalyzes the initial step of β-oxidation of long-chain fatty acids with a chain length of 14 to 20 carbons.

Manifestations Infants with the severe form of VLCAD deficiency typically present in the first months of life with cardiomyopathy, arrhythmias, hypotonia, hepatomegaly, and hypoglycemia.

Management Hypoglycemia should be treated with glucose infusion and avoided by frequent feeding. Diet restrictions with a low-fat formula and supplemental medium-chain triglycerides should be initiated early. Cardiac dysfunction is reversible with early intensive supportive care and diet modification.[11]

Table 2
Acylcarnitine profiles and genes in fatty acid oxidation defects

Fatty Acid Oxidation Defect	Genes	Acylcarnitine Profile
Very long chain acyl-CoA dehydrogenase (VLCAD) deficiency	ACADVL	Elevated C16 (hexadecanoylcarnitine), C14 (tetradecanoylcarnitine), C14:1 (tetradecenoylcarnitine), and C12 (dodecanoylcarnitine).
Medium-chain acyl-CoA dehydrogenase (MCAD) deficiency	ACADM	Elevated C6 (hexanoylcarnitine), C8 (octanoylcarnitine), C10 (decanoylcarnitine), and C10:1 (decenoylcarnitine).
Short chain acyl-CoA dehydrogenase (SCAD) deficiency	ACADS	Elevated C4 (butyrylcarnitine).
Long-chain hydroxyacyl-CoA dehydrogenase (LCHAD) deficiency	HADHA	Elevated C14OH (hydroxytetradecenoylcarnitine), C16OH (hydroxyhexadecanoylcarnitine), C18OH (hydroxystearoylcarnitine), and C18:1OH (hydroxyoleylcarnitine).
Carnitine palmitoyltransferase I (CPTI) deficiency	CPT1A	Elevated total carnitine; and decreased C16 (hexadecanoylcarnitine), C18 (octadecanoylcarnitine), and C18:1 (octadecenoylcarnitine).
Carnitine palmitoyltransferase II (CPTII) deficiency	CPT2	Decreased total carnitine; and elevated C16 (hexadecanoylcarnitine) and C18:1 (octadecenoylcarnitine).
Systemic primary carnitine deficiency	SLC22A5	Decreased total carnitine

Medium-chain acyl-CoA dehydrogenase deficiency

Medium-chain acyl-CoA dehydrogenase (MCAD) is responsible for the initial dehydrogenation of fatty acids with a chain length between 4 and 12 carbons.

Manifestations Infants with MCAD deficiency usually present between ages 3 and 24 months with hypoketotic hypoglycemia, vomiting, hepatomegaly elevated transaminases, lethargy, and seizures. Sudden and unexplained death can be the first manifestation of MCAD deficiency.

Management Hypoglycemia should be treated with glucose infusion and avoided by frequent feeding. Uncooked cornstarch also can be used to prevent the hypoglycemia.[12]

Fructose-1,6-Bisphosphatase Deficiency

Deficiency of fructose-1,6-bisphosphatase (FBPase), a key enzyme in gluconeogenesis, impairs the formation of glucose from all gluconeogenic precursors, including dietary fructose.

Manifestations

Infants with FBPase deficiency can present during the first week of life with lactic acidosis, hypoglycemia, ketosis, hepatomegaly, seizures, irritability, lethargy, hypotonia, apnea, and coma.

Diagnosis

Diagnosis is confirmed by enzyme assay and *FBP1* gene sequencing.

Management

The acute presentation can be treated with glucose infusion and bicarbonate to control hypoglycemia and acidosis. Maintenance therapy aims at avoiding fasting by frequent feeding and uncooked starch use. Restriction of fructose and sucrose is also recommended.[13]

Glycogen Storage Disease Type 1

Glycogen storage disease type 1 (GSD I) is caused by the deficiency of glucose-6-phosphatase (G6Pase) activity. The lack of liver G6Pase activity leads to inadequate conversion of glucose-6-phosphate into glucose through normal glycogenolysis and gluconeogenesis pathways, resulting in severe hypoglycemia and the accumulation of glycogen and fat in the liver and kidneys.

Manifestations

Some neonates with GSD I present with severe hypoglycemia; however, the common age of presentation is 3 to 4 months with hypoglycemia, lactic acidosis, hepatomegaly, hyperuricemia, hyperlipidemia, growth failure, and hypoglycemic seizures. Hypoglycemia and lactic acidosis can develop after a short fast (2–4 hours).

Diagnosis

Diagnosis can be confirmed by enzyme assay and sequencing of the *G6PC* gene.

Management

The acute presentation should be treated with glucose infusion and bicarbonate to control the hypoglycemia and the acidosis. Maintenance therapy aims to maintain normal glucose levels by frequent feeding, the use of uncooked starch, and intragastric continuous feeding if needed. The diet should be low in fat, sucrose, and fructose and high in complex carbohydrate.[14]

INBORN ERRORS OF METABOLISM WITH HYPERAMMONEMIA

It is essential to measure ammonia in every sick neonate whenever septic workup is considered. Hyperammonemia can be caused by IEMs or acquired disorders (**Box 8**). The presence of respiratory alkalosis or metabolic acidosis can help in guiding

---

Box 8
Differential diagnosis of hyperammonemia

- IEM
  - Urea cycle enzyme defects
    - N-Acetylglutamate synthase (NAGS) deficiency
    - Carbamoylphosphate synthase 1 (CPS 1) deficiency
    - Ornithine transcarbamoylase (OTC) deficiency
    - Argininosuccinate synthase (ASS) deficiency (citrullinemia)
    - Argininosuccinate lyase (ASL) deficiency (argininosuccinic aciduria)
    - Arginase deficiency
  - Transport defects of urea cycle intermediates
    - Mitochondrial ornithine transporter (HHH syndrome)
    - Aspartate-glutamate shuttle (citrin) deficiency
    - Lysinuric protein intolerance
  - Organic acidemias
    - Propionic acidemia
    - Methylmalonic acidemia
  - Fatty acid oxidation disorders
    - Medium-chain acyl-CoA dehydrogenase deficiency
    - Systemic primary carnitine deficiency
    - Long-chain fatty acid oxidation defects
  - Pyruvate carboxylase deficiency
  - Tyrosinemia type 1
  - Galactosemia
  - Ornithine aminotransferase deficiency
  - Hyperinsulinism-hyperammonemia syndrome
  - Mitochondrial respirator chain defects
- Acquired disorders
  - Transient hyperammonemia of the newborn
  - Diseases of the liver and biliary tract
    - Herpes simplex virus infection
    - Biliary atresia
    - Liver failure
  - Severe systemic neonatal illness

- ■ Neonates sepsis
- ■ Infection with urease-positive bacteria (with urinary tract stasis)
- ■ Reye syndrome
- ○ Medications
  - ■ Valproic acid
  - ■ Cyclophosphamide
  - ■ 5-pentanoic acid
  - ■ Asparaginase
- • Anatomic variants
  - ○ Vascular bypass of the liver (porto-systemic shunt)
- • Technical
  - ○ Inappropriate sample (eg, capillary blood)
  - ○ Sample not immediately analyzed

the evaluation (**Fig. 5**). Ammonia can cause brain damage through several mechanisms. The major one is causing cerebral edema by affecting the aquaporin system and water and potassium homeostasis in brain. Hyperammonemia also can disrupt ion gradients, neurotransmitters, transport of metabolites, and mitochondrial function in brain.

Urea Cycle Disorders

Urea cycle is the principal mechanism for the clearance of waste nitrogen resulting from breakdown of protein and other nitrogen-containing molecules through the conversion of ammonia to urea. Urea cycle disorders (UCDs) result from defects in urea cycle enzymes leading to the accumulation of ammonia and other precursor metabolites (see **Fig. 3**). UCDs are among the most common IEMs. They are inherited as autosomal recessive conditions, with the exception of OTC deficiency, which is an X-linked disorder.

Manifestations

Infants with severe forms of UCDs typically present during the first few days of life with poor feeding, vomiting, hyperventilation, hypothermia, seizures, apnea, hypotonia, lethargy, and coma.

Diagnosis

In neonatal-onset UCDs, ammonia levels are usually higher than 300 μmol/L and are often in the range of 500–1500 μmol/L. Other laboratory abnormalities include respiratory alkalosis secondary to hyperventilation, low urea, mild elevation of transaminases, and coagulopathy. Plasma amino acid profile and urinary orotic acid can help in reaching the diagnosis (see **Fig. 5**). The diagnosis is confirmed by enzyme assay and molecular genetic testing (**Table 3**).

Acute management

Treatment of acute presentation includes the following:
1. Decreasing the production of ammonia from protein intake and breakdown. Suppression of catabolism can be achieved through the use of glucose infusion, insulin infusion, and intralipid administration. Protein intake can be completely

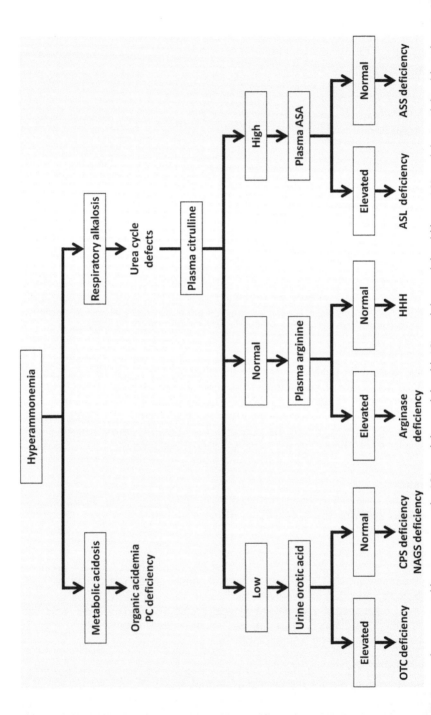

Fig. 5. Approach to neonatal hyperammonemia. ASA, argininosuccinic acid; ASL, argininosuccinic acid lyase; ASS, argininosuccinic acid synthetase; CPS, carbamylphosphate synthase; HHH, hyperornithinemia-hyperammonemia-homocitrullinuria; NAGS, N-acetyl glutamate synthase; OTC, ornithine transcarbamylase; PC, pyruvate carboxylase.

Table 3
Enzymatic and molecular genetic diagnosis of urea cycle defects

Urea Cycle Disorder	Gene	Tissue for Enzyme Assay
N-acetylglutamate synthase (NAGS) deficiency	NAGS	Liver biopsy
Carbamoylphosphate synthetase I (CPS 1) deficiency	CPS1	Liver biopsy
Ornithine transcarbamylase (OTC) deficiency	OTC	Liver biopsy
Argininosuccinate synthase (ASS) deficiency (citrullinemia)	ASS1	Fibroblasts
Argininosuccinate lyase (ASL) deficiency (argininosuccinicaciduria)	ASL	Fibroblasts
Arginase deficiency	ARG1	Red blood cells

restricted for 24 to 48 hours, followed by introducing an essential amino acid formula to maintain the appropriate levels of essential amino acids, which is necessary to reverse the catabolic state.

2. Removing ammonia. Ammonia elimination can be enhanced by the use of the intravenous ammonia-scavenging drug (Ammonul), which contains both sodium benzoate and sodium phenylacetate and is given as a loading dose of 250 mg/kg over 60-120 minutes followed by the same dose over 24 hours as a maintenance infusion. L-arginine hydrochloride is used with Ammonul as loading and maintenance as well. The L-arginine doses are 200 mg/kg for loading and similar dose for maintenance in carbamoylphosphate synthase (CPS) deficiency and OTC deficiency; and 600 mg/kg in argininosuccinate synthase (ASS) deficiency and argininosuccinate lyase (ASL) deficiency. L-arginine hydrochloride is not used in arginase deficiency. Hemodialysis is the only method for rapid removal of ammonia from blood and should be considered if ammonia is very high (>500 μmol/L). However, while preparing for dialysis, the glucose, insulin, and ammonia scavenger therapy should be maintained.

3. Reduce the risk for neurologic damage by avoiding fluid overload and treating seizures that can be subclinical.

Long-term management

Maintenance therapy includes the following:

1. Protein-restricted diet. In general, infants require 1.2 to 2.0 g protein/kg with half of the required protein provided from essential amino acids formula and half from regular infant formula.

2. Oral ammonia scavenger medications include sodium benzoate (250–400 mg/kg/d) and sodium phenylbutyrate (250–500 mg/kg/d).

3. Replacement of arginine (200-600 mg/kg/d for ASS and ASL deficiencies) and citrulline (100–200 mg/kg/d for OTC and CPS deficiencies).

4. Carbamyl glutamate (Carbaglu) is a synthetic analogue for N-acetylglutamate, which is the natural activator of CPS1. Therefore, Carbaglu is very effective in N-acetyl glutamate synthase (NAGS) deficiency and can be tried in individuals with CPS1 deficiency.

5. In children with severe types of UCDs, liver transplantation can be considered.[15,16]

INBORN ERRORS OF METABOLISM WITH NEONATAL SEIZURE

The possibility of IEMs should always be considered in neonates with unexplained and refractory seizures (see **Box 1**).[17]

Biotinidase Deficiency

Biotinidase is essential for the recycling of the vitamin biotin, which is a cofactor for several essential carboxylase enzymes.

Manifestations

Untreated children with profound biotinidase deficiency usually present between ages 1 week and 10 years with seizures, hypotonia, metabolic acidosis, elevated lactate, hyperammonemia, and cutaneous symptoms, including skin rash, alopecia, and recurrent viral or fungal infections.

Diagnosis

The diagnosis is established by assessing the biotinidase enzyme activity in blood. Sequencing of *BTD,* the gene coding biotinidase enzyme, can also be performed.

Management

Acute metabolic decompensation can be treated by glucose and sodium bicarbonate infusions. Symptoms typically improve with biotin (5–10 mg oral daily) treatment. Children with biotinidase deficiency who are diagnosed before developing symptoms (eg, by newborn screening) and who are treated with biotin do not develop any manifestations.[18]

Pyridoxine-Dependent Epilepsy

Pyridoxine-dependent epilepsy occurs due to the deficiency of antiquitin enzyme in the lysine metabolism pathway. Antiquitin functions as a piperideine-6-carboxylate (P6C)/α-aminoadipic semialdehyde (AASA) dehydrogenase, therefore its deficiency results in the accumulation of AASA and P6C. The latter binds and inactivates pyridoxal phosphate, which is a cofactor in neurotransmitters metabolism.

Manifestations

Newborns with pyridoxine-dependent epilepsy present soon after birth with irritability, lethargy, hypotonia, poor feeding, and seizures that are typically prolonged with recurrent episodes of status epilepticus.

Diagnosis

The diagnosis is established clinically by showing a response to pyridoxine. Administering 100 mg of pyridoxine IV while monitoring the electroencephalogram (EEG) can result in cessation of the clinical seizures with corresponding EEG changes generally over a period of several minutes. If a clinical response is not demonstrated, the dose can be repeated up to 500 mg. Oral pyridoxine (30 mg/kg/d) can result in cessation of the seizures within 3 to 5 days. The diagnosis can be confirmed biochemically by demonstrating high levels of pipecolic acid, ASAA, and P6C, and molecularly by detecting mutations in *ALDH7A1*, the gene coding antiquitin.

Management

In general, seizures are controlled with 50 to 100 mg of pyridoxine daily.[19]

Pyridoxal Phosphate-Responsive Epilepsy

Pyridoxal phosphate-responsive epilepsy results from deficiency of pyridox(am)ine phosphate oxidase (PNPO), an enzyme that interconverts the phosphorylated forms of pyridoxine and pyridoxamine to the biologically active pyridoxal phosphate.

Manifestations

Infants with pyridoxal phosphate–responsive epilepsy typically present during the first day of life with lethargy, hypotonia, and refractory seizures that are not responsive to pyridoxine.

Diagnosis

Diagnosis is established by the demonstration of cessation of seizure with pyridoxal phosphate administration (50 mg orally) with corresponding EEG changes usually within an hour. Glycine and threonine are elevated in plasma and cerebrospinal fluid (CSF), whereas monoamine metabolites and pyridoxal phosphate are low in CSF. Mutational analysis for *PNPO* gene is available.

Management

Seizures can usually be controlled with pyridoxal phosphate 30-50 mg/kg/d divided in four doses.[20]

Glycine Encephalopathy (Nonketotic Hyperglycinemia)

Glycine encephalopathy occurs due to the deficiency of glycine cleavage enzyme resulting in glycine accumulation in all tissues including the brain. Glycine increases neuronal excitability by activating the N-methyl D-aspartate (NMDA) receptors.

Manifestations

Neonates with glycine encephalopathy typically present in the first hours to days of life with progressive lethargy, poor feeding, hypotonia, seizures, myoclonic jerks, and apnea.

Diagnosis

Biochemical diagnosis is based on the demonstration of elevated plasma glycine level and the CSF-to–plasma glycine ratio (samples of plasma and CSF should be obtained at approximately the same time for accurate calculation of the ratio). Molecular genetic testing is available for *GLDC*, *AMT*, and *GCSH*, the 3 genes coding the glycine cleavage enzyme subunits. Enzymatic activity in liver tissue also can be measured.

Management

No effective treatment is available. Sodium benzoate (250–750 mg/kg/d) can be used to reduce glycine levels. The NMDA receptor antagonists dextromethorphan, ketamine, and felbamate can result in improvement in seizure control. However, these treatments have been of limited benefit to the ultimate neurodevelopmental outcome.[21]

INBORN ERRORS OF METABOLISM WITH HYPOTONIA

Hypotonia is a common symptom in sick neonates. Some IEMs can present predominantly as hypotonia in the neonatal period (see **Box 1**).

Mitochondrial Disorders

Mitochondria are found in all nucleated human cells and generate most of the cellular energy in the form of ATP through the respiratory chain complexes. Mitochondria contain extrachromosomal DNA (mitochondrial DNA [mtDNA]). However, most mitochondrial proteins are encoded by the nuclear DNA (nDNA). Mutations in mtDNA or mitochondria-related nDNA genes can result in mitochondrial diseases that arise as a result of inadequate energy production required to meet the energy needs of various organs, particularly those with high energy demand, including the central nervous system, skeletal and cardiac muscles, kidneys, liver, and endocrine systems. Defects in nDNA genes are inherited in autosomal recessive, autosomal dominant, or X-linked manners, whereas mtDNA is maternally inherited.

Manifestations

Manifestations of mitochondrial diseases can start at any age. Neonates with mitochondrial diseases can present with apnea, lethargy, coma, seizures, hypotonia, spasticity, muscle weakness and atrophy, cardiomyopathy, renal tubulopathy, hepatomegaly, liver dysfunction or failure, lactic acidosis, hypoglycemia, anemia, neutropenia, and pancytopenia. Some infants with mitochondrial diseases display a cluster of clinical features that fall into a discrete clinical syndrome (**Box 9**). However, there is often considerable clinical variability, and many affected individuals do not fit into one particular syndrome.

Diagnosis

Biochemical abnormalities in mitochondrial diseases include lactic acidosis, ketosis, and elevated tricarboxylic acid cycle intermediates in urine organic acid analysis. The histology of affected muscles typically shows ragged red fibers that represent peripheral and intermyofibrillar accumulation of abnormal mitochondria. The enzymatic activity of respiratory chain complexes can be assessed on skeletal muscle, skin fibroblast, or liver tissue. Molecular testing for mtDNA content and sequencing for mtDNA and known mitochondrial-related nDNA genes also can be performed.

Management

Currently, there are no satisfactory therapies available for the vast majority of mitochondrial disorders. Treatment remains largely symptomatic and does not significantly alter the course of the disease.[22,23]

Box 9
Mitochondrial syndromes associated with neonatal presentation

- Pearson syndrome:
  - Sideroblastic anemia
  - Neutropenia
  - Thrombocytopenia
  - Exocrine pancreatic dysfunction
  - Renal tubular defects
- Barth syndrome:
  - Concentric hypertrophic cardiomyopathy
  - Skeletal myopathy
  - Neutropenia
  - Affects male individuals (X-linked)
- Hepatocerebral mitochondrial DNA depletion syndromes
  - Hepatic dysfunction or failure
  - Hypotonia
  - Seizures
  - Lactic acidosis
  - Hypoglycemia

Zellweger Syndrome

Zellweger syndrome is a disorder of peroxisomal biogenesis. Peroxisomes are cell organelles that possess anabolic and catabolic functions, including synthesizing plasmalogens, which are important constituents of cell membranes and myelin, β-oxidation of very long chain fatty acids (VLCFA), oxidation of phytanic acid, and formation of bile acids.

Manifestations

Neonates with Zellweger syndrome typically present with distinctive facial features (see **Box 5**), poor feeding, severe weakness and hypotonia, widely split sutures, seizures, hepatomegaly, jaundice, elevated transaminases, short proximal limbs, and stippled epiphyses.

Diagnosis

Biochemical abnormalities include elevated phytanic acid and VLCFA and low plasmalogens. Many proteins are involved in peroxisomal biogenesis. Therefore, complementation analyses allow the determination of which protein is defective and molecular genetic analysis for the responsible gene can be performed for molecular confirmation.

Management

There is no effective treatment and management is largely symptomatic.[24]

INBORN ERRORS OF METABOLISM WITH HEPATIC MANIFESTATIONS

Several IEMs can have hepatic manifestations in the neonatal period (see **Box 2**). Galactosemia is the most common metabolic cause of liver disease in neonates.

Galactosemia

Galactosemia occurs due to deficiency of the galactose-1-phosphate uridyltransferase (GALT) that catalyzes the conversion of galactose-1-phosphate and uridine diphosphate (UDP)-glucose to UDP-galactose and glucose-1-phosphate. When GALT enzyme activity is deficient, galactose-1-phosphate and galactose accumulate. Galactose is converted to galactitol in cells and produces osmotic effects resulting in cell dysfunction.

Manifestations

Symptoms of classic galactosemia occur in neonates within days of ingestion of lactose (glucose-galactose disaccharide) through breast milk or standard lactose-containing formulas. These manifestations include poor feeding, vomiting, diarrhea, failure to thrive, hypoglycemia, jaundice, hepatomegaly, elevated transaminases, coagulopathy, ascites, liver failure, renal tubulopathy, lethargy, irritability, seizures, cataracts, and *Escherichia coli* neonatal sepsis.

Diagnosis

The biochemical profile of galactosemia includes elevated galactose in plasma, galactose-1-phosphate in erythrocytes, and galactitol in urine. Diagnosis is confirmed by measuring GALT enzyme activity in erythrocytes and sequencing the *GALT* gene.

Management

Lactose-free formula should be started during the first 3 to 10 days of life for the signs to resolve and the prognosis to be good.[25,26]

Tyrosinemia Type I

Tyrosinemia type I occurs due to deficiency of fumarylacetoacetate hydrolase (FAH), which functions in the catalytic pathway of tyrosine. FAH deficiency results in the accumulation of fumarylacetoacetate and its derivative succinylacetone, both of which form glutathione adducts thereby rendering cells susceptible to free radical damage. In addition, fumarylacetoacetate is an alkylating agent that has a widespread effect on cellular metabolism resulting in cell death.

Manifestations
Children with tyrosinemia type I can present during early infancy with vomiting, diarrhea, hepatomegaly, hypoglycemia, sepsis, liver failure with coagulopathy, ascites, jaundice, renal tubulopathy, and abnormal odor (see **Box 4**).

Diagnosis
Biochemical abnormalities include elevated urine succinylacetone and tyrosine metabolites (p-hydroxyphenylpyruvate, p-hydroxyphenyllactate, and p-hydroxyphenylacetate) and elevated tyrosine and methionine in plasma. Serum α-fetoprotein is markedly elevated. Diagnosis can be confirmed by enzyme assay and molecular genetic testing for the *FAH* gene.

Management
Nitisinone (NTBC) (1–2 mg/kg/d divided in 2 doses) blocks hydroxyphenylpyruvate dioxygenase, the second step in the tyrosine degradation pathway, and prevents the accumulation of fumarylacetoacetate and its derivative succinylacetone. Low tyrosine diet is also needed.[27]

Hereditary Fructose Intolerance

Hereditary fructose intolerance occurs due deficiency of fructose 1,6-biphosphate aldolase (aldolase B), which is part of the catabolic pathway of fructose. Fructose intake results in accumulation of fructose-1-phosphate and trapping of phosphate, leading to diminished ATP regeneration.

Manifestations
Clinical manifestations develop after the exposure to fructose from sucrose (glucose–fructose disaccharide) in soy-based formulas or later at weaning from fruits and vegetables. These manifestations include vomiting, hypoglycemia, jaundice, lethargy, irritability, seizures, coma, hepatomegaly, jaundice, elevated transaminases, coagulopathy, edema, ascites, liver failure, and renal tubulopathy.

Diagnosis
The diagnosis can be established enzymatically by measuring the aldolase B activity in liver tissue and molecularly by sequencing the *ALDOB* gene.

Management
Management is based on eliminating sucrose, fructose, and sorbitol from diet.[28]

Neonatal Intrahepatic Cholestasis Caused by Citrin Deficiency

Citrin is a mitochondrial aspartate-glutamate carrier that transports aspartate from mitochondria to cytosol (see **Fig. 3**). One of the clinical manifestations of citrin deficiency is neonatal intrahepatic cholestasis.

Manifestations
Newborn infants with citrin deficiency can present with transient intrahepatic chole-stasis, prolonged jaundice, hepatomegaly, fatty liver, elevated transaminases, hypo-proteinemia, coagulopathy, growth failure, hemolytic anemia, and hypoglycemia. Neonatal intrahepatic cholestasis caused by citrin deficiency is generally not severe, and symptoms disappear by the age of 1 year with appropriate treatment.

Diagnosis
Biochemical abnormalities include elevated plasma citrulline, arginine, threonine, methi-onine, and tyrosine. Sequencing the *SLC25A13* gene that codes citrin is available.

Management
Management includes the supplementation of fat-soluble vitamins and the use of lactose-free formula and high medium-chain triglycerides. Subsequently, a diet rich in lipids and protein and low in carbohydrates is recommended.[29]

INBORN ERRORS OF METABOLISM WITH CARDIOMYOPATHY

Some metabolic disorders can present predominantly with cardiomyopathy (see **Box 3**).

Glycogen Storage Disease Type II (Pompe Disease)

Glycogen storage disease type II (GSD II) is caused by the deficiency of the lysosomal enzyme acid α-glucosidase (GAA, acid maltase). The enzyme defect results in the accumulation of glycogen within the lysosomes in different organs.

Manifestations
Infants with the classic infantile-onset GSD II typically present in the first 2 months of life with hypotonia, muscle weakness, hepatomegaly, hypertrophic cardiomyopathy, feeding difficulties, failure to thrive, macroglossia, respiratory distress, and hearing loss.

Diagnosis
Nonspecific tests supporting the diagnosis include elevated serum creatinine kinase level and urinary oligosaccharides. The diagnosis is confirmed enzymatically by assessing GAA enzyme activity and molecularly by sequencing the *GAA* gene.

Management
Enzyme replacement therapy using alglucosidase alfa (Myozyme) should be initiated as soon as the diagnosis is established. The response to enzyme replacement therapy is better for those in whom the therapy is initiated before age 6 months and before the need for ventilatory assistance.[30]

Best Practices

- IEMs are not uncommon, neonates with IEMs usually present with nonspecific signs, and early diagnosis and institution of therapy are mandatory to prevent death and ameliorate complications from many IEMs. Therefore, a high index of suspicion for IEMs should be maintained. Consider metabolic evaluation in sick neonates and those with hypotonia, seizures, cardiomyopathy, and hepatopathy.

- After performing the initial metabolic workup, you can narrow the differential diagnosis by the following categorizations:

  ○ In metabolic acidosis with hyperammonemia, consider organic acidemia (or PC deficiency if lactate is also very high).

- o In hypoglycemia without ketosis, consider fatty acid oxidation defects or HMG CoA lyase deficiency.
- o In hypoglycemia with ketosis and elevated lactate, consider fructose-1,6-bisphosphatase deficiency and glycogen storage disease type 1.
- o In hyperammonemia with respiratory alkalosis, consider urea cycle defects.
- o In liver failure, galactosemia and tyrosinemia type I should be evaluated.
- o In cardiomyopathy, consider glycogen storage disease type II and fatty acid oxidation defects.
- When managing acute metabolic decompensation, make sure about the following:
- o Provide adequate calories, at least 20% above what is normally needed.
- o Use insulin infusion to reverse catabolism.
- o Limit the enteral feeding restriction to 24 to 48 hours and introduce enteral feeding with the appropriate formula early (after 24–48 hours).

REFERENCES

1. Campeau PM, Scriver CR, Mitchell JJ. A 25-year longitudinal analysis of treatment efficacy in inborn errors of metabolism. Mol Genet Metab 2008;95:11–6.
2. Saudubray JM, Sedel F, Walter JH. Clinical approach to treatable inborn metabolic diseases: an introduction. J Inherit Metab Dis 2006;29:261–74.
3. Leonard JV, Morris AA. Diagnosis and early management of inborn errors of metabolism presenting around the time of birth. Acta Paediatr 2006;95: 6–14.
4. Saudubray JM. Clinical approach to inborn errors of metabolism in paediatrics. In: Saudubray JM, van den Berge G, Walter JH, et al, editors. Inborn metabolic diseases diagnosis and treatment. 5th edition. New York: Springer-Verlag Berlin Heidelberg; 2012. p. 3–54.
5. El-Hattab AW, Sutton VR. Inborn errors of metabolism. In: Cloherty JP, Eichenwald EC, editors. Manual of neonatal care. 7th edition. Baltimore (MD): Lippincott Williams & Wilkins; 2011. p. 767–90.
6. Deodato F, Boenzi S, Santorelli FM, et al. Methylmalonic and propionic aciduria. Am J Med Genet C Semin Med Genet 2006;142C:104–12.
7. Seashore MR. The organic acidemias: an overview. In: Pagon RA, Adam MP, Ardinger HH, et al, editors. GeneReviews®. Seattle (WA): University of Washington, Seattle; 1993–2014.
8. Strauss KA, Wardley B, Robinson D, et al. Classical maple syrup urine disease and brain development: principles of management and formula design. Mol Genet Metab 2010;99:333–45.
9. De Meirleir L. Defects of pyruvate metabolism and the Krebs cycle. J Child Neurol 2002;17:26–33.
10. Wang D, De Vivo D. Pyruvate carboxylase deficiency. In: Pagon RA, Adam MP, Ardinger HH, et al, editors. GeneReviews®. Seattle (WA): University of Washington, Seattle; 1993–2014.
11. Arnold GL, Van Hove J, Freedenberg D, et al. A Delphi clinical practice protocol for the management of very long chain acyl-CoA dehydrogenase deficiency. Mol Genet Metab 2009;96:85–90.
12. Matern D, Rinaldo P. Medium-chain acyl-coenzyme a dehydrogenase deficiency. In: Pagon RA, Adam MP, Ardinger HH, et al, editors. GeneReviews®. Seattle (WA): University of Washington, Seattle; 1993–2014.

13. Steinmann B, Santer R. Disorders of fructose metabolism. In: Saudubray JM, van den Berghe G, Walter JH, et al, editors. Inborn metabolic diseases diagnosis and treatment. 5th edition. New York: Springer-Verlag Berlin Heidelberg; 2012. p. 157–66.
14. Wolfsdorf JI, Weinstein DA. Glycogen storage diseases. Rev Endocr Metab Disord 2003;4:95–102.
15. Summar ML, Dobbelaere D, Brusilow S, et al. Diagnosis, symptoms, frequency and mortality of 260 patients with urea cycle disorders from a 21-year, multicentre study of acute hyperammonaemic episodes. Acta Paediatr 2008;97:1420–5.
16. Summar M. Current strategies for the management of neonatal urea cycle disorders. J Pediatr 2001;138:30–9.
17. Wolf N, Garcia-Cazorla A, Hoffmann G. Epilepsy and inborn errors of metabolism. J Inherit Metab Dis 2009;32:609–17.
18. Wolf B. Biotinidase deficiency: if you have to have an inherited metabolic disease, this is the one to have. Genet Med 2012;14:565–75.
19. Scharer G, Brocker C, Vasiliou V, et al. The genotypic and phenotypic spectrum of pyridoxine-dependent epilepsy due to mutations in ALDH7A1. J Inherit Metab Dis 2010;33:571–81.
20. Bagci S, Zschocke J, Hoffmann GF, et al. Pyridoxal phosphate-dependent neonatal epileptic encephalopathy. Arch Dis Child Fetal Neonatal Ed 2008;93:151–2.
21. Hoover-Fong JE, Shah S, Van Hove JL, et al. Natural history of nonketotic hyperglycinemia in 65 patients. Neurology 2004;63:1847–53.
22. Wallace DC. Mitochondrial diseases in man and mouse. Science 1999;283:1482–8.
23. Chinnery PF. Mitochondrial disorders overview. In: Pagon RA, Adam MP, Ardinger HH, et al, editors. GeneReviews®. Seattle (WA): University of Washington, Seattle; 1993–2014.
24. Oglesbee D. An overview of peroxisomal biogenesis disorders. Mol Genet Metab 2005;84:299–301.
25. Bosch AM. Classical galactosaemia revisited. J Inherit Metab Dis 2006;29:516–25.
26. Berry GT. Classic galactosemia and clinical variant galactosemia. In: Pagon RA, Adam MP, Ardinger HH, et al, editors. GeneReviews®. Seattle (WA): University of Washington, Seattle; 1993–2014.
27. Sniderman King L, Trahms C, Scott CR. Tyrosinemia type 1. In: Pagon RA, Adam MP, Ardinger HH, et al, editors. GeneReviews®. Seattle (WA): University of Washington, Seattle; 1993–2014.
28. Wong D. Hereditary fructose intolerance. Mol Genet Metab 2005;85:165–7.
29. Kobayashi K, Saheki T, Song YZ. Citrin Deficiency. In: Pagon RA, Adam MP, Ardinger HH, et al, editors. GeneReviews®. Seattle (WA): University of Washington; 1993–2015.
30. Leslie N, Tinkle BT. Glycogen storage disease type II (Pompe disease). In: Pagon RA, Adam MP, Ardinger HH, et al, editors. GeneReviews®. Seattle (WA): University of Washington, Seattle; 1993–2014.

Newborn Screening

Susan A. Berry, MD

KEYWORDS

- Newborn screening • Inherited metabolic disorders
- Early hearing detection and intervention • Critical congenital heart disease

KEY POINTS

- Newborn screening is a triumph of public health because of early identification of screened disorders permitting prompt initiation of therapy.
- Every newborn in the United States should have access to newborn screening for a recommended uniform screening panel of conditions.
- Uniform application of newborn screening in the neonatal intensive care unit requires attention to protocols ensuring completion of this essential test both with regard to assuring initial testing and for repeat testing required to assure diagnosis in premature and low-birth-weight infants.

WHAT IS NEWBORN SCREENING?

In 2013, practitioners, public health departments, and families in the United States celebrated 50 years of newborn screening. Beginning in 1963 with screening for phenylketonuria (PKU), now all 50 states, US territories, and the US military, and many countries around the world test newborns for conditions not evident on physical examination that, if not diagnosed and treated, result in disability, disease, or death. Predominantly, screening is undertaken by analysis of blood collected on filter paper spots; it also includes point-of-service tests for hearing loss and critical congenital heart disease (CCHD). Many of the conditions ascertained through newborn screening are inborn metabolic disorders, but screening also ascertains congenital hypothyroidism, congenital adrenal hyperplasia, severe T-cell immunodeficiency (severe combined immunodeficiency [SCID]), cystic fibrosis, and hemoglobinopathies. To a large extent, the disorders found by newborn screening are genetic conditions. The primary goal of newborn screening is the prevention of significant morbidity and mortality related to the screened disorders. The undertaking of newborn screening has been identified as a public health priority, and newborn screening programs are

Disclosure: None.
Department of Pediatrics, University of Minnesota, 420 Delaware Street Southeast MMC75, Minneapolis, MN 55455, USA
E-mail address: berry002@umn.edu

primarily the responsibility of state departments of health in the United States or national or regional health agencies in other countries.

NEWBORN SCREENING AND PUBLIC HEALTH

The general concept for justification of newborn screening is that improving outcomes for affected children is productive for society as well as for the individual child.[1] The practice of newborn screening was initiated with the underlying assumption that prevention of significant morbidity and mortality in infants due to detectable diseases was a responsibility of public health agencies. Public health organizations can be granted the authority for universal screening and have the potential for efficiency and quality control needed to ensure that every baby has an equal chance to receive this critical test. Departments of health also often have infrastructure that can facilitate continuing surveillance to ensure continued access to care and monitoring of outcomes (although this is not a potential that has been uniformly realized[2,3]). Newborn screening is thus a public health responsibility and the action of screening is a process, not an event. Screening is not simply the performance of the newborn heel prick that allows drops of blood to be spotted on filter paper and tested. Screening should be understood rather as a system, beginning with the sampling, including delivery of samples to the Department of Health; testing, analysis, and reporting of test results; communication of the results to the family, primary provider, and specialist; follow-up diagnostic testing and initiation of therapy; and long-term follow-up to assure the promise of newborn screening (**Fig. 1**).[4] Newborn screening involves the partnership of many participants such as the baby's parents, hospital providers, and the associated laboratory teams; primary providers; and specialists with departments of health to monitor and assure proper functioning of all aspects of the system. Improvements and efficiencies that allow better functioning of the system are important to continue to protect infants from the consequences of the screened conditions and to realize the societal benefits of early identification and treatment.

Because blood spot testing is undertaken in departments of health, tests used for newborn screening need to be rapid, cost-efficient, and suitable to scaling for high-throughput analysis. Sample size is small, and tests need to be developed with a high degree of rigor to assure appropriate levels of detection while minimizing

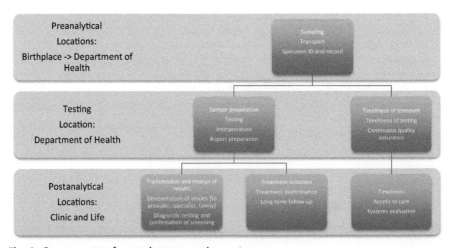

Fig. 1. Components of a newborn screening system.

false-positive results. Tests used for newborn screening are exactly that, screening tests. Although in many cases the results of tests are nearly definitive, they are not designed to be diagnostic. The results of screening are therefore primarily a prompt for initiation of further diagnostic testing, patient evaluation, and consideration of next steps, including treatment. Follow-up diagnostic testing should always be undertaken after receiving positive results of a newborn screen, even if the presumptive diagnosis is acted on and treatment initiated.

HISTORY AND PROGRESS OF NEWBORN SCREENING

The fundamental establishment of newborn screening as a target for public health good was based on early work in the management of PKU. The recognition in 1934 by Asbjörn Fölling[5] that 2 intellectually disabled siblings excreted high amounts of phenylpyruvic acid led to the understanding of PKU as a genetic inherited metabolic disorder. A fundamental rationale for early diagnosis emerged when it was observed that individuals affected with PKU had improvement in their clinical status when given formulas modified to restrict phenylalanine content.[6,7] When it also emerged that restricting phenylalanine early in life prevented the intellectual disability associated with PKU to a large extent, justification for early diagnosis came closely in association with the technological advance of Guthrie and Susi[8] who developed a simple test that could be used in screening. Not different from today's methodology, this test involved collecting neonatal blood on filter paper and doing a direct bacterial inhibition assay for phenylalanine. Massachusetts began screening for PKU as a mandatory, universal practice in 1963.

Gradually, states adopted testing for PKU and for other conditions. Wilson and Jungner[9] summarized a comprehensive rationale for criteria that could be used for inclusion of a condition in newborn screening (**Box 1**).

However, because each state determines what disorders should be included for screening, over time a broad and disparate profile of screening targets emerged even when these recommendations were generally respected. In 2006, the Maternal and Child Health Bureau (MCHB) of the Health Services Resource Administration (HRSA) and the American College of Medical Genetics published the results of an

---

Box 1
Wilson and Jungner screening criteria

1. The condition should be an important health problem.

2. There should be a treatment of the condition.

3. Facilities for diagnosis and treatment should be available.

4. There should be a latent stage of the disease.

5. There should be a test or examination for the condition.

6. The test should be acceptable to the population.

7. The natural history of the disease should be adequately understood.

8. There should be an agreed policy on whom to treat.

9. The total cost of finding a case should be economically balanced in relation to medical expenditure as a whole.

10. Case finding should be a continuous process, not just a once and for all project.

From Wilson JM, Jungner JF. Principles and practice of screening for disease. Geneva (Switzerland): World Health Organization Public Health Papers, no 34; 1968.

MCHB-commissioned project to establish standardization for state newborn screening programs. They sought establishment of a uniform screening panel and a strategy for scientific evaluation to expand the recommended panel and further sought recommendations with regard to policies and procedures for state programs and consideration of a national process for quality assurance and oversight.[10]

The Newborn Screening Saves Lives Act of 2007 was passed by the US Congress and signed into law in 2008. Provisions of this law established 7 HRSA-supported Regional Genetic and Newborn Screening Service Collaboratives and a National Coordinating Center for the Collaboratives to facilitate improvements in education and training as well as the technology of screening and establishing follow-up strategies. The law established programs to improve the newborn screening process and enhance the mandate of the Secretary's Advisory Committee on Heritable Disorders in Newborns and Children (SACHDNC). It required the creation of a clearing house; this was to be a Web-accessible organization of resources now available at the Web site *Baby's First Test*.[11] The act required quality assurance and an Interagency Coordinating Committee to facilitate coordination of activities in newborn screening within the various agencies of the Department of Health and Human Services. It established a requirement for emergency planning in the event of a public health emergency and established the Hunter James Kelly Research Program managed by the Eunice Kennedy Shriver National Institute of Child Health and Human Development (NICHD). A central outcome of this was the definition of the Recommended Uniform Screening Panel with primary and secondary conditions and a process for adding new disorders on a scientific basis.[12] Very rapidly, screening for the primary conditions on the recommended uniform screening panel was available to all US infants. As of the end of 2014, authorization for this law had expired and reauthorization was in progress.

WHO DECIDES WHAT DISORDERS ARE INCLUDED?

Based on the provisions of the Newborn Screening Saves Lives Act of 2007, the SACHDNC serves as an authority providing recommendations to the Secretary of Health and Human Services regarding potential additions to the recommended uniform screening panel. The committee follows an evidence-based process, and on agreement by the committee, recommendation for addition to the panel is forwarded to the Secretary. Following the expiration of authorization, under a new charter the committee became The Discretionary Advisory Committee on Heritable Disorders in Newborns and Children (DACHDNC), continuing the same activities. The committee encourages nomination for additional disorders to be included on the panel. Inclusion on the recommended uniform screening panel is simply that, a recommendation; states decide individually what disorders should be included. At present, all US states provide testing for the original 29 recommended primary conditions. Subsequently, the committee has approved recommendations for addition of blood spot screening for SCID and an additional point-of-service test, pulse oximetry for CCHD. States have initiated the process of testing for these additional disorders, but the process is in varying phases of implementation.[13] For some advocates, this process has seemed insufficient and state-by-state advocacy has led to inclusion of additional disorders for screening in those states.

CONDITIONS INCLUDED IN THE UNITED STATES RECOMMENDED UNIFORM SCREENING PANEL

The Recommended Uniform Screening Panel currently includes 31 primary and 26 secondary conditions (**Boxes 2** and **3**). The original 29 primary disorders were

Box 2
Recommended uniform screening panel: core conditions

Organic acid conditions

Propionic acidemia (PROP)

Methylmalonic acidemia (MUT)

Methylmalonic acidemia (Cbl A,B)

Isovaleric acidemia (IVA)

3-Methylcrotonyl-CoA carboxylase deficiency (3MCC)

Glutaric acidemia type I (GA1)

3-Hydroxy-3-methylglutaric aciduria deficiency (HMG)

β-Ketothiolase deficiency (BKT)

Holocarboxylase synthase (multiple carboxylase) deficiency (MCD)

Fatty acid oxidation disorders

Carnitine uptake defect/carnitine transport defect (CUD)

Medium-chain acyl-CoA dehydrogenase deficiency (MCAD)

Very-long-chain acyl-CoA dehydrogenase deficiency (VLCAD)

Long-chain L-3 hydroxyacyl-CoA dehydrogenase deficiency (LCHAD)

Trifunctional protein deficiency (TFP)

Amino acid disorders

Classic phenylketonuria (PKU)

Maple syrup urine disease (MSUD)

Homocystinuria (HCY)

Tyrosinemia type I (TYR)

Argininosuccinic acidemia (ASA)

Citrullinemia type I (CIT)

Endocrine disorders

Primary congenital hypothyroidism (CH)

Congenital adrenal hyperplasia (CAH)

Hemoglobin disorders

S,S disease (sickle cell anemia) (HB SS)

S, β-thalassemia (Hb S/bTh)

S,C disease (Hb S/C)

Other disorders

Biotinidase deficiency (BIOT)

Critical congenital heart disease (CCHD)

Cystic fibrosis (CF)

Classic galactosemia (GALT)

Hearing loss (HEAR)

Severe combined immunodeficiency (SCID)

From Advisory Committee on Heritable Disorders in Newborns and Children. Recommended uniform screening panel. US Dept of Health and Human Services. Available at: http://www. hrsa.gov/advisorycommittees/mchbadvisory/heritabledisorders/recommendedpanel/. Accessed October 5, 2014.

Box 3
Recommended uniform screening panel: secondary conditions

Organic acid conditions

Methylmalonic acidemia with homocystinuria (Cbl C,D)

Malonic acidemia (MAL)

Isobutyrylglycinuria (IBG)

2-Methylbutyrylglycinuria (2MBG)

3-Methylglutaconic aciduria (3MGA)

2-Methyl-3-hydroxybutyric aciduria (2M3HBA)

Fatty acid oxidation disorders

Short-chain acyl-CoA dehydrogenase deficiency (SCAD)

Medium/short-chain L-3-hydroxyacyl-CoA dehydrogenase deficiency (M/SCHAD)

Glutaric acidemia type II (GA2)

Medium-chain ketoacyl-CoA thiolase deficiency (MCAT)

2,4 Dienoyl-CoA reductase deficiency (DE RED)

Carnitine palmitoyltransferase type I deficiency (CPT-IA)

Carnitine palmitoyltransferase type II deficiency (CPT II)

Carnitine acylcarnitine translocase deficiency (CACT)

Amino acid disorders

Argininemia (ARG)

Citrullinemia type II (CIT II)

Hypermethioninemia (MET)

Benign hyperphenylalaninemia (H-PHE)

Biopterin defect in cofactor biosynthesis (BIOPT BS)

Biopterin defect in cofactor regeneration (BIOPT REG)

Tyrosinemia type II (TYR II)

Tyrosinemia type III (TYR III)

Hemoglobin disorders

Various other hemoglobinopathies (Var Hb)

Other disorders

Galactoepimerase deficiency (GALE)

Galactokinase deficiency (GALK)

T-cell–related lymphocyte deficiencies

From Advisory Committee on Heritable Disorders in Newborns and Children. Recommended uniform screening panel. US Dept of Health and Human Services. Available at: http://www. hrsa.gov/advisorycommittees/mchbadvisory/heritabledisorders/recommendedpanel/. Accessed October 5, 2014.

defined following a process based on guiding principles, a set of evaluation criteria, and solicitation of expert knowledge from the newborn screening community. Based on their overall score in this process, the core conditions were those that had the highest scores in this evaluation process. The additional secondary conditions were included because they were identified as part of the differential diagnosis of a primary disorder and were potentially clinically significant but there was a lack of sufficient knowledge base to fully justify their inclusion (insufficient information about efficacious treatment or natural history).[10] Of the conditions, 23 are identifiable by multiplex tests, either tandem mass spectrometry or hemoglobin electrophoresis. The other 6 are performed as individual tests on blood spots or are performed at the infant's bedside. Most disorders included are identified by tandem mass spectrometry, including 9 primary and 6 secondary organic acid disorders, 5 primary and 8 secondary fatty acid oxidation disorders, and 5 primary and 8 amino acid disorders. Much of the ambiguity between primary and secondary disorders emerges from the observation that the tandem mass spectrometry results yield a profile of metabolites then define a differential diagnosis of disorders requiring follow-up diagnostic testing or second tier testing for identification of an individual disorder. In addition to the disorders diagnosed by tandem mass spectrometry, hemoglobin electrophoresis identifies primary hemoglobinopathies, those hemoglobin disorders with hemoglobin S as a component. Other hemoglobin states identified in hemoglobin electrophoresis are regarded as secondary disorders. Individual tests are done for classical galactosemia, cystic fibrosis, biotinidase deficiency, hypothyroidism, congenital adrenal hyperplasia, and SCID (profound T-cell deficiency), with other T-cell deficiencies regarded as secondary targets. States have the option to follow testing strategies of their own choosing, so various strategies that yield additional secondary targets may be used (eg, states that test for galactose as the primary screening metabolite for galactosemia also identify some cases of galactokinase deficiency or galactoepimerase deficiency, secondary targets identified by that screening strategy.)

Newborn screening using point-of-service testing follows a different paradigm for evaluation than testing using blood spots but is equally critical to the outcome and long-term health of an infant. Programs in states require infrastructure to gather information about results of point-of-service testing to ensure uniform access to testing for infants. The Recommended Uniform Screening Panel includes 2 point-of-service tests and screening for hearing loss and for CCHD. Newborn hearing screening is undertaken by performing otoacoustic emissions or automated auditory brainstem responses testing at the infant's bedside with referral for further evaluation unless normal hearing is confirmed in both ears. Follow-up should include more formal hearing testing and assessment for the cause of hearing loss, including genetic testing and counseling where indicated. In 2013, the SACHDNC completed an evidence review and concluded that assessment for CCHD by pulse oximetry, identifying cyanotic heart disease, should be included as a recommended screening test. Implementation of this screening strategy remains in process in many states. Testing is undertaken using multipoint pulse oximetry, with failed testing requiring echocardiographic assessment of cardiac structure.

RESPONSIBILITIES OF THE NEONATOLOGIST IN NEWBORN SCREENING

Most infants undergoing newborn screening are normal newborns whose screening tests take place in the context of a brief hospitalization or assessment after birth at a time when they are ingesting nutrients with standard protein, fat, and carbohydrate components (most often breast milk or cow's milk–based formula). Typically, newborn screening is included as part of a standard order set and done in a routine manner, making it more likely that babies are tested because they are being cared for using standard protocols. Newborn screening is most interpretable when performed on a normally feeding infant at a standard testing time as mandated by the local state program. Unfortunately, the sick infant who requires transfer for more intensive medical care is at the highest risk for missing newborn screening or for being treated using strategies that interfere with newborn screening. Units caring for acutely ill infants, either inborn or transferred, must establish protocols to ensure that every infant in their unit is either screened at an appropriate time or has already been screened at their primary facility. Typically, newborn screening protocols recommend that screening take place between 24 and 48 hours of age. Infants in transit during those times can be missed without vigilance. Care of infants may also necessitate interventions that interfere with interpretation of screening or necessitate sampling at times not optimal for testing. Units must also develop strategies for screening and rescreening if necessary depending on such circumstances. Early red blood cell transfusion presents a particular issue for blood spot screening because of the mixture of adult blood in the baby's bloodstream. Testing for galactosemia (particularly if performed by enzymatic analysis of red blood cell galactose-1-phosphate uridyl transferase), biotinidase deficiency, and hemoglobinopathy does not produce accurate results after transfusion; in general, it is recommended that a newborn screening sample card be collected before transfusion is undertaken before the usual testing time frame to permit screening for these disorders. Infants who received in utero transfusion require clinical monitoring for these disorders and follow-up testing 90 days after the last transfusion should be undertaken. The baby should still have newborn screening testing for detection of disorders not affected by transfusion at the standard time frames. The use of steroids and certain antibiotics may also present quandaries in the diagnosis and interpretation in newborn screening as also the use of total parenteral nutrition (TPN). State departments of health typically have requirements for testing and retesting of low-birth-weight infants and infants who have undergone transfusion. Units caring for such babies must be familiar with the requirements in their specific state, and if an infant is from a neighboring state, the unit should also be aware of the requirements for follow-up for that state. Neonatal care providers also need to have a strategy to ensure that all newborn screening results are reviewed, whether positive or negative. The transition of babies during times of medical stress may present difficulty in continuity of information, but everyone caring for such a baby has a responsibility to ensure that newborn screening tests have been accomplished and results have been confirmed.

Newborn screening is not a substitute for good clinical judgment. Many of the disorders diagnosed by newborn screening may present before the results of testing are available, and the index of suspicion in an ill infant should be high and include inherited metabolic disorders in the differential diagnosis. Moreover, there are inherited metabolic disorders that present acutely in the newborn period that are not included in the newborn screening panel. Notable examples include proximal urea cycle disorders (eg, ornithine transcarbamylase deficiency, carbamyl phosphate synthetase deficiency). For this reason, newborn screening should always be regarded as an adjunct to good clinical assessment.

DIAGNOSTIC DILEMMAS IN THE LOW-BIRTH-WEIGHT OR STRESSED INFANT AFFECTING NEWBORN BLOOD SPOT SCREENING

Several disorders identified on newborn blood spot screening are significantly affected by the physical state of the baby. Testing for congenital adrenal hyperplasia by assessment of 17-hydroxyprogesterone is extremely sensitive to the gestational age of the baby, identified in most screening programs by adjusting normal values based on weight, because that measurement can be ascertained accurately as opposed to gestational age. For that reason, the weight of the baby is an important parameter by which interpretation is provided. Careful correlation with weight permits minimization of false-positive reports for this screening test.[14] The use of steroids also result in false-positive results; recording the use of steroids is required on the screening card in many states to permit accurate interpretation of results. Some programs have developed strategies for second-tier testing of additional steroid metabolites to facilitate interpretation.[15]

Screening for hypothyroidism also presents a challenge in the premature or low-birth-weight infant because of delayed maturation of the hypothalamic-pituitary-thyroid axis so that levels of thyroid-stimulating hormone (TSH), the most common screening test used, may not elevate in the face of low levels of blood thyroxine, preventing observation of a need for assessment for hypothyroidism.[16] For that reason, many state programs require additional testing at intervals after birth to further evaluate for congenital hypothyroidism in infants with low birth weight. In a term infant, sampling before 24 hours of age may result in detection of the physiologic surge of TSH, yielding a false-positive elevation.[16] State cutoffs are typically specific to the timing of the test; sampling outside those time frames can interfere with overall interpretation.

Antibiotics that are conjugated to pivalate to promote oral absorption when metabolized release this compound as part of the metabolism of these prodrugs. Pivalate in turn conjugates to carnitine, yielding a C5-acylcarnitine ester that cannot be distinguished in newborn screening from the metabolite that identifies isovaleric acidemia without additional testing.[17] For this reason, it is important that all medications being administered to the infant, including antibiotics, are reported to the newborn screening laboratory for appropriate interpretation. In a similar manner, the use of TPN can result in false-positive screening results for an amino acid disorder if the laboratory is not informed about this therapeutic intervention. The pattern of amino acid elevations can assist the laboratory in identifying the use of TPN, but a firm conclusion about interpretation requires knowledge of that treatment.

MATERNAL EFFECTS ON NEWBORN SCREENING

Newborn blood spot screening reflects the metabolic state of the infant, but in the first days of life, it also reflects the metabolic state of the baby's mother. For that reason, abnormal metabolic screening results in selected cases reflect maternal, not infant, conditions. This result is notable in the observation of elevations of levels of C5-OH carnitine, a metabolite with a broad differential diagnosis that includes 3-methyl crotonyl-CoA carboxylase deficiency. Women affected with this mild disorder of leucine metabolism may or may not have been diagnosed with the condition but untreated have low plasma carnitine levels and elevation of blood levels of metabolites typical of the disorder. An infant born to an affected mother has remarkable elevation of C5-OH carnitine level that rapidly declines after birth. For this reason, in the diagnostic assessment of a baby with this particular metabolite, in addition to diagnostic testing that facilitates its differential diagnosis, testing of the mother with organic acids and plasma acylcarnitine profile is essential for proper discrimination of whether it is the mother or the baby that is affected.[18] In a similar manner, mothers with low plasma carnitine levels because of inadequate dietary intake, abnormality in carnitine uptake,[19] or selected metabolic conditions resulting in secondary carnitine deficiency[20] have low plasma carnitine levels that is evident on newborn screening of their babies, so testing of mother is essential for interpretation of the diagnostic assessment for a baby identified with low carnitine (C0). The mother should have her plasma carnitine level measured and urine organic acids evaluated. Finally, maternal B12 deficiency can result in significant elevation of the levels of infant metabolites reflecting that deficiency. Babies whose mothers are B12 deficient may have elevated levels of C3-acylcarnitine[21]; this acylcarnitine species is among those found in more than 1 disorder, requiring a differential diagnosis. When this metabolite is identified, unless second-tier testing can confirm a specific likely diagnosis, maternal testing is also necessary, including B12 levels for both baby and mother in addition to the follow-up testing needed to discriminate among the alternative differential diagnoses for the baby associated with that metabolite.

CONTROVERSIES IN NEWBORN SCREENING

Newborn screening faces challenges because of its successes and progress. On both political and practical levels much remains to continue and improve this life-saving program. From increasing performance expectations to societal conversation regarding present and future testing, to questions about new technologies for testing and expansion of screening, newborn screening will remain in the center of debate for a long time to come.

With success, expectations of newborn screening have increased. The goal of newborn screening is to reduce morbidity and save lives, but there is a finite amount of time required for performance of the screen. After collection of the sample, there is an inevitable time delay between sample collection, transport, test performance, and reporting. Unfortunately, some of the conditions that are targets for screening may present during the intervening time. Any reductions in the efficiency of movement of the sample to the laboratory increase the window of vulnerability between sampling and result. Increasingly, the expectation for more rapid transport to the laboratory and more complete availability of laboratory services to include testing over the weekend has emerged.

The observation that most of the disorders subjected to screening are genetic conditions has resulted in concerns about privacy and family autonomy. Some privacy advocates argue that retention of newborn blood spots after screening is tantamount to creating a government DNA database. Public health advocates argue that instead safeguards protecting privacy and allowing family decision making are in place. This controversy has resulted in destruction of millions of dried blood spots retained by states in circumstances in which it was argued that the state lacked legislative authority for retention of the spots.[22,23] Public health programs require continued access to large numbers of spots for quality assurance and test development. Automatic destruction after very short periods compromises the ability of programs to continue their screening functions. It is incumbent on state programs to have clearly delineated lines of authority for retention and use of residual dried blood spots after initial testing has been completed.

Treatments for disorders identified by newborn screening are often dietary or nutritional in nature. The specialized medical foods required for treatment and supplements such as high-dose vitamins or amino acids that are necessary may not be covered by insurance. Some states provide for this in their newborn screening programs, allocating portions of funding received for screening to this necessary aspect of management for inherited metabolic diseases, but in many cases, families are responsible for substantial financial contributions to provide these essential nutrients to their children because the treatments are not covered by insurance. For the full potential of newborn screening to be realized, treatment of disorders identified by screening needs to be covered by insurance or a government-supported mechanism.

Although it is evident that screening for PKU and hypothyroidism results in substantive improvement in intellectual outcomes,[24,25] the natural history of many disorders on the newborn screening panel is incompletely defined, particularly with regard to milder phenotypes of the disorders, strategies for treatment, and ultimate long-term developmental outcomes. Despite this, it has been difficult to establish strategies to long-term follow-up programs that will ultimately define the success of newborn screening; this was recognized in the Newborn Screening Saves Lives Act of 2007 and is recognized by families and providers alike but remains an unrealized aspect of the newborn screening process.

The Long-Term Follow-Up and Treatment Subcommittee of the SACHDNC identified overarching questions that long-term follow-up systems should be able to address based on components of long-term follow-up care coordination, evidence-based treatment, continuous quality improvement, and new knowledge discovery; this should provide a framework for advancing strategies for long-term follow-up.[2]

NEWBORN SCREENING: THE FUTURE

When the expert workgroup defining the original disorders to be included in the Recommended Uniform Screening Panel concluded their efforts, they identified a group of additional disorders that did not meet their criteria for screening at that time. Chiefly, this was because there were either inadequate screening tests or because the condition did not meet other compelling criteria (treatment available, timeliness affects outcome, known benefit of early intervention.) Subsequently, interested scientists, practitioners, and families have advanced several these disorders as potential candidates for screening as these deficiencies in their candidacy are addressed. By using the nomination mechanism provided by the DACHDNC and by taking direct action with state legislatures, additional disorders are under consideration for, or have been added to, state newborn screening panels. Screening for Pompe disease (glycogen storage disease type 2), mucopolysaccharidosis (MPS) type 1 (Hurler), and adrenoleukodystrophy (ALD) are under active consideration for addition to the Recommended Uniform Screening Panel by the DACHDNC, whereas screening for ALD, Krabbe disease, Pompe disease, Fabry disease, Gaucher disease, Niemann Pick disease, and MPS1 has already been undertaken by various states by legislative fiat. Thus, in the near future it seems likely that many states will increase their screening for disorders, particularly lysosomal storage diseases.

With the advent of new technologies for rapid genome sequencing, strategies to engage direct genetic testing for newborn-screened disorders are on the near horizon. NICHD announced the award of support for projects exploring the impact of whole-genome sequencing in a newborn screening environment.[26] As new technologies emerge, new ethical and societal questions also emerge. Should disorders that have no current treatments be included in newborn screening with the hopes of eventual therapies, especially if promising new therapies are on the horizon? Is it sufficient to have early intervention as a justification for newborn screening? Is it sufficient to offer appropriate counseling for families as a justification for screening? Are the conventional strategies requiring an effective therapy and proven improvement in outcome sufficient when technology permits a rapid level of more comprehensive identification for genetic disorders? These and other questions will emerge as newborn screening advances into its next phases of development. It is important that we as a society address these questions in a forthright manner, balancing a need to know with personal autonomy for families and individuals.

REFERENCES

1. Grosse SD. Does newborn screening save money? The difference between cost-effective and cost-saving interventions. J Pediatr 2005;146(2):168–70.
2. Hinton CF, Feuchtbaum L, Kus CA, et al. What questions should newborn screening long-term follow-up be able to answer? A statement of the US Secretary for Health and Human Services' Advisory Committee on heritable disorders in newborns and children. Genet Med 2011;13(10):861–5.
3. Berry S, Brown C, Grant M, et al. Newborn screening 50 years later: access issues faced by adults with PKU. Genet Med 2013;15(8):591–9.
4. Howell RR, Terry S, Tait VF, et al. CDC grand rounds: newborn screening and improved outcomes. MMWR Morb Mortal Wkly Rep 2012;61(21):390–3.
5. Fölling A. Über ausscheidung von phenylbrenztraubensäure in den harn als stoffwechselanomalie in verbindung mit imbezillität. Hoppe-Seyler's Zeitschrift für Physiologische Chemie 1934;227(1–4):169–81.
6. Bickel H, Gerrard J, Hickmans E. Preliminary communication. Lancet 1953; 262(6790):812–3.
7. Horner FA, Streamer CW. Effect of a phenylalanine-restricted diet on patients with phenylketonuria; clinical observations in three cases. J Am Med Assoc 1956; 161(17):1628–30.
8. Guthrie R, Susi A. A simple phenylalanine method for detecting phenylketonuria in large populations of newborn infants. Pediatrics 1963;32(3):338–43.
9. Wilson JM, Jungner JF. Principles and practice of screening for disease. Geneva (Switzerland): World Health Organization; 1968. Public Health Papers, no 34.
10. American College of Medical Genetics Newborn Screening Expert Group. Newborn screening: toward a uniform screening panel and system–executive summary. Pediatrics 2006;117(5):S296–307.
11. Genetic alliance. Baby's first test. 2014. Available at: http://www.babysfirsttest. org. Accessed October 5, 2014.
12. Newborn Screening Saves Lives Act of 2007. Available at: http://www.gpo.gov/fdsys/pkg/PLAW-110publ204/html/PLAW-110publ204.htm. Accessed October 5, 2014.
13. Association of Public Health Laboratories. NewSTEPs: core Recommended Uniform Screening Panel (RUSP) conditions screened by state. 2014. Available at: https://newsteps.org/sites/default/files/Core%20Recommended%20Uniform%20Screening%20Panel%20Conditions%20Screened%20by%20State-5-2014.pdf. Accessed October 6, 2014.
14. Allen DB, Hoffman GL, Fitzpatrick P, et al. Improved precision of newborn screening for congenital adrenal hyperplasia using weight-adjusted criteria for 17-hydroxyprogesterone levels. J Pediatr 1997;130(1):128–33. Accessed October 6, 2014.
15. Lacey JM, Minutti CZ, Magera MJ, et al. Improved specificity of newborn screening for congenital adrenal hyperplasia by second-tier steroid profiling using tandem mass spectrometry. Clin Chem 2004;50(3):621–5.
16. Buyukgebiz A. Newborn screening for congenital hypothyroidism. J Clin Res Pediatr Endocrinol 2013;5(Suppl 1):8–12.
17. Shigematsu Y, Hata I, Tanaka Y. Stable-isotope dilution measurement of isovalerylglycine by tandem mass spectrometry in newborn screening for isovaleric acidemia. Clin Chim Acta 2007;386(1):82–6.

18. Koeberl DD, Millington DS, Smith WE, et al. Evaluation of 3-methylcrotonyl-CoA carboxylase deficiency detected by tandem mass spectrometry newborn screening. J Inherit Metab Dis 2003;26(1):25–35.

19. Schimmenti LA, Crombez EA, Schwahn BC, et al. Expanded newborn screening identifies maternal primary carnitine deficiency. Mol Genet Metab 2007;90(4): 441–5.

20. Crombez EA, Cederbaum SD, Spector E, et al. Maternal glutaric acidemia, type I identified by newborn screening. Mol Genet Metab 2008;94(1):132–4.

21. Sarafoglou K, Rodgers J, Hietala A, et al. Expanded newborn screening for detection of vitamin B12 deficiency. JAMA 2011;305(12):1198–200.

22. Fikac P. State to destroy newborns' blood samples. Houston Chronicle. 2009. Available at: http://www.chron.com/news/houston-texas/article/State-to-destroy-newborns-blood-samples-1599212.php. Accessed October 5, 2014.

23. Olson J. Minnesota must destroy 1 million newborn blood samples. StarTribune: Health. 2014. Available at: http://www.startribune.com/lifestyle/health/239952831. html. Accessed October 5, 2014.

24. Camp KM, Parisi MA, Acosta PB, et al. Phenylketonuria scientific review conference: state of the science and future research needs. Mol Genet Metab 2014; 112(2):87–122.

25. Grosse SD, Van Vliet G. Prevention of intellectual disability through screening for congenital hypothyroidism: how much and at what level? Arch Dis Child 2011; 96(4):374–9.

26. NIH program explores the use of genomic sequencing in newborn healthcare. NIH: Eunice Kennedy Schriver National Institute of Child Health and Human Development. 2013. Available at: https://www.nichd.nih.gov/news/releases/Pages/090413-newborn-sequencing.aspx. Accessed October 5, 2014.

Index

Note: Page numbers of article titles are in **bold face** type.

A

Abdominal wall defects, 253, 257
Absence of heterozygosity, 229
Acheiropody, 297
Achondroplasia, 266, 268, 305–306, 311–312, 369
Acidosis, metabolic, in inborn errors of metabolism, 415.419–425
Acrocardiofacial syndrome, 295
Acrodermatoungual-lacrimal-tooth (ADULT) syndrome, 295
Acrodysplasia, 294
Acrofrontofacionasal dysostosis, 294
Acromelic dysplasia, 297
Acromelic frontonasal dysostosis, 294
Acromesomelic disorders, 304
Acromesomelic dysplasia with genital anomalies, 293
Acrorenal syndrome, 295
Acrorenal-ocular syndrome, 291
Adams-Oliver syndrome, 246, 285–286
Adrenoleukodystrophy, 343
17α-Hydroxylase deficiency, 407
Alagille syndrome, 254, 381
Ambiguous genitalia. *See* Disorders of sexual development.
Amelia, 282, 297
American Cleft Palate-Craniofacial Association, 332
American College of Medical Genetics and Genomics, 234–235, 443–444
American Heart Association, genetic testing recommendations of, 383
Amniocentesis, for genetic testing, 231
Amniotic bands, 285–286
Androgens
    defects in, 406–407
    excess of, 401–403
Anemia
    Diamond-Blackfan, 291
    Fanconi, 256–257, 291
Aneuploidy syndromes, 267–268, 273–274
Aneuploidy testing, 231
Angelman syndrome, 221, 236
Anonychia, in limb deficiency disorders, 295
Anorectal malformations. *See* VACTER/VACTERL association.
Aorta, coarctation of, 254
Aortic arch, interrupted, 254
Aortic stenosis, supravalvular, 355
Apert syndrome, 330

Clin Perinatol 42 (2015) 455–467
http://dx.doi.org/10.1016/S0095-5108(15)00054-8
0095-5108/15/$ – see front matter © 2015 Elsevier Inc. All rights reserved.

perinatology.theclinics.com

Moving?

Make sure your subscription moves with you!

To notify us of your new address, find your **Clinics Account Number** (located on your mailing label above your name), and contact customer service at:

Email: journalscustomerservice-usa@elsevier.com

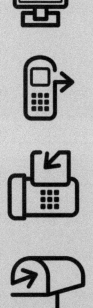

800-654-2452 (subscribers in the U.S. & Canada)
314-447-8871 (subscribers outside of the U.S. & Canada)

Fax number: 314-447-8029

Elsevier Health Sciences Division
Subscription Customer Service
3251 Riverport Lane
Maryland Heights, MO 63043

*To ensure uninterrupted delivery of your subscription, please notify us at least 4 weeks in advance of move.

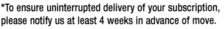